CONTEMPORARY ISSUES IN HEALTH AND SOCIAL CARE POLICY AND PRACTICE

This accessible text presents a comparative analysis of health and social care policy and practice from around the world, with learning points drawn out for the UK. It supports readers to improve practice by reflecting on differences and similarities in the policies of other OECD countries.

Divided into two parts, the book opens with a focus on core concepts in health and social care policy and practice such as service user involvement, the promotion of wellbeing, health inequalities, funding, and integrated care. The differing philosophical, socio-political, and historical perspectives that underpin these key areas in different countries are explored, in order to develop a greater understanding of the UK system. The second part of the book takes a close look at a range of specific contemporary issues, such as end-of-life care, long-term conditions, homelessness, refugee and migrant health, disability, domestic abuse, substance use, and women in prison. These in-depth case study chapters enable readers to identify best practices and challenges in relation to specific areas of health and social care policy and practice.

Ideal for undergraduate students studying health and social care policy from a range of disciplinary backgrounds, this practical text provides a deeper understanding of complex health and social care issues, and supports the development of a global and comparative skill set.

Julia Morgan is an associate professor for public health and wellbeing. She has previously worked on a child development study, and for several non-government organisations which support families with young children and community participation. Her primary research interests focus upon social justice and inequality; nomadic and Indigenous peoples; Gypsy, Roma and Travellers; rural and remote health; loneliness; gender; maternal and child health; community development; and wellbeing among people who are imprisoned. She is currently researching ADHD late diagnosis in adult women. She is the co-editor, with Vincent La Placa, of the Routledge book *Social Science Perspectives on Global Public Health*.

Vincent La Placa is associate professor of public health and policy and associate head of school for student success in the School of Human Sciences, University of Greenwich. He has been a senior research consultant at the Department of Health (now DHSC) where he managed the qualitative strand of the Healthy Foundations Life-stage Segmentation Model, one of the largest pieces of qualitative research conducted across UK government. He co-edited the book *Social Science Perspectives on Global Public Health* with Julia Morgan, published in 2023. He is an honorary fellow of Eurasia Research's Teaching, Education and Research Association.

Contemporary Issues in Health and Social Care Policy and Practice

A Comparative Introduction

Edited by
Julia Morgan
and Vincent La Placa

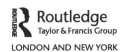

Routledge
Taylor & Francis Group

LONDON AND NEW YORK

Designed cover image: Getty Images

First published 2025
by Routledge
4 Park Square, Milton Park, Abingdon, Oxon OX14 4RN

and by Routledge
605 Third Avenue, New York, NY 10158

Routledge is an imprint of the Taylor & Francis Group, an informa business

© 2025 selection and editorial matter, Julia Morgan and Vincent La Placa;
individual chapters, the contributors

British Library Cataloguing-in-Publication Data
A catalogue record for this book is available from the British Library

ISBN: 978-1-032-38124-4 (hbk)
ISBN: 978-1-032-38123-7 (pbk)
ISBN: 978-1-003-34360-8 (ebk)

DOI: 10.4324/9781003343608

Typeset in Sabon
by KnowledgeWorks Global Ltd.

Maureen Lawson (nee Moran Fleming) (1936–2023), much loved mother to Julia, Gregory and Joseph, and grandmother to Olivia.

Christopher Pettifer (1972–2012) and Rosemary Pettifer (1961–2022), much loved and missed.

Contents

List of Figures

List of Tables

List of Boxes

Contributors

Nadya Belenky is a senior lecturer in public health at the University of Greenwich and a research fellow with the Cecil G. Sheps Center for Health Services Research at the University of North Carolina. She is a health services researcher and an epidemiologist and is interested in access to health care services and how access disparities can lead to inequalities in health outcomes.

Caroline Bradbury-Jones is a professor of gender based violence and health. She has a clinical background as a registered nurse, midwife and health visitor in the UK. Caroline has undertaken extensive research in the field of violence against women and girls and published widely about the issue. A particular focus has been on health professionals' understandings of domestic violence. Caroline is the founder and lead of the Risk, Abuse and Violence (RAV) research programme at the University of Birmingham.

Genevieve Breau is a lecturer in public health at the University of Greenwich, London. Her main area of interest is health promotion for adults with intellectual disabilities, with a special focus on promoting cancer screening to address health inequalities in this group.

Floor Christie-de Jong is an associate professor in public health in the School of Medicine at the University of Sunderland, United Kingdom. Floor has worked with different migrant populations and her research focuses on health inequalities in cancer and its screening, particularly for ethnic minority groups.

Johanna Fischer is a postdoctoral researcher at the University of Bremen (Germany) within the research project 'Global Dynamics of Long-Term Care Policies'. Her research focuses on comparative and global social policy with particular attention to long-term care systems.

John Foster is professor of addiction and mental health at University of Greenwich. He has been researching drug and alcohol abuse since 1996. His work initially focused on alcohol and drug dependency. His recent publications have concerned drug and alcohol policy and the COVID-19 lockdown.

Lotta Hackett is senior teaching fellow of public health and programme lead for BSc (Hons) public health in the School of Human Sciences, University of Greenwich. She teaches on the BA (Hons) health and social care; MSc global public health and BSc (Hons) public health degrees.

Charlotte Jeavons is head of the School of Human Sciences at University of Greenwich. She has a PhD in (dental) public health, was awarded honorary membership of the Faculty of Public Health, fellowship of the College of General Dentistry and in 2024 will be the first dental care professional to be elected as president of BASCD.

Vincent La Placa is associate professor of public health and policy and associate head of school for student success in the School of Human Sciences, University of Greenwich. He has been a senior research consultant at the Department of Health (now DHSC) where he managed the qualitative strand of the Healthy Foundations Life-stage Segmentation Model, one of the largest pieces of qualitative research conducted across UK Government. He co-edited the book *Social Science Perspectives on Global Public Health* with Julia Morgan, published in 2023. He is an honorary fellow of Eurasia Research's Teaching, Education and Research Association.

Kai Leichsenring is executive director at the European Centre for Social Welfare Policy and Research, Vienna (Austria). With a background in political sciences and organisational development consultancy he is a well-known expert in comparative and applied social policy research in ageing, health and long-term care.

Paul McCrone is professor of healthcare economics at the University of Greenwich. His work has included both UK and international studies and he has received funding from agencies including NIHR, Wellcome, ESRC, MRC, and the EU. Paul has published over 300 papers. He was formerly co-director of the NIHR Mental Health Policy Research Unit.

Julia Morgan is an associate professor for public health and wellbeing. She has previously worked on a child development study, and for several non-government organisations which support families with young children and community participation. Her primary research interests focus upon social justice and inequality; nomadic and Indigenous peoples; Gypsy, Roma and Travellers; rural and remote health; loneliness; gender; maternal and child health; community development; and wellbeing among people who are imprisoned. She is currently researching ADHD late diagnosis in adult women. She is the co-editor, with Vincent La Placa, of the Routledge book *Social Science Perspectives on Global Public Health*.

Maria Morgan is a specialist in dental and generic public health. Maria is a past president of BASCD and a fellow of the Faculty of Public Health. In 2021 Maria was enrolled on the British Dental Association Roll of Distinction honouring her outstanding services to UK dentistry and in 2024 she was awarded the FPH service medal for her outstanding contribution to the faculty.

Panagiotis Pentaris is an associate professor of social work & thanatology (death studies), with international education and practice experience in disaster work and end of life care. Panagiotis is the director of research and research studies for the Department of Social, Therapeutic and Community Studies at Goldsmiths, University of London, UK, where he is also acting as deputy head, as well as the lead for social work programmes.

Nicholas Pleace is director of the Centre for Housing Policy, an interdisciplinary research group at the University of York which was founded in 1990. Nicholas has spent over three decades working with the homelessness sector and is a member of the European Observatory on Homelessness.

Dana Sammut is a registered nurse and first-year PhD student in the Centre for Healthcare and Communities at Coventry University. Her research interests include gender-based and workplace violence, and her doctoral research explores violence against healthcare workers. Alongside her studies, she holds a part-time role at a domestic abuse service.

Cassandra Simmons is a researcher in the health and care team at the European Centre for Social Welfare Policy & Research, based in Vienna (Austria). An economist by training, her research focuses on the sustainability and equitable development of long-term care systems, with a concentration on financing, inequalities in access and use, informal care, among others.

Betsy Thom is professor of health policy and co-director of the Drug and Alcohol Research Centre at Middlesex University. She is an honorary professor in the Department of Psychology and Behavioural Sciences, Aarhus University, Denmark. Her research includes cultural and social aspects of drug and alcohol policy and practice.

Jackie Yaskey is senior lecturer and academic portfolio lead for social work in the School of Human Sciences at the University of Greenwich. She is a registered social worker with experience in children's safeguarding and has been a supervising and assessing social worker for both local authority and independent sector fostering agencies.

Acknowledgements

Thank you to all the authors who have contributed to this edited book. Thanks also to Grace McInnes and Madii Cherry-Moreton from Routledge for all your support; and to the copy editors for ensuring consistency throughout.

PART I

CHAPTER 1

Introduction

....

Julia Morgan and Vincent La Placa

INTRODUCTION

This chapter outlines the primary aims of the book and defines health and social care. The 38 countries of the OECD are introduced, and the importance of comparative analysis is explored including difficulties which arise when comparing diverse countries. An overview of some health and social care issues are focused upon including the impact of COVID 19 on health and social care systems and the importance of a well-trained and supported workforce. Finally, the outline of the book is discussed. Part I of the book focuses on core concepts in health and social care policy and practice such as typologies and theories of welfare regimes, health and social care financing, wellbeing, health inequalities, partnership working including integrated care, and service user involvement. Part II then continues by focusing on specific health and social care topics, exploring issues across OECD countries or selected OECD countries using a comparative lens. Specific topics focused upon in Part II are homelessness, domestic violence and abuse, substance use policies, health inequalities and people with learning disabilities, women in prison, end of life care, dental services, long term care services, health policies in OECD countries for refugees and migrants, and loneliness.

The primary aim of this book is to offer students an opportunity to explore health and social care policy and practice across Organisation for Economic Co-operation and Development (OECD) countries (or across selected OECD countries) and to assist students to develop skills and knowledge to understand complex health and social care systems. Health and social care are crucial to providing a fair and just society and are areas that all of us will encounter at some time in our lives. Health and social care can refer to many activities that support health, well-being, need and quality of life for adults and children, which can take place in a range of settings including prisons. Adult social care, for example, tends to include services, provided by social work including safeguarding and a range of publicly or privately funded care providers, who support adults (and their carers) with physical or learning

DOI: 10.4324/9781003343608-2

disabilities, physical or mental health conditions, other long-term conditions, or support needs to live their lives as independently as possible.

This can include services for people who are homeless, or those who experience domestic violence and abuse. Social care normally takes place in the home, community or in residential care facilities and can be formally provided through a range of private, statutory, or voluntary organisations, or informally provided through an individual's family, community, or friends. Across the United Kingdom (UK) social care, like health care, is a devolved matter, this means that the four countries of the UK (England, Northern Ireland, Scotland, Wales), each may have their own policies with differing types of provision. Local authorities are responsible for social care in England, Wales, and Scotland but in Northern Ireland health and social care trusts are responsible (Dodsworth and Oung, 2023). Social care in the UK is not free at the point of contact but is means tested which can result in many people not being able to access the care that they require (King's Fund, 2020).

However, there are differences within the four devolved nations with England tending to offer less generous packages. Countries across the 38 countries of the OECD may use different terminology to refer to social care including social welfare, social protection, social policy, personal care workers, or long-term conditions. While other countries may not distinguish between health and social care services with social care being provided within the health system. However, in relation to health systems, social care systems and services tend to be underfunded and are often positioned as of secondary importance (Glasby, 2019; Glasby et al., 2023). Moreover, demographic changes in terms of increases in the numbers of older people across the OECD, which is projected to rise from 17% in 2019 to 27% by 2050, coupled with the current deficit in long term care workers, means that more investment is needed in this area to meet both current and future demand (OECD, 2021b).

Healthcare, however, refers to services which aim to promote, restore, or maintain health. This can include activities such as preventative health services, diagnosis treatment, and rehabilitation, provision of services in hospitals and in the community at the primary, secondary and tertiary levels, as well as other activities such as the supply and production of medical drugs. These activities can be provided by a range of multisectoral organisations including the public sector, private for-profit and private not-for-profit organisations, public-private partnerships, as well as within communities and families. Healthcare in the devolved nations of the UK is provided in a wide range of settings including in the community, in hospitals and in people's homes normally through the National Health Service with private providers also evident. While healthcare in the UK tends to be free at the point of contact (funded through taxation), there are out-of-pocket expenses, in England for example, for prescriptions, dental services and eye care. This means that fees, normally subsidised, will be charged unless a person is exempt from payment. Health system financing differs across OECD countries with some countries funding health systems through general taxation such as Nordic countries, UK, Australia, Canada, and New Zealand while others opt for social insurance such as Germany and Japan with the USA being funded through private insurance and government supported schemes such as Medicaid (OECD, 2021a).

Across the OECD, health and social care systems employ substantial numbers of workers with more than 15% of all jobs in the Netherlands and Nordic countries being in these sectors (OECD, 2021a). Over 75% of workers in health and social care in OECD countries are women (OECD, 2021a) with this number rising to 90% in long term care jobs (OECD, 2019a); with many women in long term care jobs earning less than men for the same role (OECD, 2023a). Many health and social care jobs tend to be poorly paid (International Labour Organization, 2018) with some long-term care workers, across the OECD, earning 70% of the national hourly wage (OECD, 2023a). Working conditions and pay can thus be seen to contribute to difficulties in recruiting and retaining staff. There are differences, however, between job roles with nurses, for example, earning more than the average for all workers across the OECD. Nevertheless, there are differences between countries again with nurses earning less in Switzerland, Lithuania, France, Latvia, and Finland and earning more in Chile, Mexico, Israel, and Luxembourg (OECD, 2019b; OECD, 2021a). In the UK nurses earn less than the average wage (OECD, 2019b) with salaries falling in real terms by over 5% between 2010 and 2018 (OECD, 2021a).

Informal carers contribute significantly to health and social care and are often invisible with little support (Sibley et al., 2023). For example, one in nine Australians are an informal carer with many having to give up employment to provide care (Deloitte, 2020), in Lithuania, Greece and Poland most long term care, due to a lack of provision and possibly because of a focus on family care, is more likely to be provided by family members (OECD, 2022; OECD, 2023a), while in the UK, seven percent of the population are informal carers with nine percent of these caring for more than one person (Department for Work and Pensions, 2023). Exploring the Family Resources Survey for the UK shows that individuals in the age range 55 to 64 years were more likely to be informal carers. In relation to gender women overall were more likely to provide informal care (9% women compared to 6% men) this was especially the case for women who were aged 25 to 74 years old. However, both men and women aged between 16-24 and 75+ were as likely as each other to be informal carers. Interesting, child carers until the aged of 15 were all female (Department for Work and Pensions, 2023).

COVID-19 highlighted numerous vulnerabilities within health and social care systems across many countries in the OECD with histories of chronic underinvestment and understaffing impacting on the responses of these systems to the crisis (King's Fund, 2020; CQC, 2020; Rocard et al., 2021; BMA, 2022; European Union, 2022; OECD, 2023b). For example, the OECD highlights that long term care (LTC) sectors were not prepared in relation to infection control procedures, were not prioritised in relation to PPE and testing, had poor data collection on the numbers impacted by COVID-19, and that there was weak integration between LTC settings and health systems impacting directly on the health of service users in LTC (Rocard et al., 2021). In England and Wales approximately four times as many deaths from COVID-19 occurred in care homes as opposed to hospitals during the period March to April

2020, with excess deaths in care homes estimated to be approximately 20,000 (Burki, 2020). While in the European region approximately half of deaths from COVID-19 in 2020 were in long term care facilities (Kluge, 2020). The wellbeing of long-term care residents was also impacted by the stringent lockdown measures which were introduced in these facilities, including cancellation of activities and visitors, with research from the Netherlands highlighting increases in loneliness, behavioural issues and depression among residents (Van der Roest et al., 2020). Reports have also indicated that COVID-19 has had long term impacts on health and social care provision with post-pandemic increases in waiting times for treatment, assessment and services struggling to meet demand and need (CQC, 2021; OECD, 2023b).

COMPARING COUNTRIES ACROSS THE OECD

The Organisation for Economic Co-operation and Development (OECD) is an organisation which focuses on economic development and world trade and consists of 38 member countries (see Table 1.1 for a list of countries). Together with governments, policy makers and citizens, it establishes evidence-based international standards and solutions to current social, economic and environmental challenges. Most OECD countries can be found in Europe, with the majority being defined as high-income countries.

Comparing health and social care policy and practice across OECD countries enables an exploration of patterns, similarities, and differences in how health and social care is provided across a range of countries. Analysis of how different countries address health and social care concerns can lead to a deeper understanding of complex health and social care issues and can highlight issues such as how countries respond to ageing populations and long-term care needs. Moreover, deeper understanding of health and social care across countries may improve national practice and policy, enabling policy makers and practitioners to reflect upon taken for granted knowledge and practice to improve outcomes for service users by comparing different approaches. Many countries may have differing philosophical, socio-political, and historical traditions which have impacted policy and practice in relation to health and social care systems. By exploring health and social care across OECD countries, this may lead to a greater understanding of the UK system, and its own history, and an understanding of the differing trajectories of other systems.

TABLE 1.1 List of OECD Countries

Australia	Austria	Belgium	Canada	Chile
Columbia	Costa Rica	Czechia	Denmark	Estonia
Finland	France	Germany	Greece	Hungary
Iceland	Ireland	Israel	Italy	Japan
Korea	Latvia	Lithuania	Luxembourg	Mexico
Netherlands	New Zealand	Norway	Poland	Portugal
Slovak Republic	Slovenia	Spain	Sweden	Switzerland
Türkiye	United Kingdom	United States		

There are challenges, however, in comparing countries across the OECD such as a lack of data for countries, different definitions of care, and differing ways of providing care. Divergent economic and cultural factors also make for a challenge in comparisons although evidence suggests a convergence across countries throughout the OECD in relation to health and social care policies, expenditure, and structural organisation of services. Convergence is the process through which societies display tendencies to grow more alike and develop similarities in terms of social, political, and economic structures and policy and practice processes (Bennett, 1991). Emulation of one another is caused, for example, by the need of Governments and elites to harmonise and share expertise, through to insecurities about the costs and potential risks of innovating differently or alternatives to current practice. Convergence is also encouraged by processes of Globalisation (La Placa and Knight, 2023) which increase tendencies to converge and lessen differences in the face of threats and events which are globally apparent. Indeed, discernible across much of the evidence in this book, is a dual convergence of increased expenditure on health and social care across the OECD and that of diversifying and marketising much of the latter. Regardless of the challenges, comparative analysis of health and social care policy and practice brings about substantial benefits in our understandings of health and social care and there is no doubt that OECD countries can and do maintain some form of independence and discretion in the face of increasing policy convergence.

OUTLINE OF CHAPTERS

The book is divided into two parts. Part I focuses on core concepts in health and social care policy and practice such as typologies and theories of welfare regimes (Chapter 2), health and social care financing (Chapter 3), wellbeing (Chapter 4), health inequalities (Chapter 5), partnership working including integrated care (Chapter 6), and service user involvement (Chapter 7). Part 2 then continues by focusing on specific health and social care topics, exploring issues across OECD countries or selected OECD countries using a comparative lens. Specific topics focused upon in part 2 are homelessness (Chapter 8), domestic violence and abuse (Chapter 9), substance use policies (Chapter 10), health inequalities and people with learning disabilities (Chapter 11), women in prison (Chapter 12), end of life care (Chapter 13), dental services (Chapter 14), long term care services (Chapter 15), health policies in OECD countries for refugees and migrants (Chapter 16), and loneliness (Chapter 17). In Chapter 18, the book concludes that firstly, OECD countries are subject to important global developments, such as ageing populations, health inequalities, and globalisation, among others. Secondly, there is a dual convergence of both increasing expenditure upon health and social care and processes of marketisation and diversity in provision across the OECD. Thirdly, health and social care research, policy and practice, requires adaptation to increasing complexity and change and responses. Each chapter has research points and reflective exercises to consolidate learning.

REFERENCES

Bennett, C. J. (1991). What Is Policy Convergence and What Causes It? *British Journal of Political Science*, 21 (2): 215–233. www.jstor.org/stable/193876

BMA. (2022). *Delivery of Healthcare During the Pandemic*. London: BMA.

Burki, T, (2020). England and Wales see 20 000 Excess Deaths in Care Homes. *The Lanc*et, 395 (10237): 1602. https://doi.org/10.1016/S0140-6736(20)31199-5.

CQC. (2020). State of Care 2019/20. Available at: www.cqc.org.uk/publications/major-report/state-care-201920 (Accessed: 15 January 2024).

CQC. (2021). State of Care 2020/2021. Available at: www.cqc.org.uk/publication/state-care-202021 (Accessed: 16 February 2024).

Deloitte. (2020). The Value of Informal Care in 2020. Available at: www2.deloitte.com/au/en/pages/economics/articles/value-of-informal-care-2020.html (Accessed: 18 February 2024).

Department for Work and Pensions. (2023). Family Resources Survey: Financial Year 2021 to 2022. Available at: www.gov.uk/government/statistics/family-resources-survey-financial-year-2021-to-2022/family-resources-survey-financial-year-2021-to-2022 (Accessed: 16 January 2024).

Dodsworth, E. and Oung, C. (2023). Who Organises and Funds Social Care? In E. Dodsworth and C. Oung (eds), *Adult Social Care in the Four Countries of the UK*. Explainer Series. London: Nuffield Trust.

European Union. (2022). *State of Health in the EU: Companion Report 21*. Luxembourg: European Union.

Glasby, J. (2019). *The Short Guide to Health and Social Care*. Bristol: Policy Press.

Glasby, J., Farquharson, C., Hanson, L. and Minkman, M. (2023). Building a Better Understanding of Adult Social Care. *BMJ* 382. doi:10.1136/bmj-2022-073720

International Labour Organization. (2018). *Care Work and Care Jobs for the Future of Decent Work*. Geneva: ILO.

King's Fund. (2020). How Covid-19 has Magnified Some of Social Care's Key Problems. Available at: www.kingsfund.org.uk/publications/covid-19-magnified-social-care-problems (Accessed: 15 January 2023).

Kluge, H. H. P. (2020). Statement – Invest in the Overlooked and Unsung: Build Sustainable People-Centred Long-Term Care in the Wake of COVID-19. Available at: www.who.int/europe/news/item/23-04-2020-statement-invest-in-the-overlooked-and-unsung-build-sustainable-people-centred-long-term-care-in-the-wake-of-covid-19 (Accessed: 20 February 2024).

La Placa, V. and Knight, A. (2023). Globalisation and Global Public Health. In V. La Placa and J. Morgan (eds), S*ocial Science Perspectives on Global Public Health*. London: Routledge, 17–28.

OECD. (2019a). Women are Well-Represented in Health and Long-Term Care Professions, but Often in Jobs with Poor Working Conditions. Available at: www.oecd.org/gender/data/women-are-well-represented-in-health-and-long-term-care-professions-but-often-in-jobs-with-poor-working-conditions.htm (Accessed: 15 January 2024).

OECD. (2019b). *Health at a Glance 2019: OECD Indicators*. Paris: OECD Publishing.

OECD. (2021a). *Health at a Glance 2021: OECD Indicators*. Paris: OECD Publishing.

OECD. (2021b). Key Insights & Proposed Solutions from the Future of Care and the Caregiving Workforce: Lessons and Insights from the COVID-19 Experience. www2.oecd.org/health/Caregiving-Workforce-Workshop-Report-Oct2021.pdf (Accessed: 16 January 2024).

OECD. (2022). *Integrating Services for Older People in Lithuania*. Paris: OECD Publishing.

OECD. (2023a). *Beyond Applause? Improving Working Conditions in Long-Term Care*. Paris: OECD Publishing.

OECD. (2023b). *Ready for the Next Crisis? Investing in Health System Resilience.* OECD Health Policy Studies. Paris: OECD Publishing.

Rocard, E., Sillitti, P. and Llena-Nozal, A. (2021). *COVID-19 in Long-Term Care: Impact, Policy Responses and Challenges.* OECD Health Working Papers, No. 131. Paris: OECD Publishing.

Sibley, M., Hallam, L. and Robins, S. (2023). Invisible no More: Unpaid Care Giving in the Shadow of Covid-19. *BMJ, 382.* doi:10.1136/bmj-2022-073053

Van der Roest, H. G., Prins, M., van der Velden, C., Steinmetz, S., Stolte, E., et al. (2020). The Impact of COVID-19 Measures on Well-Being of Older Long-Term Care Facility Residents in the Netherlands. *Journal of the American Medical Directors Association, 21*(11): 1569–1570. https://doi.org/10.1016/j.jamda.2020.09.007

CHAPTER 2

Theories of Social Policy and Welfare States

....

Vincent La Placa and Lotta Hackett

INTRODUCTION

This chapter will explore models and theories of the development of social policies and welfare states across OECD countries. It draws attention to the different typologies of welfare regimes across the OECD and proceeds to discuss four core theories of welfare states and the strengths and weaknesses of the theories. The four theories are 'structuralism', 'Marxism', 'pluralism', and 'postmodernism'. The first two theories are broadly structuralist and the latter two focus more on plurality, multiplicity, and discourse, in their approach to social policy and welfare states. The chapter ends with a focus upon the concept of 'globalisation', its impact upon current social and welfare policies, particularly around convergence of welfare states, and its implications for theories of and research on social policies across OECD countries.

SOCIAL POLICY AND WELFARE STATES ACROSS THE OECD

Social and welfare policies are often referred to as systems whereby the State undertakes to protect the health and wellbeing of its citizens, particularly people in financial or social need, often through redistribution of wealth and resources across populations. This is achieved by means of grants, pensions, and other benefits, and is a recognisable phenomenon across the OECD. The size of welfare states varies significantly across OECD countries. Spending on welfare and social services is around 30% in France. However, Austria, Belgium, Denmark, Finland, Germany, Italy, Norway, and Sweden assign more than a quarter of their gross domestic product (GDP) to health and social support (OECD, 2020a). In contrast, social spending in countries such as Chile, Colombia, Costa Rica, Ireland, Korea, Mexico and Türkiye, comprise less than 15% of GDP (OECD, 2020a). Welfare expenditure encompasses cash benefits, direct in-kind provision of goods and services, and tax breaks with

DOI: 10.4324/9781003343608-3

social purposes. Benefits may be targeted at low-income households, older individuals, the disabled, sick, unemployed, or younger individuals. Forms of welfare states are often linked to economic and social developments with countries. States which industrialised earlier, after the Second World War, for example, the United States of America (USA), United Kingdom (UK) and European Union (EU), spend more. Prevailing ideologies around, for instance, poverty, and wealth distribution, 'structural constraints and facilitators' and various levels of 'economic development', contribute to how social policies and welfare states are defined and resourced. For example, comparatively, healthcare systems between the USA and EU exist on a continuum of more private and market orientated provision on one hand, and more state orientated approaches, on the other. Others, such as France and Germany, span both models, emphasising provision of social insurance, as well as the former approaches (Russell, 2018).

All OECD countries are confronted by ageing populations, which exercise upward pressure on spending through demands for healthcare and income support in retirement, for instance. However, current economic downturns restrain social spending increases, but may enhance capital and resources allocated to, for instance, unemployment and social assistance payments (OECD, 2020b). The COVID-19 pandemic since 2020/2021 has compounded significant increases in social spending (OECD, 2020a), as demands on welfare and healthcare systems augmented, and a varied array of social and economic support was implemented to relieve individuals of the most negative impacts of lockdowns and economic contractions. In addition, debates about globalisation influence responses to welfare expenditure and the forms it assumes. Russell (2018) asserts that since the emergence of the 'post 1989 world order', where advanced capitalism and free markets became the dominant economic

TABLE 2.1 Liberal Market and Coordinated Market Economy Regime Types

Type	Characteristics
Liberal market regimes (e.g., USA, UK, Canada, Australia, New Zealand, and Ireland)	In liberal market regimes, companies primarily coordinate their endeavours by means of hierarchies and free market mechanisms, with less state intervention instead, for instance, government, and trades union agents, individuals, and activities.
Coordinated market economy regimes (e.g., Germany, France, Japan, Sweden, and Austria)	Coordinated market economies rely more strongly on non-market mechanisms of interaction in the coordination of their relationships with groups and individuals. For instance, they exhibit higher levels of state intervention and expenditure within institutional arrangements, in more interaction with civil society. Sometimes, they are referred to as 'organised capitalist societies, which develop strong civil societies, around, for instance, social movements and voluntary organisations (La Placa and Corlyon, 2014a).

model, it has developed the emergence of two ideological approaches towards social policy and welfare. One, conceives higher taxes and generous social benefits as befitting capitalism, normally associated to varying degrees, with the UK and EU; the other perceives capitalism as generating an ideological approach which promotes lower taxes and less generous welfare, associated more, with the USA. Hall and Soskice (2001) argue that capitalist economies veer towards one of two forms of capitalism, based upon structured institutional arrangements between liberal market and coordinated market economy regime types.

The model is often criticised for presenting ideal types of capitalist economies and institutional arrangements as opposed to empirical realities, which often comprise overlapping characteristics of both; as well as negation of how state and economic agents and individuals can subjectively alter and produce changes within a given institutional arrangement (Crouch, 2005). Esping-Andersen (1990) formulated a typology of 18 OECD welfare states based upon three tenets: 'decommodification' (the extent to which an individual's welfare is orientated towards the market; 'social stratification' (the influence of welfare states in maintaining or reducing socio-economic social stratification) and the 'private–public mix' (the influences of the state, the family, the voluntary sector and the market in welfare provision). The operationalisation of the above tenets, mostly using decommodification indexes, leads to the division of welfare states into three ideal regime types. These are liberal, conservative, and social democratic regimes. Table 2.2 outlines the type and their characteristics.

TABLE 2.2 Liberal, Conservative, and Social Democratic Regime Types

Type	Characteristics
Liberal regimes	Liberal regimes are characterised by minimal state provision of welfare, and often apply strict entitlement criteria, with welfare more means-tested and recipients subject to stigma. For instance, often there is a distinction asserted between the 'deserving' and 'undeserving' poor, with less sympathy for the latter, often portrayed as 'scroungers' or 'shirkers', for example, the UK and USA.
Conservative regimes	Conservative regimes are characterised by their 'status differentiating' welfare programmes in which benefits are often earnings-related, administered through the employer, and biased towards maintaining existing social patterns. The family's role is also emphasised, and the state/collective redistributive element is lessened, for example, Spain and Italy.
Social democratic regimes	Social democratic regimes represent the smallest group, according to Esping-Andersen (1990). Welfare provision is founded upon universal and more generous benefits, a commitment to full employment and income protection, and a highly interventionist state used to promote equality through a redistributive framework, such as the Scandinavian countries.

Esping-Andersen (1990) argue, however, that despite the differences between the regimes, all tended towards a convergence of increasing welfare expenditure, including the more Conservative regimes, where the family assumes a fundamental ancillary role in social protection. The model is also often criticised for delineating a too narrow view of welfare regimes and fails to adequately consider the diverse ways in which policies are realised, for example, the use of public expenditure versus supply side policy instruments to redistribute wealth (Castles and Mitchell, 1993). Similarly, Santos and Simoes (2021) revised Esping-Andersen's (1990) framework based upon the work of Hein et al. (2021) and grouped 36 OECD countries in different welfare models by combining public social spending and redistributive policies data with socio-economic indicators (see Table 2.3). Their focus assumes four specific indicators: trade union density; employment protection legislation; public social spending (as a share of GDP) and redistribution effectiveness. Six classifications were produced

TABLE 2.3 Six Classifications of Welfare Regimes by Santos and Simoes (2021)

Type	Characteristics
Social-democratic/Nordic	Social-democratic/Nordic welfare provision is extensive, and it exhibits higher shares of welfare spending. Trade Union activity is higher compared to the others as is employment protection. Countries included are Denmark, Finland, Iceland, Norway, and Sweden.
Continental/corporative/ conservative	Continental/corporative/conservative models also have extensive welfare state spending but show signs of convergence with the Social-democratic/Nordic model. Countries included are Austria, Belgium, France, Germany, Japan, Korea, Luxembourg, The Netherlands, and Switzerland.
Anglo Saxon/liberal	Anglo Saxon/liberal are more market orientated and less collectivist, displaying lower levels of expenditure although this is increasing. Countries included are Australia, Canada, Ireland, New Zealand, UK, and USA.
Mediterranean/southern European	Mediterranean/southern European regimes spend lower on welfare expenditure with lower rates of Trade Union activity and redistributive policies. However, the tendency is to increased expenditure due to increasing unemployment as economies are exposed to recession. These regimes tend to be a balance of individualist and collectivist tendencies. Countries included are Greece, Italy, Portugal, and Spain.
Central & eastern European	These are like Mediterranean/southern European models and faced with similar structural and economic issues. As a result, there is more pressure from civil society to increase expenditure towards continental/corporative/conservative levels. Countries included are Czechia, Estonia, Hungary. Latvia. Lithuania, Poland, the Slovak Republic, and Slovenia.
Others	These currently display much lower levels of expenditure and social protection with less developed welfare states and benefits. Countries included are Chile, Israel, Mexico, and Türkiye.

by Santos and Simoes (2021), although they argue that there is a tendency across the different regimes to increase expenditure on welfare and social protection.

This chapter will now consider theoretical perspectives on social policies and welfare states and proceeds to focus on the role of 'globalisation' afterwards.

THEORETICAL PERSPECTIVES ON SOCIAL POLICY AND WELFARE STATES ACROSS THE OECD

Since the Second World War, welfare states across the OECD have become a common and recognisable empirical feature of its social and political systems. For instance, expenditure across OECD countries has increased immensely since the 1950s/1960s with all countries developing converging social benefits and healthcare systems as a discernible part of welfare systems, despite different approaches and forms of welfare. Empirical realities activate use of theoretical perspectives to explain historical, political, and explanatory models of their existence, and how a particular form of social policy and welfare states, emerge in relation to broader structural and social determinants. The chapter will now proceed to consider four core theories of welfare states: 'functionalism', 'pluralism', 'Marxism', and 'postmodernism'.

Structural Functionalism

Historically, the earliest approaches to social policies and welfare states tended to emerge from a structuralist functionalist approach. This accentuates the development of welfare states as a response to meet the complex requirements of societies at a specific stage of, for instance, 'industrialisation,' 'modernisation' or 'advanced' capitalism. The structural functionalist theory of welfare states is elaborated upon by Kerr et al. (1960) who argued that 'total industrialisation', as an empirical feature of modern societies, is explained through the actual course of transition from a preceding 'agricultural' or 'commercial' society, towards the 'industrial' one. The emergence of an industrial workforce, based upon factory and shift patterns, precipitates welfare states to provide minimum standards of health and social security such as, sickness benefits and unemployment insurance. Consensus emerges that society bears responsibility for the welfare of workers in productive activity, especially as the close family and kinship relations, associated with the agrarian stage, declines, due to greater movement of people from the land (Galbraith, 1963; Wilensky, 1975).

Durkheim (1893/1964) similarly argued that technological development created distinct categories of workers and skills specialisation, which created division between socio-economic groups, and reduced social solidarity. As a result, reformist social policies, were necessary to enhance social solidarity, and mitigate the effects of the disruption and dislocation engendered by industrial capitalism. Like Marxism, structural changes, promote the emergence of class relations and protectionism for the industrial classes, as a key component in organising social policies. Gough (1978) argued that structural functionalism promoted an enlightened response to the material poverty and inequalities of the industrial revolution, whereby structural changes, enabled forms of limited moral and political consciousness, emphasising needs and protection, within what capitalist ideology permitted. Social policies, then emerge consensually and organically, to resolve problems within a newly structured social organisation, led by industrialism, demographic, and technological changes. This explains the shift to welfare states and convergence across the advanced capitalist countries to accommodate diverse family structures and care for older people as the extended family weakens under industrialisation.

Gough (1978) criticised this approach for being too structuralist and questioned assumptions that welfare is created for positive reasons, and, for ignoring the historical and contextual basis of welfare development. For example, since 1945, UK expenditure on welfare increased, because of economic and moral decisions resulting from the Second World War, and memories of inter-war economic decline, which led to welfare retrenchment at the time. Rimlinger (1971) argued that the nature of the political system and culturally shaped norms and values as to economics and morality is as significant as industrialisation and class relations. For instance, countries with more individualistic cultures and less altruistic attitudes to social mobility and work were less likely to develop large welfare states as opposed to those that emphasise collectivism and strong national identities. Flora and Heidenheimer (1981) perceived welfare states as general traits of 'modernisation', whereby the social and economic divisions, characteristic of modern capitalism, precipitated the social and political mobilisation of various social economic groups, to lobby for and against, different forms of social spending and welfare. The chapter now proceeds to the Marxist theory of welfare.

Marxism

If structural functionalism accentuates the positive functions which welfare development and social expenditure assumes, to ensure the stable functioning of industrial societies, the Marxist approach, (while also supporting a structuralist understanding of the welfare state), emphasised instead that welfare spending was a contradictory process tending towards economic, social, and political crisis. For Marxists, historical relations do not play out in one unilinear trajectory towards progress, rationality, and modernisation, outside of conflict between one's materialist location in the class structure, where a dominant economic class consistently subordinates and oppresses another (Marx, 1867/1990). History is a succession of qualitatively distinct stages of 'modes of production', and not one unilinear development, whereby each stage transitions to another, until the communist stage emerges (termed 'historical materialism'). Table 2.4 delineates the modes of production and their characteristics.

Each stage then determines class conflict, and the types of societies, which structurally evolve (Marx, 1867/1990; Gough, 1978). For Marxists, current welfare states constitute a particular function of contemporary capitalism (stage four) and are perceived as part of contemporary class relations and capitalist mode of production, used to repress, and control the current working class or 'proletariat' by the owners of the means of production or 'bourgeoisie'. O'Connor (1973) contended

TABLE 2.4 Modes of Production in Marxist Theory

Mode of Production	Characteristics
Primitive communism (agrarian times)	These are known as 'hunter–gatherer' societies or 'primitive' communist societies. They are mostly agrarian. Societies are not run by a political nation state and there is no observable property, money, or social classes. Due to their limited means of production (hunting and gathering) everyone was only able to produce enough to sustain themselves. Therefore, there was no profit or exploitation.
Slave society (ancient times)	Slave societies are characterised by use of slavery and minor private property; production for use is the primary form of production between citizens and slaves. Surplus from agriculture is distributed to the citizens, who exploit slaves who toil in the fields.
Feudalism (from Roman times to eighteenth century)	Feudalism comprises class relations between an entrenched nobility and serfdom. Simple commodity production existed in the form of artisans and merchants. This merchant class would increase and eventually transform into the bourgeoisie.
Capitalism (from nineteenth century onwards)	Capitalism emerges when the rising bourgeois class becomes large enough to institute a shift in the productive forces to large scale industrial production which employ the emerging working classes (proletariat) in large-scale industrial and factory settings. Workers are exploited for profit and immiserated as a result.
Communism	Communism materialises when the proletariat overthrow the bourgeoisie class and create a society based upon equality, where people only produce commodities which they need to equally distribute as opposed to for profit. Previous class relations evaporate as exploitation and inequality disappear.

that capitalism serves two distinct and mutually contradictory objectives, that of 'accumulation' and 'legitimisation'. Welfare states abet both in prolonging the continuation, stability, and effective operation of the economic system and in enhancing the integration of social classes within it, as well as the stabilisation of social order to legitimise it and control workers. Simultaneously, it also abets the oppression and subordination of the working classes. O'Connor (1973) asserted that because of the contradictory character of capitalism, welfare state expenditure serves accumulation and legitimisation functions simultaneously. For example, welfare transfers and benefits pacify the poor and prevent resistance to social and economic inequalities. Expenditure on health and social care also assists capitalism in the promotion of the false assumption that welfare maintains a healthy, hardworking, and productive workforce, and the belief that individuals and groups are somehow 'looked after', shielded from poverty, and comprise a stake in the economy.

The State's intervention in health and social care protects capitalism and promotes biomedical ideology to maintain class structures and systems of domination, which conceals the social and economic foundations of health and illness inequalities (Waitzkin, 1978; Bengtsson, 2017; Moncrieff, 2022). Social and welfare systems increasingly assist in augmenting capitalist domination and the subordination of the working class; while conversely, contributing to its demise as the working class increasingly become more 'class conscious' and realise the actual and material role, which it assumes in maintaining their subordination (Cowling, 1985). Marxist explanations of social and welfare systems are often perceived as strongly recognising that often illness and disease is not a bio-medical phenomenon, for example, 'mental illnesses, but the results of the increasingly precarious nature of people's working lives and the endemic stress, poverty, oppression, and low wages associated with capitalism and material class relations (Moncrieff, 2022; Das, 2023). However, Marxist explanations are often also too narrow in that they are over reliant on concepts of class and the economy to explain health and illness, and their effects, are often only implied by Marxist theorists (Das, 2023).

The structural approach assumed by Marxism also aligns it with Structural Functionalism, lessening the distinction. Social and economic transitions and paradigms are structurally determined, and thinking about welfare and health and social care systems reflects the limited mode of thought which the transition permits. However, as Das (2023) asserts, the 'social determinants' model, often dominant in current health and social care practice, comprises its origins in Marxism, albeit tentatively. Given the structural and materialist bias of Marxism, pluralism has emerged and provided the foundations for more empirical based studies of the policy making process, as regards social policies and welfare.

Pluralism

The key tenet of the pluralist approach is that power is widely diffused throughout the political system. Consequently, conflict between different and competing groups in the policy making process, is effectively managed, without any group exerting a dominant influence over the political system (Dahl, 1961; Galbraith, 1969). The state also remains neutral and ensures no group dominates sufficiently, thereby ensuring that policy is approached through a multiple perspective and emerges through the contribution of a wide range of individual thought, action, and influence. Social and welfare policies, as a result, are often approached empirically through a case study perspective and pluralism is sceptical that an overall meta-narrative can explain each case, as is the case with, for instance, structural functionalism and Marxism. For example, the emergence of the National Health Service (NHS) in the UK was the result of debate, competing compromise, and engagement, across the British Medical Association (BMA), local authorities, the insurance lobby, voluntary hospitals, including charities, and the civil service (Gough, 1978), with medical professionals, however, exercising greater influence. However, by the 1980s and 1990s, as concepts of 'choice' and 'accountability' emerged as key policy challenges, other interest groups, such as patient consultation groups, and the then Department of Health (DH) rapidly expanded their influence and power upon service innovation and performance (Alaszewski and Brown, 2012).

The functioning of policy making, according to pluralism, occurs outside any materially structured class relations, so ensures against dominance of one group over another. Distribution of power resources in capitalist democracies can vary between groups and policy networks and power alters interchangeably. Political institutions and elections assume a significant role in the processing of conflicts of interest-based groups and parties. For Korpi (1989), this perspective can partially and empirically explain the growth of welfare and health and social services across OECD countries, especially the often dominant and countervailing power of left-wing interests, and social democratic parties, which have broadly supported increased welfare, since the 1930s. Pluralism is often criticised for its lack of recourse to dominant class and power structures and for negating arguments around who frames the policy agenda and defines the dominant norms, values, and priorities (Gough, 1978). As Miliband (1969) and Gramsci (1971) have asserted, dominant values and ideologies are embedded within political and social systems, which legitimate the social order, and become internalised by a population, often unconsciously. However, a key strength is that it assumes a methodological individualist approach which enables a case-by-case study of policy formulation to social policy and welfare. It also views individual action and behaviour within its context and can accommodate potential conflict and shifting power balances (Gough, 1978).

As a result, whereas structural functionalism is often criticised for 'reification' and objectification of social structures and determinants, Gough (1978) argues that pluralism proceeds too much in the opposite direction, that of 'subjectification' of social action. For Gough (1978) a Marxist approach which could bridge both poles and focus upon how human subjective action is constructed within the confines and restrictions of class-based societies would prove more fruitful in an analysis of social policies and welfare states. However, emerging throughout the 1970s and 1980s, postmodernism, with its rejection of grand theory and meta-narratives, argued that societies and policy making processes were more complex than assumed, even by pluralists. Progress and emancipation required revision in the light of new theoretical and empirical realities, as well as scepticism of modern grand theories, such as the ones above.

Postmodernism

Postmodernism dismisses the view that 'emancipatory' politics and policies can be explained through unitary explanatory theoretical frameworks, typical of modernity, which emerged through the Enlightenment and scientific revolutions, and which subsequently established concepts of 'truth' and 'facts' (Lyotard, 1984; Jameson, 1991; Seidman and Wagner, 1992). Rather, truth, as far as there can be, and social ontology, is contextual, relative, and socially and discursively contingent. Postmodernists also repudiate foundationalism and essentialism, the idea that knowledge and beliefs are constructed through a single foundation, or one source of truth, typical of modern thought. Understanding social phenomena invariably involves multiple interpretations of change and deconstruction of grand theory. 'Difference' and 'multiplicity' is embraced, often emphasising 'identity' politics, for example, 'oppressed' groups, such as welfare claimants and minority users of services, and the multiple discourses, which construct and destabilise action and identities, over time.

Unlike, for instance, structural orientated theories, postmodern societies are in a constant process of creation and contingencies and cannot be reduced to stabilised social structures and pre-determined stages of historical development. Even pluralist theory is perceived as static and unitary by postmodernists, in that it is reduced to an essential and singular assumption that power and influence is distributed through competitive politics. For postmodernists, concepts of health, welfare, and social care, are often perceived as products of modern singular and essentialist thought which reduces multiplicity. Modern thought also incorrectly assumes that collective responsibility, and the creation of large progressive bureaucratic systems of welfare, are possible, or even desirable. Modern belief in the progress of social and welfare policy often obfuscated the deleterious effects and consequences, which such interventions often had upon minorities and oppressed groups, as medical professionals' and social workers' knowledge was institutionalised and hierarchised above patients' and service users' needs. For example, historically, psychiatric discourses have stigmatised individuals with mental health issues, often subjecting them to cruel treatments, institutionalisation, and lack of rights. Instead, for postmodernists, the emphasis pertains to creation of health and welfare through new practices and discourses, relevant to postmodernity, and the conditions of uncertainty, cultural relativity, and contingency (Peter, 1996).

Social and welfare policies are continuously constructed and deconstructed through language and discourse and cannot be perceived as solid structures beyond the subjectivities of its creators. For example, Lindström (2020) argued, that in Sweden, the COVID-19 global pandemic, produced a reaction against modernist discourses of welfare and health and social care. Overconfidence in collective notions of herd immunity, and traditional empirical evidence-based medicine, was replaced by emerging concepts of individual responsibility in managing the pandemic, which engendered contextual and individual solutions, such as re-evaluation of traditional medicine, as opposed to collectively prescribed interventions. Chevannes (2002) using a broadly postmodernist perspective, ascertained that health and social care professionals' assessments of older people was based upon contexts, which locate them in roles, where they mostly perceive themselves as acting for state, voluntary, or private agencies, and not in roles where they collaborate with older people to help serve their needs. Professionals categorise older people into two groups or 'classes,' i.e., those having 'health needs' as distinct from those with 'social care' needs. The techniques employed magnitude to an exercise of power by professionals over older people, to categorise and control them, and negate their perceived needs.

Powell (2023) advocates that postmodernist concepts cater to decisions for how service users' needs are met or not; how assessment of needs impinges upon power and surveillance, and the extent to which service users' 'voices' are heard. For instance, regarding older people and aging, a postmodern gerontology, can disclose the diversity of service users, and the varied social and cultural representations and experiences of aging and older people's identities. It traverses the modernistic bio-medical equation of 'aging as decline' and enables alternative perspectives on how clients and professionals construct discourses of old age- which are contingent upon continuous engagement with meaning and discourse (Powell and Gilbert, 2009). However, postmodernism has been criticised for elevating conservatism and deterring collective responsibility and social action. Any theory which refuses and delegitimises concrete concepts of, for instance, 'equality,' 'freedom' and 'social justice' as merely discursive social constructs (and not empirically 'real') is perceived as inimical to the welfare, social justice, and solidarity. If health and social care, for instance, cannot be adequately defined and institutionalised across countries, its rationale is diminished, and its functions cannot be adequately evaluated through empirical research, one of the core principles of theory (Hartley, 2022). Rather, postmodernism can often, it is argued, constitute alignment with 'neoliberalism', by framing concepts of welfare, health, and social care, as questions of 'difference,' 'diversity', and 'choice' (Hartley, 2022), rather than collective solidarity and care. Thus far, this chapter has focused upon four core theories to explain social policies and welfare states in OECD countries. It now proceeds to a focus upon the concept of globalisation and its relevance to social policies and welfare states across the OECD.

GLOBALISATION, THEORY, AND RESEARCH

The emergence of globalisation has had a major impact across theoretical debates and research around economies, societies, and welfare states across the OECD, especially given some of the more structured models alluded to earlier, and their impact on further research into health and social care models and social policies. For example, Esping-Andersen (1990) and Hall and Soskice (2001) did not assume adequate focus upon how globalisation impacted their frameworks; although such debates were not as prevalent at the time of their development. While globalisation is a contested concept, it often refers to a rapid development and expansion of a network of independencies and connections, characteristic of modern life, across politics, economics, culture, and technology. Modern life compresses and wanes as geographical, social, and economic boundaries dissipate and people, information, products, and knowledge, spread across boundaries, reducing distance between individuals and countries (Chirico, 2014; La Placa and Knight, 2023). From a Marxist perspective, it is advocated that global homogenisation legitimises the imposition of neoliberal tendencies and free markets, cost cutting and asset-stripping, particularly in the Global South. As a result, wages and living conditions globally are pushed down, as competition for investment increases. Welfare funding is reduced to accommodate this, and economies are forced to restructure in capital's interests, thus increasing class inequalities. Similarly, Simmonds (2021a) argues that globalisation encourages states towards a neoliberal outlook, whereby responsibility for health and social care shifts from the state to the individual, as economies are forced to restructure and reduce costs, and services are privatised and outsourced to private organisations to profit and reduce costs further. This reinforces the health and social inequalities which welfare states were originally designed to eradicate.

Globalisation is also associated with theories of 'late modernity' and 'risk society,' where societies and relations become more 'fluid', 'dislocated', 'risky', and 'unpredictable' across all strata of society, as the social, personal, and economic certainties of traditional modernity recede (Beck, 1992; Giddens, 1984; 1990; La Placa and Corlyon, 2014b). Social and welfare reform, accordingly, focuses on the individual. It exists to equip individuals with the skills and capacities to deal with the socio-economic risks inherent in a global risk society, for example, jobs reskilling and enhanced education, as opposed to collective wealth redistribution and social solidarity. Hence, globalisation shifts perspectives on the functions of social policy- as economies and societies face more competition, changes in employment markets, and limited ability to tax corporations, and fund social expenditure, because of globalisation.

Some empirical studies demonstrate a negative relationship between globalisation and the welfare state while others suggest adverse or non-significant outcomes (Rudra and Haggard, 2005; Burgoon and Schakel, 2022). Its impact, however, can be neither uniform nor unidirectional because of the contextual differences in the economies of welfare states, with much evidence suggesting convergence. Social policies reflect qualitative differences in configurations of welfare, suggesting that national welfare regimes themselves may influence the impact of globalisation on welfare states. Kim and Zurlo (2009) empirically studied the impact of economic globalisation on 18 high-income countries and concluded that welfare regimes respond differently to its impact, and therefore, mediate the relationship between globalisation and welfare policy. Globalisation negatively affected welfare provision and expenditure in 'social democratic' regimes, but marginally in 'liberal' and 'conservative' regimes, largely because the former displayed higher levels of spending initially. There was also a tendency to reduce labour market-related spending, while expanding social service-related spending, but overall, countries maintained significant leverage to make decisions in the face of global economic restructuring, risk, and free markets. Wu et al. (2023) found that welfare states enhance the 'quality' of welfare, for example, increasing coverage of benefits to protect groups and individuals against unemployment and competition, suggesting no significant retrenchment of welfare globally.

Santos and Simoes (2021) considered what difference welfare models make for how globalisation influenced the composition of social expenditure within given welfare states. Using data for 36 OECD countries from 1990–2018, they explored whether and how different welfare state models influence the impact of the economic, social, and political dimensions of globalisation on social expenditure programmes across the OECD. The influence of globalisation upon social spending varies across welfare models in intensity but overall, it encouraged higher expenditure within countries. For instance, those countries which currently exhibited high welfare expenditure and collectivist ideologies, such as social democratic/Nordic countries, continued to pursue, for example, active labour market policies and increased spending on housing.

Further examination suggested that health and education spending, for example, were not affected, even in countries with historically lower expenditure on welfare such as in Canada, UK, and USA, where there is a wider emphasis on markets and individualism.

The fact that globalisation does not undermine a welfare regime's ability to pursue increased welfare expenditure and promote social protection, according to Santos and Simoes (2021) suggests a convergence in welfare regimes to stronger protection across OECD countries and where discretionary social and welfare policy can improve the social and economic outcomes of globalisation. Pressure from voters and civil society acting independently also exert influence upon welfare regimes as much as exogenous economic factors such as globalisation. Hence, despite differences between, for example, individualist and collectivist tendencies to welfare, the overall evidence is that expenditure has increased across the OECD with enhanced opportunity to mitigate the impact of economic contraction as well internal and external pressure to control costs and expenditure. Simmonds (2021a; 2021b), however, counters this with the argument that the pervasiveness of neoliberalism, due to globalisation, facilitates a different type of convergence among welfare states, despite evidence of discretionary policies and independence in terms of expenditure. This convergence occurs around the fact that health and social care services are consistently forced to adapt to market mechanisms and efficiency-motivated state interventions. This facilitates market competition and customer choice, and wider disparities in access to services (Simmonds, 2021b).

The emergence of globalisation as a significant driver around, for instance, convergence, is also a challenging issue regarding theorising its causes and effects across the OECD. As La Placa and Knight (2023) contend, globalisation is often approached as a totalising and structural system, which interacts with other homogeneous structural hierarchies such as 'colonialism', 'racism', 'homophobia', and 'social exclusion'. However, this renders a significant gap between ontology and empirically confirming the existence of such large-scale social structures, across time and space, countries, and continents, and lived experiences and actions (Stones, 1996; La Placa and Knight, 2023). It also reduces the significance of historical complexity and the contextual experiences and qualitative empirical differences involved. Empirical demonstrations of systems theorising of totalising social structures (and their production) are challenging too. Also, grand theories of globalisation, (often influenced by Marxism), have been re-aligned with similarly problematic totalising theories such as 'post-colonialism' and 'decolonisation', as well as 'convergence', engendering links between welfare and globalisation precarious, and difficult to demonstrate empirically (La Placa and Knight, 2023).

Moreover, debates are also now challenged by concepts of 'de-globalisation' (La Placa and Knight, 2023), whereby the social and economic interdependencies and relations, created through Globalisation, are reduced and reconfigured, and sometimes, referred to as 'de-risking'. For instance, rivalry between the USA, its allies, and China, the Russian invasion of Ukraine, increased trade policy restrictions and the reverberations of the global pandemic (which threatened and interrupted global production and supply chains) may well mean actions towards, and expenditure upon social welfare, are reconfigured. Russia's withdrawal from the deal enabling Ukraine to safely export grain through the Black Sea in the summer of 2023 comprised negative effects across OECD countries as food and energy supply prices increase, adding to the burdens of dealing with climate and environmental changes (BBC, 2023). This will have significant ramifications for policies, as globalisation processes potentially recede, and explanatory models are reconfigured as a response to empirical realities and policy drivers.

CONCLUSION

This chapter has drawn attention to the different typologies of welfare regimes across the OECD which often influence social and welfare policies in specific OECD countries. It then explored the development of OECD welfare states and social policy and discussed four theories of the development of social policies and welfare states across OECD countries: 'structural functionalism'; 'Marxism'; 'pluralism', and 'postmodernism'. The chapter ended with a focus upon the concept of Globalisation and its implications for theories of and research on social policies and welfare across OECD countries.

RESEARCH POINTS AND REFLECTIVE EXERCISES

- Reflect upon how far welfare states differ across the OECD and the impact of this on the health and wellbeing of OECD citizens?
- What do you think will be the impact of globalisation and de-globalisation on welfare states across OECD countries?

REFERENCES

Alaszewski, A. and Brown, P. (2012). *Making Health Policy: A Critical Introduction*. Cambridge: Polity.

BBC. (2023). Russia's Grain Deal Exit is a Stab in the Back – Kenya. Available at: www.bbc.co.uk/news/world-europe-66223280 (Accessed: 1 August 2023).

Beck, U. (1992). *Risk Society: Towards A New Modernity*. London: Sage.

Bengtsson, S. (2017). Out of the Frame: Disability and the Body in the Writings of Karl Marx. *Scand. J. Disabil. Res*, 19 (2): 151–160. https://doi.org/10.1080/15017419.2016.1263972

Burgoon, B. and Schakel, W. (2022). Embedded Liberalism or Embedded Nationalism? How Welfare States Affect Anti-Globalisation Nationalism in Party Platforms. *West European Politics*, 45 (1): 50–76. https://doi.org/10.1080/01402382.2021.1908707

Castles, F. and Mitchell, D. (1993). Worlds of Welfare and Families of Nations. In F. Castles (ed.), *Families of Nations: Patterns of Public Policy in Western Democracies*. Aldershot: Dartmouth, 93–128.

Chevannes, M. (2002). Social Construction of the Managerialism of Needs Assessment by Health and Social Care Professionals. *Health and Social Care in the Community*, 10 (3): 168–178. https://doi.org/10.1046/j.1365-2524.2002.00355.x

Chirico, J. (2014). *Globalization: Prospects and Problems*. London: Sage.

Cowling, M. (1985). The Welfare State as a Reproduction Condition of Capitalism: What Does This Explanation Tell Us?. *International Journal of Sociology and Social Policy*, 5 (1): 68–78. https://doi.org/10.1108/eb012979

Crouch, C. (2005). *Capitalist Diversity and Change: Recombinant Governance and Institutional Entrepreneurs*. Oxford: Oxford University Press.

Dahl, R. A. (1961). *Who Governs? Power and Democracy in an American City*. New Haven: Yale University Press.

Das, R. J. (2023). Capital, Capitalism and Health. *Critical Sociology*, 49 (3): 395–414. https://doi.org/10.1177/08969205221083503

Durkheim, É. (1893/1964). *The Division of Labour in Society*. Glencoe, IL: Free Press.

Esping-Andersen, G. (1990). *The Three Worlds of Welfare Capitalism*. London: Polity.

Flora, P. and Heidenheimer, A. J. (1981). *The Development of Welfare States in Europe and America*. New Brunswick: Transaction Books.

Galbraith, J. K. (1963). *American Capitalism: The Concept of Countervailing Power*. Harmondsworth: Penguin.

Galbraith, J. K. (1969). *The New Industrial State*. Harmondsworth: Penguin.

Giddens, A. (1984). *The Constitution of Society*. Cambridge: Polity Press.

Giddens, A. (1990). *The Consequences of Modernity*. Cambridge: Polity Press.

Gough, I. (1978). Theories of the Welfare State: A Critique. *International Journal of Health Services*, 8 (1): 27–40. https://doi.org/10.2190/W1U7-NXMM-YUCQ-PVJ1

Gramsci, A. (1971). *Selections from the Prison Notebooks*. New York: International Publishers.

Hall, P. A. and Soskice, D. (2001). *Varieties Of Capitalism: The Institutional Foundations of Comparative Advantage*. Oxford: Oxford University Press.

Hartley, T. (2022). Who Killed Social Welfare?. *The British Journal of Social Work*, 52 (7): 4436–4449, https://doi.org/10.1093/bjsw/bcac056

Hein, E., Meloni, W. P. and Tridico, P. (2021). Welfare Models and Demand-Led Growth Regimes Before and After the Financial and Economic Crisis. *Rev Int Polit Econ*, 28 (5): 1196–1223. https://doi.org/10.1080/09692290.2020.1744178

Jameson, F. (1991). *Postmodernism: Or, The Cultural Logic of Late Capitalism*. Durham, NC: Duke University Press.

Kerr, C., Dunlop, J. T., Harbison, F. and Myers, C. A. (1960). *Industrialism and Industrial Man: The Problems of Labor and Management in Economic Growth*. Cambridge, MA: Harvard University Press.

Kim, T. K. and Zurlo, K. (2009). How Does Economic Globalisation Affect the Welfare State? Focusing on the Mediating Effect of Welfare Regimes. *Int J Soc Welfare*, 18: 130–141. https://doi.org/10.1111/j.1468-2397.2008.00575.x

Korpi, W. (1989). Power, Politics, and State Autonomy in the Development of Social Citizenship: Social Rights During Sickness in Eighteen OECD Countries Since 1930. *American Sociological Review*, 54 (3): 309–28. https://doi.org/10.2307/2095608

La Placa, V. and Corlyon, J. (2014a) Social Tourism and Organised Capitalism: Research, Policy and Practice. *Journal of Policy Research in Tourism, Leisure and Events*, 6 (1): 66–79. https://doi.org/10.1080/19407963.2013.833934

La Placa, V. and Corlyon, J. (2014b), Barriers to Inclusion and Successful Engagement of Parents in Mainstream Services: Evidence and Research, *Journal of Children's Services*, 9 (30): 220–234. https://doi.org/10.1108/JCS-05-2014-0027

La Placa, V. and Knight, A. (2023). Globalisation and Global Public Health. In V. La Placa and J. Morgan (eds), *Social Science Perspectives on Global Public Health*. London: Routledge, 17–28.

Lindström, M. (2020). The COVID-19 Pandemic and the Swedish Strategy: Epidemiology and Postmodernism. *SSM – Population Health*, 11: 100643. https://doi.org/10.1016/j.ssmph.2020.100643

Lyotard, J. F. (1984). *The Postmodern Condition*. Manchester: Manchester University Press.

Marx, K. (1867/1990). *Capital Volume 1*. London: Penguin.

Miliband, R. (1969). *The State in Capitalist Society*. London: Weidenfeld and Nicholson.

Moncrieff, J. (2022). The Political Economy of the Mental Health System: A Marxist Analysis. *Front. Sociol*, 6: 771875. https://doi.org/10.3389/fsoc.2021.771875

O'Connor, J. (1973). *The Fiscal Crisis of the State*. New York: St Martin's Press.

OECD. (2020a). *Social Expenditure (SOCX) Update 2020: Social Spending Makes Up 20% of OECD GDP*. Paris: OECD.

OECD. (2020b). *Supporting Livelihoods During the COVID-19 Crisis: Closing the Gaps in Safety Nets: OECD Policy Responses to Coronavirus (COVID-19)*. Paris: OECD.

Peter, L. (1996). Three Discourses on Practice: A Postmodern Re-Appraisal. *The Journal of Sociology and Social Welfare*, 11 (1): 23–48. https://doi.org/10.15453/0191-5096.2327

Powell, J. L. and Gilbert, T. (2009). *Aging and Identity: A Dialogue with Postmodernism*. New York: Nova Science.

Powell, J. L. (2023). *Postmodern Health, Care and Aging*. New York: Nova Science Pub.

Rimlinger, G. V. (1971). *Welfare Policy and Industrialization in Europe, America and Russia*. New York: Wiley.

Rudra, N. and Haggard, S. (2005). Globalisation, Democracy and Effective Welfare Spending in the Developing World. *Comparative Political Studies*, 38 (9): 1015–1049. https://doi.org/10.1177/0010414005279258

Russell, J. W. (2018). *Double Standard: Social Policy in Europe and the United States*, 4th edn. Lanham: Rowman and Littlefield.

Santos, M. and Simoes, M. (2021). Globalisation, Welfare Models and Social Expenditure in OECD Countries. *Open Economic Review*, 32: 1063–1088. https://doi.org/10.1007/s11079-021-09646-2

Seidman, S. and Wagner, D. (1992). *Postmodernism and Social Theory*. Oxford: Blackwell.

Simmonds, B. (2021a). Globalisation, Neoliberalism and Welfare State Models: A Comparative Analysis. In B. Simmonds (ed.), *Ageing and the Crisis in Health and Social Care: Global and National Perspectives*. Bristol: University Press, 24–43. doi:10.46692/9781447348726.004

Simmonds, B. (2021b). Failing Health and Social Care in the UK: Austerity, Neoliberal Ideology and Precarity. In B. Simmonds (ed.), *Ageing and the Crisis in Health and Social Care: Global and National Perspectives*. Bristol: University Press, 44–59.

Stones, R. (1996). *Sociological Reasoning: Towards a Past-Modern Sociology*. Basingstoke. Macmillan Press.

Waitzkin, H. (1978). A Marxist View of Medical Care. *Ann Intern Med*, 89 (2): 264–278. https://doi.org/10.7326/0003-4819-89-2-264.

Wilensky, H. (1975). *The Welfare State and Equality*. Berkeley, CA: University of California Press.

Wu, W., Zhang, L., Mahalik, M. K., Wan, Q., Gozgor, G., et al. (2023). Revisiting the Globalisation-Welfare State Nexus: What About the Quality of the Social Welfare?. *Economic Research-Ekonomska Istraživanja*, 36 (3). https://doi.org/10.1080/1331677X.2022.2147978

CHAPTER 3

Health and Social Care Funding across the OECD

....

Paul McCrone

INTRODUCTION

Health and social care systems exist to maintain, improve, and maximise health through the fair provision of appropriate services, treatment, and support. To achieve this in a world of resource scarcity requires an effective approach to financing to ensure acceptable levels of care provision in a way that represents substantial value for money. These broad aims arguably apply to any system of care, but the actual way systems have been developed differs between countries. This chapter describes pertinent issues around health and social care financing and specifically the key approaches that have been developed for this: the Bismarck model, the Semashko model, the Beveridge model, and the residual model. Alongside discussion of these, attention is also given to their key attributes: funding through taxation, insurance schemes, and out-of-pocket payments. Focus is given to OECD countries, while recognising that key historical insights and current developments also need to draw upon developments outside this collection of developed countries. It will become apparent that while the systems are distinctive, differences between specific countries are blurred, and rigid adherence to a particular funding model may not be helpful.

HEALTH AND SOCIAL CARE SYSTEMS

Health and social care systems exist to address needs that people have throughout their life course, but it must be recognised that 'formal' health and social care is not the only contributor to improvements in health and the ability to play a full part in society. Systems can be organised in a variety of ways at the level of the individual, their family, community, workplace, or government, and we might argue that to some extent, systems might exist across all these domains. The World Health Organization (WHO) defines a health system as one that includes 'all the activities

DOI: 10.4324/9781003343608-4

whose primary purpose is to promote, restore or maintain health' (WHO, 2000). A system of social care could be similarly defined, but with a focus on the promoting, improving, and maintaining the ability to function in society. Clearly, there is overlap between the two concepts. Although health and social care needs apply throughout the life course, it is effectively recognised that in societies where the population is on average getting older, there are likely to be growing and interconnected health and social care needs requiring interventions and solutions through systems. Whether these systems are organised by individuals, independent (voluntary and private) organisations, employers, or governments is open for debate. However, what is obvious is that provision and organisation of support entails resources, and as such, funding care is a key aspect of any health and social care system. The aims of care systems are generally to maximise health, ensure high quality of care, enable access that is equitable, and to achieve this while containing costs (Or et al., 2010). The emphasis placed on these aims varies between countries.

To some extent each country in the world has its own unique healthcare system, but these can be broadly categorised into four types. While some aspects of care systems will be country-specific, there are also similarities with variations of the Beveridge and Bismarck models predominating in OECD countries. A third type of system, the Semashko model was ubiquitous across eastern Europe until the early 1990s. Since then, those responsible for reform in these countries have looked to the Beveridge or Bismarck models for inspiration. The fourth category is the residual model, which places most emphasis on the funding through private insurance and out of pocket payments. While these systems are clearly distinctive, a common feature (other than systems that are focused on out-of-pocket payments) is that risk is 'pooled' which is accepted as necessary given uncertainty about future health needs. How this risk pooling is operationalised is perhaps the key consideration of healthcare reform debates.

RESOURCE SCARCITY AND COST CONTAINMENT

The orthodox view is that resources (whether professionals, land, or money) required to provide care usually are limited in their supply (i.e., there is resource scarcity), and almost always have alternative uses (i.e., they have an 'opportunity' cost). Given resource scarcity and competing demands for resources, choices must be made about the best use for those resources. While much of this may seem obvious, the issue over resource scarcity is somewhat nuanced. Workforce constraints are certainly evident, especially in the short term, but finance may be diverted from other sectors or borrowed as was seen during the COVID-19 pandemic.

Widespread concerns exist over the level of health spending, but the extent to which such concerns are justified is contentious. The content of spending needs to be considered rather than just measured in monetary terms. For example, if spending on pharmaceutical products increases simply because of increased prices demanded by companies, then this is quite different to costs increasing due to more people with a previously untreated condition, receiving appropriate therapy. We also need to consider the belief, expounded by the American economist William Baumol, that as societies develop, many products become relatively cheaper due to productivity improvements (Baumol, 2012). However, health and social care are labour intensive 'industries' which cannot enjoy similar productivity improvements. This inevitably means that costs increase in these sectors relative to others and we should expect, and perhaps even welcome, increased proportions of GDP going towards health and social care.

Studies have borne out the conclusions of Baumol (2012). For example, in an analysis of health expenditure in the European Union between 2013 and 2017, Rokicki et al. (2021) found that the strongest determinant of spending was the level of economic development. While this appears to support the Baumol (2012) argument, it could also reflect inefficiencies in systems, as they evolve, and excess profits that are made by private companies.

Despite the arguments put forward by Baumol (2012) and others, the prevailing view of politicians and other decision-makers appears to be that we should be concerned by the high and increasing costs of health and social care and cost-containment strategies should be introduced. 'Cost' clearly has a negative connotation. Most of us would wish to avoid costs wherever possible, and if not, then we would wish to reduce their perceived impact by moving them into the future (the economic concept of 'discounting'). However, the issue is more nuanced once we start to consider what we mean by 'cost'.

Sometimes, the argument is straightforward. For example, if a doctor prescribes a patient with a branded drug that is identical in every important way to a generic drug other than its price, then that can be seen as a cost to be avoided. What though of costs that are incurred by increasing treatment coverage for people with a particular condition? We know that treatment rates for depression, for example, are sub-optimal and that by reducing treatment gaps we are likely to see increased healthcare costs (Strawbridge et al., 2022; McCrone et al., 2023). Presumably, that increased level of treatment has benefits which may well justify the extra cost incurred. Similarly, should we view increased costs of social care for an ageing population negatively? Cost of care can be considered as the monetary representation of the inputs that are provided. If we feel that such care inputs are unnecessary, ineffective, inappropriate, or excessive, then we might justifiably restrict their use, but we do need to emphasise that it is often care inputs we are trying to address when we talk of 'cost-containment'. This does not mean that we do not address cost increases, but rather that we investigate them to determine their causes. If the arguments of Baumol (2012) are correct, then a future society, where increasing proportions of gross domestic product is accounted for by health and social care may be entirely reasonable if other products, goods, and services have become easily affordable due to productivity increases.

HEALTH AND SOCIAL CARE FUNDING MODELS

Four broad systems of healthcare organisation have emerged since the later nineteenth century: the Bismarck model, the Semashko model, the Beveridge model, and the residual model. To some extent we can categorise countries as drawing on one of these models although distinctions are blurred, and most countries may operate a hybrid system. Whichever model is chosen, the objectives of healthcare systems tend to be to provide good access to modern effective care that represents fair value for money (Smółka, 2022). One of the driving forces behind current debates about healthcare reform is the desire to achieve universal healthcare coverage without people facing financial hardship.

Beveridge Model

The Beveridge report of 1942 laid out the foundations for the provision of social support in the UK following the second world war, and the principles on which the provision should be based (Beveridge, 1942). The report identified 12 key provisions to support citizens of all ages throughout their lives. Interestingly, only one of these provisions was specifically health-related: 'Medical treatment covering all requirements will be provided for all citizens by a national health service' (p. 11). The report emphasises the role of the state in providing financial, health, and social support when needed, but also indicates the need for individual responsibility: 'Restoration of a sick person to health is a duty of the State and the sick person, prior to any other consideration' (p. 159).

Three fundamental characteristics of the Beveridge model of healthcare are: (1) there is a national system of healthcare provision (e.g., through a national health service), (2) provision is mainly publicly organised rather than privately, and (3) funding comes primarily through revenue collected by the government. Within the OECD examples of countries following the Beveridge model are the UK, Italy, Spain, Sweden, Denmark, Norway, Finland, and Canada (Lameire et al., 1999).

The Beveridge model emphasises health and social care funding from central government, with the sources of such funding generally considered to be tax revenues and borrowing. This presents economic and political challenges to governments who may be reluctant to either increase taxes or borrowing. If reliance is placed on funding through taxation, and if tax increases are to be avoided, then the only solution is to increase tax revenues through economic growth. If the economy grows, more people should be in work and earning more, and hopefully companies make more profits, all serving to raise tax revenues. This is a risky option as growth is not guaranteed. The challenge is even more apparent when we consider the fact that in times of economic downturn health and social care needs are likely to increase. To add to the complexity of the situation, as the population ages, there will potentially be greater health and social care needs, and fewer people in the workforce. To maintain health spending in times of economic downturn, governments can borrow, but they are clearly reluctant to do this due to the adverse connotations of going further into debt. Governments though are not households and can comfortably operate with a high level of debt, which, represents a surplus elsewhere (e.g., pension funds).

Bismarck Model

A key feature of the Bismarck model (named after the German chancellor who reformed healthcare in the late nineteenth century) is the funding of care through social health insurance (SHI) schemes. These are generally linked to employment, with employees and employers paying into a fund managed by an external (usually not for profit) agency. Family members are generally covered by the scheme and provision for those not in the workforce comes from central government. There are differences between countries in how SHI operates, but four common aspects are evident: (1) SHI is an employment-based system, which (2) links entitlement to healthcare with contributions to the scheme from employees who (3) represent their families, who are also covered, and (4) the scheme is to some extent separate from the government (Olsen, 2017). Regarding the latter feature, governments may subsidise the scheme and act as a 'safety net' for those not in work. In some countries, there is a single scheme, while elsewhere schemes compete for members. Opt-outs may also be possible if employees prefer to pay into a private health insurance scheme.

The partial separation of SHI schemes from the government may be seen as appropriate, particularly if we wish to ensure that healthcare is 'de-politicised'. This though may make reasonable regulation of schemes challenging and some degree of government influence may not be a negative feature. Under enrolment may be common. Contributions to schemes can be regressive and SHI can lead to adverse risk-selection (Wagstaff, 2010).

Semashko Model

Following the 1917 revolution in Russia, a system of centrally planned and financed healthcare was introduced by Nikolai Semashko. This model ensured free care at the point of delivery with an emphasis on the hospital treatment of acute problems, and with healthcare professionals being employed directly by the state (Ariaans et al., 2021). There was no place for the market in healthcare delivery and this may be perceived as having limited incentives to innovate and improve quality. Furthermore, there was relatively little primary care provision and hospitals tended to be condition specific (Antoun et al., 2011). Even now, healthcare in Russia gives much emphasis to specialist care rather than provision by generalists (Sheiman et al., 2018).

The Semashko model aimed to provide universal healthcare from central budgets and with top-down coordination and control. However, the history of the system shows that it was severely underfunded (Sheiman et al., 2018), and healthcare funding received less emphasis than that on the military and industrial development. The dominance of the Soviet Union saw similar systems established in countries across eastern Europe from the second world war until the collapse of communism. While criticism of the Semashko model is widespread and may to some extent be justified, it is important to look at it in the context of a change from a country that did not have a unified healthcare system, and had very high mortality and morbidity rates, compared to other European countries (Krementsov, 2017). Some countries (for example, Czechia) clearly experienced improvements in public health following the introduction of the system. However, as Heinrich (2022) points out, while the Semashko model may well have been suited to the situation in the Soviet Union between the wars, it struggled more in meeting the needs of a rapidly growing industrial society.

The legacy of the Semashko model cannot be easily dismissed. The idea (even if not continuously achieved) of universal coverage, free care at the point of delivery, and planning by the state permutates discussions about healthcare reform across the world. Arguably, the differences between this model and the Beveridge model are not always substantial and moves towards a more market orientated system have regularly been resisted. A common distinction made between the Beveridge and Semashko models is that the former relies on tax revenues to fund care while the latter funds care from central government budgets. This difference may not actually be that meaningful given that countries such as the UK do not wait for taxes to be collected before spending.

Residual Model

The role of the individual and the private sector is emphasised in the residual model. Individuals are expected to take out private health insurance to pool risk or to finance care out of their own pockets. Insurance companies compete for customers with variation in what they will cover, and risk of illness influences premiums paid. The USA is often described as using this residual system, although in fact the state-run insurance schemes (Medicare and Medicaid) are key players in the system. Concerns over the extent to which individuals were covered by existing schemes led to Barack Obama putting forward legislation (the Affordable Care Act) which aimed to achieve insurance coverage for all, to reduce healthcare costs, and to improve care quality. The Act made it mandatory to take out insurance and the refusal to insure those with existing conditions was outlawed. The Act resulted in a halving of the number of uninsured Americans, but inequalities remained and 29 million were still uninsured by 2017 (Gaffney and McCormick, 2017). Opposition to the Act has been substantial and this remains a deeply contested area of public policy in the USA and as Dalen et al. (2015) point out, the opposition by many to a greater role for government in the provision of healthcare will hinder increasing coverage for all.

One of the disadvantages of insurance-based schemes, whether social health insurance or private health insurance, is the existence of 'moral hazard'. This occurs in two forms (Culyer, 2005). First, the very fact that someone is insured may influence behaviour which can increase the need for health care. For example, if I am insured against the risks associated with a particular activity or sport, then I may be more likely to engage in it; thus, increasing the likelihood of some adverse event occurring. Similarly, I may not worry too much about lifestyle choices such as drinking or smoking if I know that my health insurance scheme will cover me if I become unwell. Second, if I pay into a scheme then I may feel more justified in using services (which I perceive I have paid for) even if the need is not really justified. Of course, some aspects of moral hazard can extend to tax-based systems as well. With such a system, there may though be an underlying level of moral hazard, and this is then increased for those who also are covered by insurance schemes.

Funding schemes differ according to freedom to pay into them and coverage eligibility. Whether or not people pay into health insurance schemes is usually their own choice. The amount paid in though will depend on the level of risk that the insurance company deems to exist, and as such, it can prove prohibitive for those with chronic conditions. Social health insurance is usually compulsory for employees (although private insurance may be taken out as an alternative) but there is no consideration of risk. Tax-based systems are compulsory whether or not alternative schemes are also utilised and again there is no explicit consideration of risk. There is substantial variation between countries in financing schemes, but it is not apparent that performance differs substantially (Morris et al., 2012).

HEALTHCARE FINANCING IN THE OECD

A simplified way of classifying OCED countries is by examining the proportion of health expenditure that is covered by different funding sources. From Figure 3.1, we can see that Canada, Denmark, Finland, Iceland, Ireland, Italy, Latvia, Norway, Portugal, Spain, Sweden, the UK, Australia, and New Zealand all have in excess of 60% of health expenditure covered directly by central government. This is a necessary, but not sufficient, condition for following the Beveridge model. By contrast, countries with a strong focus on compulsory social health insurance schemes (a key characteristic of Bismarck schemes) include Columbia, Costa Rica, Belgium, Czechia (the Czech Republic in Figure 3.1), Estonia, France, Germany, Hungary, Lithuania, Luxembourg, Poland, Slovak Republic (Slovakia in Figure 3.1), Slovenia, and Japan. However, it is important to recognise that central governments will to

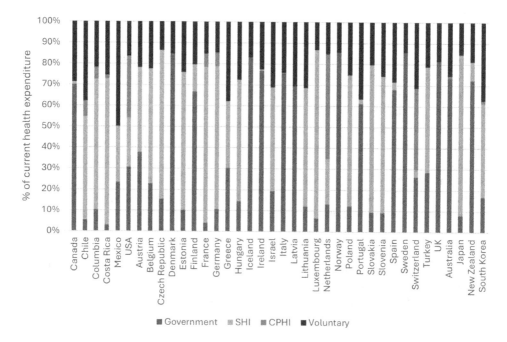

FIGURE 3.1 Distribution of Current Health Expenditure in OECD Countries by Funding Source

Source: WHO Global Health Expenditure Database (https://apps.who.int/nha/database)

a greater or lesser extent subsidise these schemes, making the distinction between the models less clear. The countries with a relatively high reliance on either compulsory private health insurance or voluntary payments (which also include into private health insurance schemes and out of pocket payments) are Mexico, Chile, the USA, the Netherlands, and Switzerland. However, even these countries have a strong role for other forms of financing including the state. Most OECD countries have a small proportion of health expenditure that is accounted for by household out of pocket payments. However, this is at most 3% of the total.

Almost all the other countries in the OECD have private sector involvement in financing healthcare and require individuals to cover some of the costs of care (e.g., payments for primary health care in France and Germany, and dental services and prescriptions in the UK). The use of charges for some aspects of care (especially in social care) can serve as a way of raising revenue and can also reduce excess demand for care. However, it is also regressive in that those on higher incomes will find it easier to pay charges and care that is necessary may be avoided. Outside of the OECD, we see a large focus on out-of-pocket payments in many low-income countries, further indicating that systems develop as economies evolve.

The amount of GDP accounted for by healthcare expenditure in 2021 or 2022 (depending on data availability) is highest in the USA, Germany, Austria, the Netherlands, and Switzerland (Figure 3.2). While there is not a clear relationship between the model of financing and this measure, it is interesting that none of these

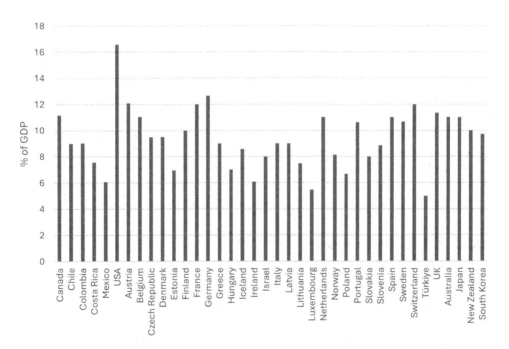

FIGURE 3.2 Healthcare Expenditure as Percentage of Gross Domestic Product (2021 or 2022)

Source: WHO Global Health Expenditure Database (https://apps.who.int/nha/database)

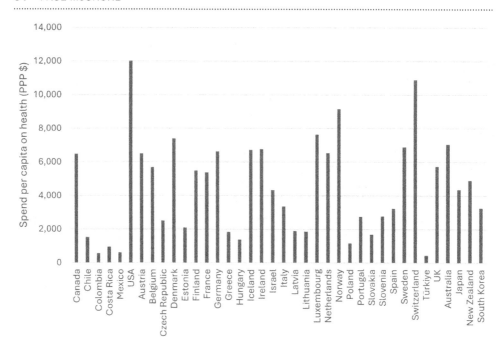

FIGURE 3.3 Health Expenditure Per Capita in 2021 (PPP $)

Source: WHO Global Health Expenditure Database (https://apps.who.int/nha/database)

four countries operate what we might consider to be a Beveridge model. The lowest proportion of GDP allocated to health is in Mexico and Türkiye, and while this may suggest a link with economic development, it is also the case that Luxembourg has a low spend on health as a proportion of output.

It is perhaps more informative to focus on the actual amount that is spent on health per head of population, with adjustment made for purchasing power parity (PPP). From Figure 3.3, we see that this was highest in the USA, Switzerland, Norway, and then Luxembourg. The countries with lowest levels of per capita spend do tend to be those with lower levels of economic development. Again, there is no obvious difference between countries with a strong focus on central government funding and those relying more on social health insurance schemes.

SOCIAL CARE FINANCING IN THE OECD

Social care is more loosely defined than healthcare and substantial heterogeneity exists in terms of its provision and financing across the OECD. We can broadly define social care as being that which supports people in activities of everyday living. This can be long-term care for those 'limited in their ability to function independently, on a daily basis and over an extended period of time' (Halásková et al., 2017), but also care for similar reasons provided for a limited period. This clearly requires careful consideration of context. Population characteristics, demographic changes, the expectations placed on families etc. will all differ between countries and influence the role that government has in providing and funding social care. In some countries, funding for social care is like that for healthcare, although with less of a role for insurance schemes, and with greater emphasis on means testing, and charges to recipients. Interestingly, the Beveridge model described earlier, while largely associated with systems, such as the NHS in the UK, had a key focus on social care from its inception. Another distinction with social care is the emphasis place on monetary transfers from the state to individuals and families for the purchase of care.

While disentangling social care and health care is not straightforward, the OECD does produce helpful statistics on the provision of long-term care across member countries. Long-term care is predominantly for older adults, and while social care has wider coverage it is the increase in the proportion of older adults in society that is seen as placing disproportionate pressure on care systems. There is a debate about the actual impact that ageing has on medical and other care costs and there is evidence that proximity to death is a more important indicator of health care needs and associated costs than ageing itself (Zweifel et al., 1999). Such a view is echoed elsewhere (Seshamani and Gray, 2004). However, while this is likely to be the case for medical care, for social care, they point out that ageing may still be crucial (Breyer and Lorenz, 2021).

Using published data relating to 25 OECD countries, Ariaans et al. (2021) derived six long-term care types. These were (1) residual public system (Czechia, Latvia, Poland) where supply of services was relatively low and there was limited private expenditure; (2) private supply system (Finland, Germany) with medium to high supply and high levels of private expenditure; (3) public supply system (Denmark, Ireland, Norway, Sweden) which had high service supply and medium to low private expenditure; (4) evolving public supply system (Japan, Korea [identified as South Korea in Figures]) which had medium to low supply medium to low private expenditure; (5) need-based supply system (Australia, Belgium, Switzerland, Luxembourg, the Netherlands, Slovak Republic, Slovenia) with both medium to high supply and private expenditure; and (6) evolving private need-based system (France, Israel, Spain, United Kingdon, United States) which had medium to low supply and medium to high private expenditure. New Zealand and Estonia could not be easily categorised alongside other countries. The authors suggested that the best performing model was the evolving private need-based system, while the worst, was the Residual public system.

Interestingly, Ariaans et al. (2021) also suggest that the typology of long-term care models does not necessarily reflect how care is funded. For example, some countries may finance care through social insurance (Germany, the Netherlands, Luxembourg, Japan, and Korea) and yet have very different models of care provision. Furthermore, while regional distinctions do apply, these are arguably less obvious now. The Nordic countries for example have long been recognised as examples where social care has been largely state provided and financed with an emphasis on universalism, but demographic changes (specifically the ageing population) have led to increased funding from individuals and their families for some services (Rostgaard et al., 2022).

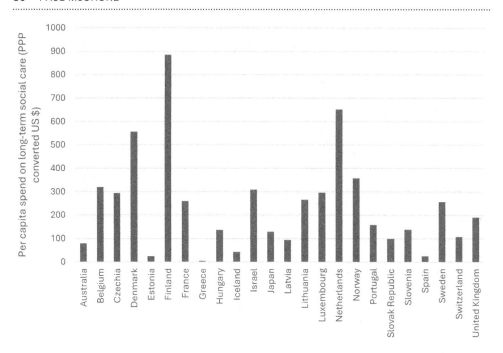

FIGURE 3.4 Spending Per Person on Long-Term Social Care in Selected OECD Countries

Source: OECD Data Explorer (https://data-explorer.oecd.org)

Note: Figures are in 2015 constant prices except for: Japan (2015), Australia (2020), Greece (2020).

Spending on long-term care shows substantial variation between OECD countries (Figure 3.4). The highest per capita spend in 2015 prices is in Finland, followed by the Netherlands and Denmark. Relatively little is spent in Greece, Estonia, and Spain. However, defining long-term care is not without challenges and there is of course crossover with long-term medical care. As such these variations need to be treated with some caution.

It is revealing that while most countries in the OECD provide healthcare for free at the point of delivery or with a small co-payment, the same is not the case for social care. Means testing is common with social care as shown by the work of Ariaans et al. (2021) who investigated the long-term care systems of 25 OECD countries. Of these, 14 used a form of means testing to determine long-term care eligibility. Of the 11 that did not use means testing, four were identified. They also report private expenditure as a percentage of the total for these 25 countries. In four countries (Estonia, Denmark, Switzerland, and the UK), this exceeded 30%, while in four (Czechia, Poland, Slovak Republic, and Slovenia) it was below 5%.

FUNDING SYSTEMS COMPARED

It is challenging to make adequate comparisons of healthcare funding models using quantitative data. Previous work has found few differences in health outcomes between tax-based and social health insurance-based systems, but that the former tend to be better at containing costs (confusingly conflated with being more efficient) while satisfaction with care provided is generally better with the latter (Van Der Zee and Kroneman, 2007). In their own analyses, the authors found that the social health insurance systems were slightly better in terms of mortality rates and life expectancy but had higher costs. They also suggested (like the previous studies they describe) that this form of model also produces enhanced levels of satisfaction. However, as was previously pointed out, earlier cost containment is contentious and can result in care being reduced. This is far from an efficient outcome. It may though be easier to achieve in a tax-funded system, but then the argument for greater levels of satisfaction, and indeed health outcomes, may be to raise the level of spending by central government in line with the arguments put forward by Baumol (2012).

An in-depth analysis of different healthcare funding models was conducted by the influential Health Foundation think tank to inform the debate about policy in the UK (Thorlby and Buzelli, 2024). They compared four systems (Italy, Spain, Sweden, and the UK) that followed the Beveridge model in funding care predominantly from tax revenue with three countries operating a Bismarckian social health insurance scheme (France, Germany, and the Netherlands). Key conclusions were that (1) while the three social health insurance schemes all spent more per head than the UK, so did Sweden; (2) distinctions were becoming unclear as social health insurance schemes had increasing levels of central government regulation and control and tax-based systems incorporated 'market' features such as a split between commissioning and provision, (3) the operating costs of the tax-based systems are lower; and (4) user charges exist in both types of model. Overall, the authors found no reason for the UK to switch to a system of social health insurance.

CONCLUSIONS

There is no doubt in the OECD, the dominant forms of financing healthcare, and to some extent social care, are tax-based systems, and social health insurance schemes. However, we need to be cautious about assuming that the funding model translates into substantial differences in the provision and organisation of care, as both models of financing are ways of pooling risk, and both incorporate a strong role for the state (Kutzin, 2001). Countries developing healthcare systems from a relatively low base can draw guidance from those in existence elsewhere. It is less obvious that moving from a tax-based system to a social health insurance system would be accompanied by substantial gains. The fact that systems do differ leads understandably to the question as to which is better (Van Der Zee and Kroneman, 2007).

Given that within each model, there are country-level idiosyncrasies and contexts, it is likely to be a question that cannot be definitively answered. Perhaps more intriguing is the near disappearance of the Semashko model. The characteristics of this system (universal health coverage, state coordination and provision, and absence of market influences) are those that advocates of the Beveridge and Bismarck continue to be influenced by. Perhaps the main limitation of the Semashko model was that it received insufficient funding required to meet the needs of the population.

This is also a characteristic of other systems (particularly those with *a priori* determined budgets) and strongly suggests that the actual system is not the main issue, but rather the political will that exists to prioritise sufficient resources for health and social care.

RESEARCH POINTS AND REFLECTIVE EXERCISES

• In what ways do you think that health and social care funding schemes may change as economies develop?
• Beveridge-type models arguably encourage cost-containment. Is this a reasonable aim of a healthcare system?
• It has been suggested that health and social care systems in some countries are unsustainable. Is more openness to market forces the answer to this problem?

REFERENCES

Antoun, J., Phillips, F. and Johnson, T. (2011). Post-Soviet Transition: Improving Health Services Delivery and Management. *Mount Sinai Journal of Medicine*, 78 (3): 436–448. https://doi.org/10.1002/msj.20261

Ariaans, M., Linden, P. and Wendt, C. (2021). Worlds of Long-Term Care: A Typology of OECD Countries. *Health Policy*, 125 (5): 609–617. https://doi.org/10.1016/j.healthpol.2021.02.009

Baumol, W. J. (2012). *The Cost Disease: Why Computers Get Cheaper and Health Care Doesn't*. New Haven, CT: Yale University Press.

Beveridge, W. (1942). *Social Insurance and Allied Services: Report by Sir William Beveridge*. London: His Majesty's Stationery Office.

Breyer, F. and Lorenz, N. (2021). The 'Red Herring' After 20 Years: Ageing and Health Care Expenditures. *European Journal of Health Economics*, 22 (5): 661–667. https://doi.org/10.1007/s10198-020-01203-x

Culyer, A. J. (2005). *The Dictionary of Health Economics*. Cheltenham: Edward Elgar.

Dalen, J. E., Waterbrook, K., & Alpert, J. S. (2015). Why Do so Many Americans Oppose the Affordable Care Act? *The American Journal of Medicine*, 128 (8), 807–810. https://doi.org/10.1016/j.amjmed.2015.01.032

Gaffney, A. and McCormick, D. (2017). The Affordable Care Act: Implications for Health-Care Equity. *The Lancet*, 389 (10077): 1442–1452. https://doi.org/10.1016/S0140-6736(17)30786-9

Halásková, R., Bednář, P. and Halásková, M. (2017). Forms of Providing and Financing Long-Term Care in OECD Countries. *Review of Economic Perspectives*, 17 (2): 159–178. https://doi.org/10.1515/revecp-2017-0008

Heinrich, A. (2022). The Emergence of the Socialist Healthcare Model After the First World War. In F. Nullmeier, D. González de Reufels and H. Obinger (eds), *International Impacts on Social Policy: Short Histories in Global Perspective*. London: Palgrave Macmillan, 35–46.

Krementsov, N. (2017). The Promises, Realities, and Legacies of the Bolshevik Revolution, 1917-2017. *American Journal of Public Health*, 107 (11): 1693–1694. https://doi.org/10.2105/AJPH.2017.304092

Kutzin, J. (2001). A Descriptive Framework for Country-Level Analysis of Health Care Financing Arrangements. *Health Policy*, 56: 171–204. https://doi.org/10.1016/S0168-8510(00)00149-4

Lameire, N., Joffe, P. and Wiedemann, M. (1999). Healthcare Systems- An International Review: An Overview. *Nephrology Dialysis Transplantation*, 14 (6): 3–9. https://doi.org/10.1093/ndt/14.suppl_6.3

McCrone, P., Young, A. H., Zahn, R., Eberhard, J., Wasserman, et al. (2023). Economic Impact of Reducing Treatment Gaps in Depression. *European Psychiatry*, 66 (1): e57. https://doi.org/10.1192/j.eurpsy.2023.2415

Morris, S., Devlin, N., Parkin, D. and Spencer, A. (2012). *Economic Analysis in Health Care*, 2nd edn. London: Wiley.

Olsen, J. A. (2017). *Principles in Health Economics and Policy*. Oxford: Oxford University Press.

Or, Z., Cases, C., Lisac, M., Vrangbk, K., Winblad, U., et al. (2010). Are Health Problems Systemic? Politics of Access and Choice Under Beveridge and Bismarck Systems. *Health Economics, Policy and Law*, 5 (3): 269–293. https://doi.org/10.1017/S1744133110000034

Rokicki, T., Perkowska, A. and Ratajczak, M. (2021). Differentiation in Healthcare Financing in EU Countries. *Sustainability*, 13 (1): 251. https://doi.org/10.3390/su13010251

Rostgaard, T., Jacobsen, F., Kröger, T. and Peterson, E. (2022). Revisiting the Nordic Long-Term Care Model for Older People—Still Equal? *European Journal of Ageing*, 19 (2): 201–210. https://doi.org/10.1007/s10433-022-00703-4

Seshamani, M. and Gray, A. (2004). Ageing and Health-Care Expenditure: The Red Herring Argument Revisited. *Health Economics*, 13 (4): 303–314. https://doi.org/10.1002/hec.826

Sheiman, I., Shishkin, S. and Shevsky, V. (2018). The Evolving Semashko Model of Primary Health Care: The Case of the Russian Federation. *Risk Management and Healthcare Policy*, 11: 209–220. https://doi.org/10.2147/RMHP.S168399

Smółka, J. (2022). Institutional Analysis of Healthcare Systems in Selected Developed Countries. In M. A. Weresa, C. Ciecierski, and L. Filus (eds), *Economics and Mathematical Modeling in Health-Related Research*. Leiden: Brill, 228. Available at: https://brill.com/display/book/9789004517295/BP000012.xml (Accessed: 1 August 2023).

Strawbridge, R., McCrone, P., Ulrichsen, A., Zahn, R., Eberhard, J., et al. (2022). Care Pathways for People with Major Depressive Disorder: A European Brain Council Value of Treatment Study. *Eur Psychiatry*, 65 (1): 1–21. https://doi.org/10.1192/j.eurpsy.2022.28.

Thorlby T. and Buzelli, L. (2024). *Is the Grass Really Greener?* London: The Health Foundation.

Van Der Zee, J. and Kroneman, M. W. (2007). Bismarck or Beveridge: A Beauty Contest Between Dinosaurs. *BMC Health Serv Res*, 7 (94). https://doi.org/10.1186/1472-6963-7-94

Wagstaff, A. (2010). Social Health Insurance Reexamined. *Health Economics*, 19 (5): 503–517. https://doi.org/10.1002/hec.1492.

WHO. (2000). *Health Systems: Improving Performance*. Geneva: World Health Organization.

Zweifel, P., Felder, S. and Meiers, M. (1999). Ageing of Population and Health Care Expenditure: A Red Herring? *Health Economics*, 8 (6): 485–496. https://doi.org/10.1002/(SICI)1099-1050(199909)8:6<485:AID-HEC461>3.0.CO;2-4

CHAPTER 4

Towards a Definitional Framework of Wellbeing in Health and Social Care Research, Policy, and Practice

....

Vincent La Placa

THE CONCEPT OF WELLBEING: AN INTRODUCTION

Recent interest in health and social care policy and practice has witnessed a shift away from traditional remedial orientated focus, and ill-health definitions, in terms of 'absence' of disease, towards one of universal access to services, conducive to the concept of wellbeing, and the humanisation of care (Knight and McNaught, 2011; Fisher, 2019). Ideas of wellbeing traditionally occurred within the philosophy of ethics, particularly around how 'one ought to live' and the virtues of 'discovering' happiness and satisfaction (Haybron, 2008; La Placa et al., 2013). Positive psychology (invariably biased towards positivistic and psychological concepts) then attempted to integrate subjective states and objective elements, such as family, community, and the built environment, which therefore influenced individuals' active ability to cope, thrive, and construct resilience on the subjective level, and attain positive 'quality of life'. However, these analyses of wellbeing never adequately articulated the range of specialist areas of research and practice, requisite to comprehend positive states of existence in specific domains, among different populations, and contexts (McNaught, 2011; La Placa and Knight, 2023).

The concept of wellbeing across health and social care has also been used to distinguish traditional concepts of 'health' around the 'physical' and the presence or absence of disease, to encompass a more holistic, and all-embracing concept of health and wellbeing. Table 4.1 outlines the definitions of wellbeing of the World Health Organization (WHO) and of the United Nations (UN).

Historically, where wellbeing was referred to, it was perceived through the lens of economics and material wellbeing, equating wellbeing with material and measurable indicators, for instance, employment, income, economic growth, and increases

DOI: 10.4324/9781003343608-5

TABLE 4.1 Definitions of Wellbeing: WHO and UN

Organisation	Definition
World Health Organization (WHO)	The connection of wellbeing to health and social care is indicated in the WHO 1948 constitution, 'Health is a state of complete physical, mental and social wellbeing and not merely the absence of disease or infirmity' (WHO, 2021).
United Nations (UN)	The third goal of the 17 United Nations' Sustainable Development Goals (UNSDGs) also refers to 'Good Health and Wellbeing', the promotion of healthy lives, and wellbeing (United Nations Development of Economic and Social Affairs, 2021)

in gross domestic product (GDP) (La Placa and Knight, 2014a). As regards, the Organisation for Economic Co-operation and Development (OECD) countries particularly, decades of economic growth, and financial stability, encouraged this view. However, this is changing significantly, given the previous financial crises, COVID-19, and the potential instability of potential 'de-globalisation'. The latter is where countries become less dependent upon one another, rupturing previous supply chains, which once guaranteed stable production and delivery of, for example, energy, pharmaceuticals, and food supplies (La Placa and Knight, 2023) and will impact healthcare, social care, and levels of wellbeing. However, the increasing use of and interest in wellbeing has diversified and enhanced the concept to transcend the purely material (measured through economic statistics and indicators) and focus beyond this to the social, psychological, and environmental domains.

La Placa and Knight (2014a; 2017; 2023) have argued that the shift to a more multi-faceted approach reflects changes in late modern societies, where increased individualisation, enhanced use of technology, and construction of more complex personal narratives and biographies, compared with traditional societies, furthers it use in health and social care discourses and practices. As a result, globally, wellbeing is a contested concept, both definitionally and theoretically, despite its increasing use in health and social care policies. The multi-faceted approach is also mirrored in WHO's (2016; 2022) approach that wellbeing be perceived and used through 'objective' and 'subjective' dimensions; the former embracing, for instance, material wellbeing and population-based health and wellbeing, the latter, individuals' experiences and constructions of health and wellbeing in interaction with, for instance, families, communities, and the broader society.

As a result, the OECD has also moved beyond assessing wellbeing, as mainly the measurable functioning of the economy, to a more diverse focus upon individual experiences, and living conditions of people and households, known as the 'beyond GDP approach' (OECD, 2020). Measuring and enhancing wellbeing is a core priority, which the OECD is pursuing through various streams of work, notably the OECD Better Life Initiative, which seeks to measure advancement of wellbeing across OECD countries (OECD, 2020). The concept of wellbeing is also being applied across national policy initiatives in OECD countries to reflect its increasing usefulness, its distinction from traditional concepts of health; and in designing policies and interventions, to enhance wellbeing, and integrate into health and social care systems. For example, in 2009, the Commission on the Measurement of Economic Performance and Social Progress submitted its report to the then French President, Nicolas Sarkozy, during a conference at the Sorbonne in Paris (Stiglitz et al., 2009). The Commission recommended widening the scope of the traditional indicators used to measure 'economic progress' to include measures of quality of life, inequality, and wellbeing, sustainable development, and the environment.

In the UK, wellbeing was initiated on to the policy agenda with a consultation process, termed 'Measuring National Wellbeing' (Office for National Statistics, 2010), asking people 'What Matters?' to understand what should be included in measures of national wellbeing. The opinions and indicators generated were used in surveys conducted by the UK Office for National Statistics (ONS) to measure wellbeing and evaluate the impact of government policy upon it including public health, community learning, local government, occupational health, transport, and environmental policies. In 2019, New Zealand unveiled its first 'Wellbeing Budget'. This approach was designed around the New Zealand Treasury's 'Living Standards Framework' (LSF), a national measurement framework, employed to consider the intergenerational wellbeing impacts of policies and proposals. Various OECD countries have also designed national wellbeing frameworks to collect data on wellbeing and inform policy. These frameworks define identified outcomes or broad objectives, related to wellbeing, and track progress publicly, based on a dashboard of indicators, from the Australian Treasury's 'Wellbeing Framework' developed in 2004, through to most recently, the 'New Zealand Living Standards Framework' in 2018; the 'Iceland Indicators of Wellbeing' in 2019 and Canada's 'Quality of Life Framework' in 2021. The latter uses prosperity; health; society; and good governance as core wellbeing indicators (Canadian Index of Wellbeing, 2016; Department of Finance Canada, 2021).

WELLBEING AND HEALTH AND SOCIAL CARE

The concept of wellbeing has also assumed a central tenet in providing public health and social care services and needs assessment across the OECD. Across OECD countries, ageing populations and increasing numbers of people with chronic diseases have shifted the focus of healthcare services away from acute care and to emphasis upon longer episodes of healthcare needs. This has precipitated a debate around the need for integrated health and social care delivery systems and interventions which are able to address consistent, coordinated, and effective care delivery throughout individuals' life courses and to enhance wellbeing and quality of life (OECD, 2023). Health and social care systems have steadily increased numbers of health and social care workers as a result. For example, in 2019, 10% of jobs were in health or social care, up from less than 9% in 2000. In Nordic countries and the Netherlands, more than 15% of all jobs are health and social work related. From 2000 to 2019, the share of health and social care workers increased in all countries except the Slovak Republic and Sweden (OECD, 2021b). The numbers also increased rapidly over the past two decades in Japan (by over 5%) and in Ireland and Luxembourg by 4% (OECD, 2021b).

Health and social care refer to the healthcare infrastructure and the forms it assumes, for example, private and public care. As was implied earlier, health is perceived as a function of welfare, which depends on a range of factors including biological, environmental, nutrition and living standards. Healthcare focuses on providing medical care to individuals and communities, often in terms of diagnosis and treatment and encompasses services, such as hospital and primary care and public health (Kelly et al., 2023). In policy terms, it is often framed around access and impact upon health and social inequalities. Social care focuses upon the daily activities of living, for instance, feeding and basic hygiene maintenance, but also maintaining individuals'' independence, promoting social interaction, protection from vulnerable environments and coping with complex individual and contextual relationships. It is delivered through social work, personal care, and social support (Kelly et al., 2023). Healthcare services are provided by the National Health Service (NHS) in the UK, free at the point of use. Social care services, on the other hand, are run by local authorities, for example, authorised to provide diverse levels of care, depending on income and circumstances, or can be privately purchased, if not.

A healthcare need is associated with treatment, control or prevention of a disease, illness, disability of injury and the aftercare necessary as a result. Social care needs primarily refer to those around need of assistance in terms of, for example, ability to be independent, maintenance of daily living activities; interaction with other individuals and environments, as well as reducing vulnerability to specific circumstances and events, often involving safeguarding (Masterson et al., 2022). In the UK, the Care Act (2014) specifies wellbeing as one of the core responsibilities for care providers as well as prevention and protection and asserts its importance, not only in matching needs to a specific service, but as an intrinsic concept in designing needs assessment and planning processes in conjunction with carers and service users and in enhancing important outcomes to both. Table 4.2 outlines nine principles of the Care Act (2014) which highlights the areas that wellbeing encompasses.

TABLE 4.2 The Nine Principles of Wellbeing in the Care Act 2014

1. Personal dignity, including treatment of the individual with respect
2. Physical mental and emotional wellbeing
3. Protection from abuse and neglect
4. Control by the individual over their day-to-day life and includes care and support provided and the ways they are provided
5. Participation in work, education, training, or recreation
6. Social and economic wellbeing
7. Domestic, family, and personal domains
8. Suitability of the individual's living accommodation
9. The individual's contribution to society

Similarly, The Social Services and Wellbeing Act (2014) in Wales also gives prominence to the concept of wellbeing within social care. The Act accentuates the wellbeing of individuals, who require care and support, and highlights that local authorities and their partners possess a statutory duty to promote wellbeing. This also includes a duty to involve individuals within decisions about needs, care, and support. Both Acts accentuate the link between wellbeing and personalised care especially, with the former perceived as essential to involvement of service users in defining their health and quality of life needs and as active participants in needs assessment and care services (La Placa and Knight, 2014b). The importance placed upon individuals' definition of wellbeing is also conceptualised as an essential element in integrating health and social care at the point of assessment and planning to produce an integrated assessment and planning experience, and which results in, for example, a single consolidated personalised care and support plan, with wellbeing at the forefront of this (Henderson et al., 2020).

DEFINITIONAL FRAMEWORKS AND INDICATORS OF WELLBEING ACROSS THE OECD

Comparatively, the enhanced use of concepts and indicators of wellbeing across OECD countries, and the recognition of it as a relevant policy tool across health and social care, has precipitated, albeit limited, the development of conceptual, indicative, and definitional approaches, to encompass and locate concepts of wellbeing. Traditionally, researchers and scholars, who have attempted to define or theorise wellbeing, have achieved this through explaining it on the more psychological level, around concepts of mental health; positive psychology; hedonic wellbeing (happiness in terms of pleasure attainment and pain avoidance; eudaemonic wellbeing (the process whereby the causes of pleasure and happiness on a subjective level are recognised); and psychological wellbeing (attempts to feel 'good' subjectively), while developing awareness of the domains which limit this, for example, lack of personal self-acceptance (Oades and Mossman, 2017; Fisher, 2019). Despite the importance of this emphasis on the psychological and the subjective, such articulations are limited in that they do not adequately attempt to bridge the divide between the subjective and psychological with, for instance, the broader structural, systemic, and economic determinants, which influence subjective development, and experiences of wellbeing, and more crucially, the relationship between the two. Addressing these issues is of significance for the credibility and democratic accountability of health and social care policies, which seek to restructure health and social care systems and practices globally (O'Donovan, 2023).

For example, the OECD Framework of Wellbeing identifies eleven definitional dimensions and indicators of wellbeing, as essential to people's lives 'here and now,' ranging from health status to subjective wellbeing, as well as more material dimensions, such as housing (OECD, 2020; 2021). In addition, four 'stocks of resources' are highlighted as important for sustaining wellbeing outcomes over time. This is highlighted in Table 4.3.

TABLE 4.3 The OECD Framework of Wellbeing

Indicators	Income and wealth; work and job quality; housing; health; knowledge and skills; environmental quality; subjective wellbeing; safety; work-life balance; social connections; civil engagement
Indicator Measured through	Averages; inequalities between groups; inequalities between top and bottom performers; deprivation
Stocks of Knowledge	Natural capital; economic capital; human capital; social capital

However, the OECD framework provides little in the way of concretely defining them and attempting an explanatory model as to where these fit within the subjective and objective schema, or potential interactions and mediations among them. OECD countries, as evidenced above, have tended towards developing categories of indicators to assess and monitor wellbeing at national level, but which are less grounded in explanatory, conceptually and definitionally rigorous frameworks. Many of the indicators also often conceptualise health and wellbeing as synonymous, produced on the social, physical, psychological, and environmental level, suggesting that wellbeing is a multi-levelled definition, but not articulated as such. As a result, researchers, practitioners, and policy makers need to be clearer in respect of potential definitional frameworks, and how they are used to articulate interventions, policy, and evaluations of wellbeing.

Fisher (2019) argued for a 'public wellbeing' approach whereby the impact of social determinants upon mental health were derived. However, this account is limited in that its focus is on how brain and cognitive processes interact with social settings (which are never adequately defined) and how this affects stress arousal due to interpretations of others' perceptions. Health and social care services, however, who assist individuals to, for instance, live more independent, and healthier lives, require broader definitional depth and analyses, and which transcends psychological health and wellbeing, only. Explanations and indications of wellbeing, developed by researchers, have also tended not to develop, and apply the concepts and processes of existing grand theory and narratives, which economists and social scientists use in research and policy. In much of the literature, there is little reference to the concepts and explanatory models of, for instance, 'feminism' (Leavy and Harris, 2019) or 'critical public theory' (Renault, 2017), despite the emphasis upon structural health inequalities and health and social care disparities, both nationally and globally. This reduces attempts to locate wellbeing research and frameworks within sufficient theoretical frameworks, which would deliver more credence in developing indicators and definitions, (often perceived as stand alone, in the current wellbeing literature).

McNAUGHT'S DEFINITIONAL FRAMEWORK OF WELLBEING

As a result, it is the author's view that McNaught's Definitional Framework of Wellbeing (Figure 4.1), which attempts to define and structure the parameters within which operational definitions of wellbeing and research can be devised, is most suited to articulating wellbeing policy and practice (McNaught, 2011; La Placa and

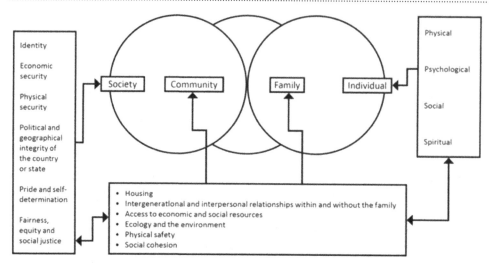

FIGURE 4.1 A Structured Framework for Defining Wellbeing

Source: Knight and McNaught (2011), reproduced with permission from Lantern Publishing

Knight, 2023). It identifies a common currency that expedites the operationalisation of wellbeing research and practice initiatives, thereby ensuring robust evaluations, and comparisons to facilitate more substantial definitions, design of indicators across populations, and establishes a guide for use, within and between, countries and communities.

The framework substantiates the claim that wellbeing constitutes an area of research and practice, characterised by objective and subjective domains, as researchers and practitioners, can affect more significant evaluations of wellbeing, if this is accounted for. The framework widens wellbeing to various domains beyond individual and psychological subjectivity to incorporate the family, community, and society and a range of environmental, geographic, socio-economic, and political dimensions (McNaught, 2011; La Placa et al., 2013). While the individual and psychological domain is subsumed within the framework, the psychological perspective does not monopolise it, which is often the case with positive psychology. The framework provides a holistic definitional model of wellbeing, to be applied across not only populations, but defined groups of individuals across those populations. The four domains of the framework are 'individual' wellbeing, 'family' wellbeing, 'community' wellbeing, and 'societal' wellbeing. The framework can pioneer design of research, clarify meanings, and potentially be incorporated into broader theoretical frameworks, used in research.

The framework promotes wellbeing as constituted dynamically, constructed by its agents through reciprocity, between their circumstances, locality, activities, and psychological resources, including interpersonal relations with, for example, families and communities. Individuals change accounts of their lives, and manage their actions, with reference to the four domains. For example, La Placa et al. (2013)

give the example of an individual who does not feel happy with events and relations in his or her birth family and undertakes to move to another part of the family or decides to do things differently when he or she starts a family. Conversely, individuals can embrace divergent models of relationships, for instance, personal, and familial, where earlier unmet needs are fulfilled.

Individual wellbeing comprises a large element of the framework and imputes significant agency to individuals to socially construct and define wellbeing. It is influenced significantly by Diener's (2005) view that subjective wellbeing comprises both positive and negative judgements around life events and life satisfaction. However, unlike much of the literature around wellbeing, significantly influenced, by positive psychology, the model builds in a link to understand how agents' experiences and constructions of wellbeing are influenced and mediated by broader structural and circumstances.

Linked to this is the concept of *family* wellbeing, which is significantly underplayed in the OECD's framework of wellbeing (OECD, 2020; 2021). Experiences of, and positions within a given family structure, affect evaluations of wellbeing about families and relationships. Families also grant and remove specific financial and psychological resources, depending on one's location within it, for instance, love, money, and status (McNaught, 2011; La Placa and Knight, 2023). The framework organises the family as a system, comprising sub-systems of hierarchies and relationships, capable of affecting outcomes across child and adulthood experiences, and can represent a multitude of changing family structures and cultures, typical of families, across OECD countries (supporting eco-system and family systems theory to enhance its contemporary relevance). The family domain could be more universally used across OECD research and indicators, too, given the key location of individuals and households in its own indicators of wellbeing.

Community wellbeing denotes the personal, cultural, and structural resources and assets, which communities allocate, and which may or may not personally fulfil wellbeing. Again, the psychological domain is transcended to focus upon how communities, as well as families, allocate capital, resources, and assets (Roy, 2017) and recognises communities and families are constructed through broader social and economic conditions, which mediate wellbeing experiences, within and between them. The capacity to connect the mediating domains is a significant strength of the model, pulling away from positive psychologies, and unilinear biomedical definitions of health and illness. The concept of community wellbeing, often negated across the study of wellbeing, also fills an important gap in OECD, and broader global definitions, around, for example, what the OECD terms, 'key resources and dimension of future wellbeing' and highlights people's relations to specific local populations, and communities, be they, for instance, area, or ethnicity based. The inter-relation between family and community (though not exclusively) is an important tenet when focusing upon formal and informal care across OECD countries and enables policy makers to evaluate the potentially different wellbeing requirements of them. For example, informal care is often provided for individuals, residing at home, and by those living in the same household (Bergmann and Wagner, 2021). Informal care has a significant gender and socio-economic dimension wedded to it, given may informal carers are women, and a significant determinant of inequalities across families and communities, affecting distribution of resources, and therefore, wellbeing experiences.

The promotion of *societal* wellbeing is crucial to the framework, given the shift away from measuring it in terms of economic functioning, and broadening this to focusing on, for example, agents' experiences of health and social care services, systems of care, and interventions. The framework uses and mirrors Skilton's (2009) argument that broader economic, social, and political systems deliver a range of resources and relations to the State, and which affect individual, family, and community constructions of wellbeing. The framework can illustrate the broader society's leverage over subjective wellbeing in, for example, financial rewards, forms of employment, public services, and the state of the environment, which national policy encourages and devises. The emphasis upon societal wellbeing also raises fundamental questions around structural and social inequalities (Wilkinson and Pickett, 2010; Keister and Southgate, 2021) given the importance allocated to these in the OECD framework, and the impact of broader processes enveloping constructions of wellbeing and social care, such as globalisation, and global governance.

USES OF THE DEFINITIONAL FRAMEWORK OF WELLBEING

The framework postulates wellbeing as a macro concept or arrangement with clearly discernible components and relationships which can be applied across a range of theoretical and empirical research (Burns et al., 2020; Griffin et al., 2023). It continues to concede the debated nature of concepts around wellbeing, demonstrating its variegate nature; but integrates it into a framework, which provides for organisation, structure, and clarification. As a result, the framework can be used across the variation exhibited by OECD countries in tracking progress, and informing health and social care policy debates, and where individual countries often lack a formal mechanism to integrate wellbeing indicators into the policy process (OECD, 2020). For example, it may assist to globally develop analogous types of indicators, reflecting a consensus on the core determinants of wellbeing, and enable development of consistent metrics, which permit global comparisons, and capture progress towards meeting the United Nations' 17 Sustainable Development Goals (SDGs). Wellbeing measurement initiatives and indicators, when founded upon a clear conceptual and definitional framework, ensure their effective use in delineating how to think about wellbeing, and how to widen types of indicators of outcomes, which the policy process targets. This also assists decisions as to whether, for instance, this should assume the form of a specific set of indicators or whether wellbeing should be viewed as a prism, through which to examine various policies.

Simultaneously, the framework enables many opportunities to focus in-depth on areas of health and social care, which require emphasis upon wellbeing and care. For instance, informal carers can face negative consequences for their health and wellbeing, if forced to reduce or relinquish employment, putting themselves at risk of poverty and social exclusion (Schulmann et al., 2019). Given the role of an informal carer can be particularly challenging, with little choices as to the conditions, in which they undertake the role, the issue of wellbeing needs to be meticulously considered, especially where lack of formal, alternative care arrangements exist (United Nations Economic Commission for Europe, 2019). The emphasis upon objective and subjective definitions and assessments of wellbeing captures it as a phenomenon beyond behavioural change or the concern of positive psychology. La Placa et al. (2013) contend that the strength of the framework lays in its abilities to coalesce how individuals feel about their circumstances and assessment of how their objective circumstances influence them as individuals, for instance, families, and the broader society.

Theoretical frameworks, widely associated with grand theory and metanarratives, advise broad assumptions about processes of behaviour and its determinants, lead data collection, and ground planning of inventive interventions within empirical research, (which often transcends design of indicators and preliminary attempts at definition of a phenomenon). McNaught's definitional framework prepares a pathway towards the use and development of broader theoretical frameworks, which further embrace it, encompass the design of empirical research strategies and topics; and provide the evidence to ground the design effective health and social care interventions. For example, the emphasis upon change, interaction, and multi-levelled domains, locates the framework within the broader theoretical paradigm, which combines both agency and structure, or what is often termed, the 'duality' of structure and agency (La Placa et al., 2013). It locates effective agents within a web of other domains, which themselves are altered by the conscious actions and resource mobilisation of agents. The definitional framework can be used within a theoretical approach, which perceives wellbeing, for instance, as constituted through a duality of structure and agency (Giddens, 1984; Stones, 2005). Social environment and structure are both the medium and the outcome of social action as people negotiate reflexively through both in accordance with circumstances and interpretation.

The framework can also support critical theoretical perspectives, such as the Critical Public Health perspective, which focuses upon structural inequalities, and the role of social and healthcare institutions in creating 'social suffering' and enduring health disparities and inequities (Crenshaw, 1991; Renault, 2017). The conceptual underpinnings and definitions apparent in the framework are multiple and vigorous enough to support and link to a theory/theoretical framework, and guide empirical research, to illustrate both theory and research. For instance, the disruption caused by the global COVID-19 pandemic from 2020 onwards on global health and social care systems, unmasked the profound levels of socio-economic, health, and wellbeing inequalities, which exist, with evidence strongly suggesting that Black, Asian and minority ethnic (BAME) communities, adults with learning disabilities, and individuals on the lowest incomes, were disproportionately affected (Otu et al., 2020; OECD, 2021). Further research on the wellbeing of marginalised communities, and the post COVID-19 reconstruction of care systems, are likely to bestow critical perspectives to elucidate it; and draw upon McNaught's definitional framework to, for instance, guide definitions, decide requisite levels and domains of wellbeing, conceptualise the interconnections between proximal and distal determinants, and usher the appropriate research methods, to illustrate the critical perspective. La Placa and Knight (2023) also contend that while the framework does not explicitly reference 'globalisation', it currently provides an adaptable framework to remove silo and often amorphous approaches to wellbeing, on both a local, national, and potentially global scale.

CONCLUSION

This chapter examined definitional frameworks and contemporary understandings of wellbeing and argued for the usefulness of McNaught's definitional framework of wellbeing, in broadening development of wellbeing models and indicators, its uses in research, and its ability to link with, and support broader theoretical frameworks. For example, it can enhance consistent methodology used for indications of wellbeing and sustainability and create consensus around, for instance, development of indicators as a measure of wellbeing. A need for people-centred and lifeworld led care health and care support systems is acknowledged as a global priority (Galvin and Todres, 2013; WHO, 2016; Henderson et al., 2020).

Many countries face challenges in enabling safe, effective, affordable, integrated, and coordinated care, around the needs and preferences of people, who access integrated health and social care services. This includes ensuring access to appropriate services; enhancing relationships between professionals and service users; and surmounting challenges in navigating integrated systems, to ensure new and existing structures are visible and accessible (Baxter et al., 2018; Henderson et al., 2020). Furthermore, if person-centred systems are to adhere to the tenets of participatory care and governance, both nationally and globally, and enable parity between population health, wellbeing, and ill-health prevention, more focus upon wellbeing is necessary for this. The use of McNaught's structured definitional framework of wellbeing is a useful starting point to achieve this in development of wellbeing research, policy, and practice.

RESEARCH POINTS AND REFLECTIVE EXERCISES

- What do you understand by the term 'wellbeing' and how does it differ from the WHO definition?
- How can the concept of wellbeing be applied to enhance the experiences of health and social care service users post COVID 19?

REFERENCES

Baxter, S., Johnson, M., Chambers, D., Sutton, A., Goyder, E., et al. (2018). The Effects of Integrated Care: A Systematic Review of UK and International Evidence. *BMC Health Serv Res*, 18 (350). https://doi.org/10.1186/s12913-018-3161-3

Bergmann, M. and Wagner, M. (2021). The Impact of COVID-19 on Informal Caregiving and Care Receiving Across Europe During the First Phase of the Pandemic. *Frontiers in Public Health*, 6 (9): 673874. https://doi.org/10.3389/fpubh.2021.673874

Burns, D., Dagnall, N. and Holt, M. (2020). Assessing the Impact of the COVID-19 Pandemic on Student Wellbeing at Universities in the United Kingdom: A Conceptual Analysis. *Frontiers*, 5. https://doi.org/10.3389/feduc.2020.582882

Canadian Index of Wellbeing. (2016). *How are Canadians Really Doing? The 2016 CIW National Report*. Waterloo, ON: Canadian Index of Wellbeing and University of Waterloo.

Care Act. (2014). Available at: www.legislation.gov.uk/ukpga/2014/23/contents/enacted (Accessed: 14 April 2023).

Crenshaw, K. (1991). Mapping the Margins: Intersectionality, Identity Politics, and Violence Against Women of Color. *Stanford Law Review*, 43 (6): 1241–1299. https://doi.org/10.2307/1229039

Department of Finance Canada. (2021). Toward a Quality of Life Strategy for Canada. Available at: www.canada.ca/en/department-finance/services/publications/measuring-what-matters-toward-quality-life-strategy-canada.html (Accessed: 12 April 2023).

Diener, E. (2005). *Guidelines for National Indicators of Subjective Well-being and Ill-being*. Chicago, IL: University of Illinois

Fisher, M. (2019). A Theory of Public Wellbeing. *BMC Public Health*, 19 (1): 1283. https://doi.org/10.1186/s12889-019-7626-z

Galvin, K. and Todres, L. (2013). *Caring and Well-being: A Lifeworld Approach*. London: Routledge.

Giddens, A. (1984). *The Constitution of Society*. Cambridge: Polity Press.

Griffin, T., Grey, E., Lambert, J. Gillison, F., Townsend, N., et al. (2023). Life in Lockdown: A Qualitative Study Exploring the Experience of Living Through the Initial COVID-19 Lockdown in the UK and its Impact on Diet, Physical Activity and Mental Health. *BMC Public Health*, 23 (588). https://doi.org/10.1186/s12889-023-15441-0

Haybron, D. M. (2008). Philosophy and the Science of Subjective Well-being. In M. Eid and R. J. Larsen (eds), *The Science of Subjective Wellbeing*. London: Guildford Press, 17–43.

Henderson, L., Bain, H., Allan, E. and Kennedy, C. (2020). Integrated Health and Social Care in the Community: A Critical Integrative Review of the Experiences and Well-being Needs of Service Users and Their Families. *Health and Social Care in the Community*, 29 (15): 1145–1168. https://doi.org/10.1111/hsc.13179

Keister, L. A. and Southgate, D. E. (2021). *Inequality: A Contemporary Approach to Race, Class, and Gender*, 2nd edn. Cambridge: Cambridge University Press.

Kelly, Y., O'Rourke, N., Flynn, R., Hegarty, J. and O'Connor, L. (2023). Definitions of Health and Social Care Standards Used Internationally: A Narrative Review. *The International Journal of Health Planning and Management*, 38 (1): 40–52. https://doi.org/10.1002/hpm.3573

Knight, A. and McNaught, A. (2011). *Understanding Wellbeing: An Introduction for Students and Practitioners of Health and Social Care*. Banbury: Lantern Publishing.

La Placa, V. G., McNaught, A. and Knight, A. (2013). Discourse of Wellbeing in Research and Practice. *International Journal of Wellbeing*, 3 (1): 116–125. https://doi.org/10.5502/ijw.v3i1.7

La Placa, V. and Knight, A. (2014a). Wellbeing: A New Policy Phenomenon? In A. Knight, V. La Placa and A. McNaught (eds), *Wellbeing: Policy and Practice*. Banbury: Lantern Publishing, 17–27.

La Placa, V. and Knight, A. (2014b). Well-being: Its Influence and Local Impact on Public Health. *Public Health*, 128 (1): 38–42. https://doi.org/10.1016/j.puhe.2013.09.017

La Placa, V. and Knight, A. (2017). The Emergence of Wellbeing in Late Modern Capitalism: Theory, Research and Policy Responses. *International Journal of Social Science Studies*, 5 (3): 1–11. https://doi.org/10.11114/ijsss.v5i3.2207

La Placa, V. and Knight, A. (2023). Globalisation and Global Public Health. In V. La Placa and J. Morgan (eds), *Social Science Perspectives on Global Public Health*. London: Routledge, 17–28.

Leavy, P. and Harris, A. (2019). *Contemporary Feminist Research from Theory to Practice*. London: Guildford Press.

Masterson, D., Areskoug Josefsson, K., Robert, G., Nylander, E. and Kjellström, S. (2022). Mapping Definitions of Co-Production and Co-Design in Health and Social Care: A Systematic Scoping Review Providing Lessons for the Future. *Health Expectations*, 25 (3): 902–913. https://doi.org/10.1111/hex.13470

McNaught, A. (2011). Defining Wellbeing. In A. Knight and A. McNaught (eds), *Understanding Wellbeing: An Introduction for Students and Practitioners of Health and Social Care*. Banbury: Lantern Publishing, 7–22.

Oades, L. G. and Mossman, L. (2017). The Science of Wellbeing and Positive Psychology. In M. Slade, L. Oades and A. Jarden (eds), *Wellbeing, Recovery and Mental Health*. Cambridge: Cambridge University Press, 7–24.

O'Donovan, C. (2023). Accountability and Neglect in UK Social Care Innovation. *International Journal of Care and Caring*, 7 (1): 67–90. https://doi.org/10.1332/2397882 21X16613769194393

OECD. (2020). *How's Life? 2020: Measuring Well-being*. Paris OECD Publishing. https://doi.org/10.1787/9870c393-en.

OECD. (2021a). *COVID-19 and Well-being Life in the Pandemic*. Paris: OECD Publishing.

OECD. (2021b). Health and Social Care Workforce. In. *OECD Health At a Glance 2021: OECD Indicators*. Paris: OECD Publishing, 209–232.

OECD. (2023). *Integrating Care to Prevent and Manage Chronic Diseases: Best Practices in Public Health*. Paris: OECD Publishing.

Office for National Statistics. (2010). Measuring National Wellbeing. Available at: https://webarchive.nationalarchives.gov.uk/ukgwa/20160105160711/http://www.ons.gov.uk/ons/guide-method/user-guidance/well-being/index.html (Accessed: 18 April 2023).

Otu, A., Ahinkorah, B. O., Ameyaw, E. K. Seidu, A. A., and Yaya, S. (2020). One Country, Two Crises: What Covid-19 Reveals about Health Inequalities Among BAME Communities in the United Kingdom and the Sustainability of its Health System? *International Journal of Equity Health*, 19 (189). https://doi.org/10.1186/s12939-020-01307-z

Renault, E. (2017). *Social Suffering: Sociology, Psychology, Politics*. London: Rowman and Littlefield International.

Roy, M. J. (2017). The Assets-Based Approach: Furthering a Neoliberal Agenda or Rediscovering the Old Public Health? A Critical Examination of Practitioner Discourses. *Critical Public Health*, 27 (4): 455–464. https://doi.org/10.1080/09581596.2016.1249826

Schulmann, K., Reichert M., and Leichsenring, K. (2019). Social Support and Long-Term Care for Older People: The Potential for Social Innovation and Active Ageing. In A. Walker (ed.), *The Future of Ageing in Europe – Making an Asset of Longevity*. Singapore: Palgrave Macmillan, 255–286.

Skilton, L. (2009). *Working Paper: Measuring Societal Wellbeing in the UK*. London: Office for National Statistics.

Stiglitz, J. E., Sen, A. and Fittousi, J. P. (2009). Report by the Commission on the Measurement of Economic Performance and Social Progress. Available at: https://ec.europa.eu/eurostat/documents/8131721/8131772/Stiglitz-Sen-Fitoussi-Commission-report.pdf (Accessed: 13 April 2023).

Social Services and Wellbeing Act. (2014). Available at: https://socialcare.wales/resources-guidance/information-and-learning-hub/sswbact/overview (Accessed: 19 January 2024).

Stones, R. (2005). *Structuration Theory*. Basingstoke: Palgrave Macmillan.

United Nations Economic Commission for Europe. (2019). Policy Brief: The Challenging Roles of Informal Carers. Available at: https://unece.org/DAM/pau/age/Policy_briefs/ECE_WG1_31.pdf (Accessed: 13 April 2023).

United Nations Development of Economic and Social Affairs. (2021). Sustainable Development: The 17 Goals. Available at: https://sdgs.un.org/goals (Accessed: 2 August 2021).

WHO. (2016). Integrated Care Models: An Overview of Health Services Delivery Programme. Available at: www.euro.who.int/__data/assets/pdf_file/0005/322475/Integrated-care-models-overview.pdf (Accessed: 13 April 2023).

WHO. (2021). WHO Remains Firmly Committed to the Principles Set Out in the Preamble to the Constitution. Available at: www.who.int/about/who-we-are/constitution (Accessed: 18 April 2023).

WHO. (2022). *Bending the Trends to Promote Health and Well-being: A Strategic Foresight on the Future of Health Promotion.* Geneva: World Health Organization.

Wilkinson, R. and Pickett, K. (2010). *The Spirit Level: Why Equality is Better for Everyone.* London: Penguin.

CHAPTER 5

Health Inequalities

....

Nadya Belenky

INTRODUCTION

Despite consistent improvement in life expectancy and mortality rates across OECD countries, substantial health inequalities remain, and, in some countries, those inequalities are worsening (Forster et al., 2018). Health inequalities exist both between countries, such as differences in life expectancy in various countries, but also within countries, where there are often disparities in morbidity, mortality, and life expectancy, by age, gender, educational level, occupation, and income (La Placa and Morgan, 2023). This chapter will examine health inequalities across several countries belonging to the Organisation for Economic Co-operation and Development (OECD), focusing on common indicators of health inequalities, such as life expectancy and avoidable mortality. In addition, this chapter includes descriptive analyses of mortality rates attributed to behavioural health conditions across a subset of OECD countries.

HEALTH INEQUALITIES

In this chapter, health inequalities are defined as the differences in health or health determinants between people or groups (Arcaya et al., 2015). In assessing health inequalities, this chapter takes a descriptive approach, and compares key indicators across a select group of OECD countries, with a specific comparative focus on the UK. The UK is composed of four devolved countries (England, Northern Ireland, Scotland, and Wales), each of which retains responsibility for organising healthcare delivery. All four countries retain the National Health Service (NHS) model, and each country sets its own planning goals and funding priorities, which can contribute to variation in health policy and health outcomes within the UK.

Of the 38 OECD member countries, the chapter chose a subset by balancing geographic proximity to the UK with diversity in healthcare systems. To include countries that might serve as models for future policy development, it cross-referenced the

DOI: 10.4324/9781003343608-6

initial set of countries with a recent study on healthcare innovation across OECD countries, which clusters OECD countries by national health innovation (Proksch et al., 2019). The final subset of OECD countries includes Australia, Canada, Denmark, Finland, France, Germany, Ireland, Japan, Norway, Poland, Sweden, the US, and the UK. Within OECD data, the UK is compared to other OECD countries as a combined unit, rather than broken out by the 4 devolved countries within the UK. Data were retrieved from the OECD data warehouse, which includes data and metadata for relevant themes for OECD countries and selected non-member countries (OECD, 2014). Data for most countries and most indicators are available through 2021, though some of the comparisons are limited by data availability.

The key OECD indicators selected to outline health inequalities include life expectancy, self-rated health, preventable mortality, and treatable mortality. In addition to general health indicators, this chapter also examines the mortality rate attributable to behavioural health conditions. The descriptive analyses below focus preferentially on the OECD countries within the subset, if those OECD countries indicated trends over time, which were especially informative. In other words, for clarity and ease of oversight, even though the data for all OECD countries in the subset indicated above were analysed, not all figures below will include all countries in the chosen OECD subset.

INEQUALITIES IN LIFE EXPECTANCY AND SELF-RATED HEALTH

Life expectancy and self-rated health status are two key indicators of the overall health of a population. Life expectancy is defined as how long, on average, a person will live or years of life at birth. Life expectancies are calculated using current death rates, because for each new birth cohort, the actual death rates cannot be known at the time of birth. As death rates change, the actual average lifespan of a birth cohort will differ from life expectancy estimates at birth. The OECD database draws on data for life expectancy from Eurostat for European Union (EU) countries. Life expectancy is one of the most common measures of a population's health status, and consequently, is also a primary indicator for health inequality. Across countries, it is well-established that life expectancy is closely tied to deprivation (Tobias and Cheung, 2003; Singh and Siahpush, 2006; Kroll et al., 2017; Parker et al., 2020).

Previous analyses of OECD data indicate that life expectancy at birth has increased significantly in EU OECD countries between 2005-2016, and that in the same period, differences between countries have also narrowed. However, those same analyses have indicated a slowdown in improvements in life expectancy since 2011 (Ho and Hendi, 2018; Raleigh, 2019). Within-country analyses indicate widespread declines in life expectancy in 2015, generally attributed to an especially severe outbreak of influenza (Molbak et al., 2015; Pebody et al., 2018). In the UK, Dementia and Alzheimer's disease were indicated as the cause of death that was negatively and increasingly contributing to worsening life expectancy in both men and women (Raleigh, 2019).

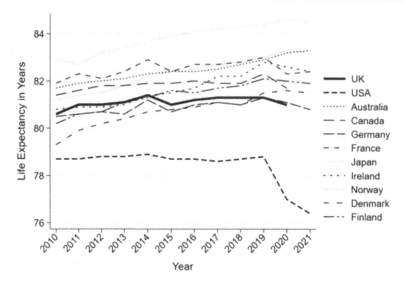

FIGURE 5.1 Life Expectancy by Country

Building on previous analyses of OECD data, these current analyses on life expectancy by country (see Figure 5.1) support previous findings on a slowdown in improvement in life expectancy. These data also outline the early effects of the COVID-19 pandemic in 2020 and 2021, where the effect on life expectancy is especially striking in the USA and aligns with recent decreases in life expectancy in France, Germany, Canada, UK, and Ireland. The findings on US life expectancy are well supported by other studies, driven by increased mortality in young and middle-aged adults (Harris et al., 2021) and compounded by inadequate policies to address social determinants of health and a lack of universal healthcare (Venkataramani et al., 2021; Woolf et al., 2022).

While trends in life expectancy are informative, this chapter goes a step further and investigates inequalities in life expectancy, by gender, across a range of OECD countries (see Figure 5.2). While several countries have notably reduced the gender gap in life expectancy (e.g., Norway, Denmark), between 2010 and 2021, the COVID-19 pandemic appears to have exacerbated gender disparities in life expectancy. Some countries showed increases in gender disparities (e.g., Sweden, Germany, France) which erased the improvements in those disparities over the last several years, while the USA witnessed a trend that had been increasing for several years, leading up to 2020 and dramatically increasing in 2020 and 2021. Other analyses of life expectancy within OECD data further show that differences in educational attainment account for approximately 10% of the differences in life expectancy (Murtin et al., 2017).

Characteristics of the US healthcare system, specifically the lack of universal coverage, combined with less equitable social welfare spending (Avendano and Kawachi, 2014) appear to leave the country exceptionally vulnerable to the strain of the COVID-19 pandemic, indicated by the substantial decrease in life expectancy, and an increase in both preventable and treatable mortality (see Figures 5.4 and 5.5). Given that healthcare spending within the US is approximately twice as high as other

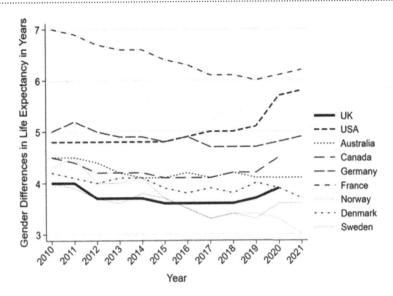

FIGURE 5.2 Gender Difference in Life Expectancy by Country

high-income countries (approximately 18% of GDP), it indicates that additional spending has not translated into a more resilient healthcare system or improvements in life expectancy (Papanicolas et al., 2018).

As a complement to life expectancy, self-rated health provides individuals' assessment of their own health. As an OECD indicator, self-rated health is intended as a composite measure of both physical and mental health. Both life expectancy and self-rated health are generally available across OECD countries. However, self-rated health allows for a more holistic measurement of health inequalities across countries, going beyond measures of survival. Finally, even though self-rated health is a subjective measurement, meaning that individuals report on their own perceived health status, self-rated health has been shown to predict morbidity and healthcare utilisation (Palladino et al., 2016).

Across all OECD countries in 2019, approximately 9% of adults reported being in poor health (see Figure 5.3), ranging from 4% to 15% (OECD, 2021) and these analyses expand on those results by describing trends over time between 2010 and 2020/2021, including a description of the effects of COVID-19 on self-rated health. As described elsewhere, self-rated health is unique in that it is a subjective measure, which means that results across countries are not directly comparable, due to a combination of methodological differences, and asymmetrical response patterns.

Within the UK, where data on self-rated health were available through 2019, it showed that, on average, 7% of the population self-rated their health as bad/very bad over 2010 and 2019. However, the time trend indicates an increase of 28% over the ten-year time period. Notably, in the USA, where self-rated health data was available through 2021, the proportion of the population that reported bad/very bad health remained stable at around 3% between 2010 and 2021, despite a pronounced

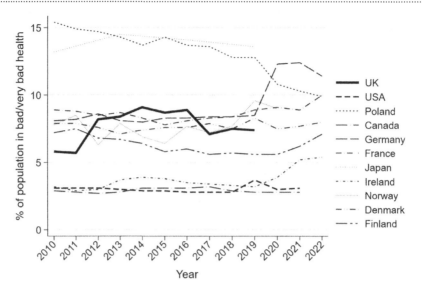

FIGURE 5.3 Self-Rate Bad/Very Bad Health by Country

decrease in life expectancy and worsening of gender disparities within that measure over 2020 and 2021. Canada's self-rated health followed a similar pattern, beginning in 2010, with similar levels of self-rated health, and maintaining those levels over the period of observation. However, this measure may be difficult to compare across countries, as both the USA and Canada, show asymmetrical response patterns towards the positive categories of self-rated health, implying a bias towards positive self-assessment. The asymmetrical response pattern is specific to self-rated health and makes it difficult to compare to OECD countries within the EU, which report symmetrical responses to questions about self-rated health (Raleigh, 2019).

For countries that included data on self-rated health during the COVID-19 pandemic (i.e., Poland, Germany, France, Denmark, and Ireland), most indicated an increase in the proportion of the population self-reporting bad or very bad health. Over the full period before 2020, however, most countries' proportion of the population reporting bad or very bad health was stable over time. Poland was the notable exception, beginning at 15% of the population reporting bad or very bad health in 2010, the highest proportion in bad or very bad health of the comparison countries, to 10% by 2022, a decrease of 36%, including strong decreases during 2020–2022. Although some of the data is not shown here, Korea, Japan, and Portugal are unique, in that all three countries have high life expectancies (between 82 and 84 years) but relatively poor self-rated health (14–15%). Countries in which life expectancy and self-rated health appear to be inconsistent, point to unique demographic and health system characteristics, specific to those countries, and support more in-depth studies on the interplay between life expectancy, and self-rated health.

There are two major limitations to self-rated health as a measure of inequality across countries. First, most OECD countries regularly conduct health surveys of their population, including questions focused on self-rated health. However, because those surveys are country-specific, the questions on self-rated health are formulated and scaled differently across countries. Second, because older people tend to report worse levels of health compared to younger people, differences between countries in average self-rated health may be driven by the age distribution within that country. For example, countries with younger populations are likely to show higher levels of self-rated health compared to countries with older populations.

INEQUALITIES IN PREVENTABLE MORTALITY AND TREATABLE MORTALITY

The chapter proceeds to expand upon traditional indicators of health inequalities such as life expectancy and self-rated health status, by examining preventable and treatable mortality across countries as an indicator of the effectiveness of healthcare within countries. Preventable mortality is defined using the 2019 OECD/Eurostat definitions as a cause of death, which can be avoided through effective intervention (either public health intervention or primary prevention); in other words, preventing the onset of diseases or injuries, before they result in incident disease and subsequently, mortality. Treatable mortality is defined as a cause of death which can be avoided through timely and effective healthcare interventions, meaning deaths which are prevented through secondary prevention and treatment for health conditions after the onset of the disease.

When there was evidence that a cause of death could be both prevented and treated, that cause of death was attributed to the preventable mortality category, on the basis that if a cause of death could be both treated and prevented, then prevention should take precedence, because it negates the need for treatment. When the evidence behind the cause of death was not predominantly either preventable or treatable, the cause of death was split across both categories, avoiding double-counting (OECD, 2022). The cross-country comparisons of preventable and treatable mortality rates (see Figures 5.4 and 5.5) are shown as annual rates per 100,000

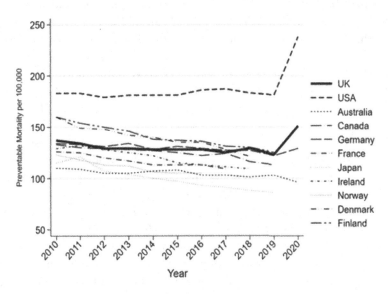

FIGURE 5.4 Preventable Mortality Rate by Country

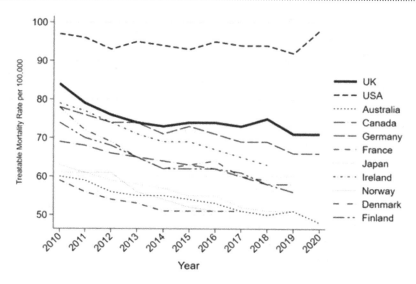

FIGURE 5.5 Treatable Mortality Rate by Country

and are standardised by age and sex. The use of standardised rates improves the validity of the comparison across OECD countries, which differ in their age and sex composition. More information on how these indicators were developed is available through the OECD (OECD, 2022).

Before 2020, preventable mortality rates appear to be declining across the OECD comparison countries (Figure 5.4), except for the USA and UK, which remain stable over time, despite UK rates being substantially lower than the preventable mortality rate in the USA. In the USA, preventable mortality rates remain around 180 preventable deaths per 100,000 until 2020, where the preventable mortality rate increases by 32% to 238 preventable deaths per 100,000 in 2020. The UK follows a similar pattern to the USA, beginning from a lower baseline preventable mortality rate, which was approximately stable at 123 preventable deaths per 100,000 until 2020. Between 2019 and 2020, the UK witnessed its preventable mortality rate increase by 23% to 151 preventable deaths per 100,000 in 2020. The increase in 2020 more than erased the 11% decrease in preventable mortality which the UK had experienced in the preceding 10 years.

The treatable mortality rate is almost universally declining across the OECD comparison countries (Figure 5.5), in addition to anchoring at lower baseline rates in all countries compared to preventable mortality (Figure 5.4). The USA represents the notable exception to this decreasing trend in treatable mortality, where the rate remains both stable and higher, comparatively, until increasing still further in 2020. Of the comparison countries, even those countries beginning with low treatable mortality rates (Japan, Norway, France, Australia) showed a decrease in treatable mortality over the years observed. As more countries publish their 2020 data, the effects of COVID-19 on preventable and treatable mortality rates will become more evident.

Avoidable mortality, the combination of preventable and treatable mortality, assumes that deaths can be avoided given appropriate medical treatment or intervention. The concept of avoidable mortality is interlinked with health inequalities because appropriate and timely medical care can assume a significant role in reducing health inequalities. Avoidable mortality has been used in other studies to measure differences in the performance of national health systems (Desai et al., 2011; Nolte and McKee, 2011). This measure must be interpreted cautiously as a surveillance tool, having shown limited validity in international comparisons (Mackenbach et al., 2013). However, it remains that avoidable mortality can be considered a measure of the potential scope for further population health gain (Tobias and Jackson, 2001) and, consequently, may be an informative tool for evidence-based health policy development.

INEQUALITIES IN BEHAVIOURAL HEALTH

In addition to examining general measures of health and health inequalities, this chapter explores inequalities specific to behavioural health across OECD countries. The global burden of behavioural health, the combination of mental health and substance use disorders, is growing, and increased by 38% between 1990 and 2010 (Whiteford et al., 2013). Behavioural health is central to individual wellbeing, in addition to being commonly comorbid with other health conditions and assumes a pivotal role in the management of those co-morbidities (Naylor et al., 2012). Mental health conditions, if left unmanaged, can exacerbate a range of comorbidities (DiMatteo et al., 2000). Consequently, inequalities in mental health outcomes are both indicators of health inequality in addition to modifying factors, which can contribute to increasing health inequalities.

The burden of behavioural health conditions is also economic, where the economic cost represents approximately 4% of GDP across the OECD countries (OECD, 2021). However, the actual cost is likely to be much higher, as behavioural health conditions can drive up the complexity and cost of treating other comorbidities (König et al., 2019). The comparative analysis of this chapter now focuses on trends in the mortality rate attributed to behavioural health conditions in selected OECD countries.

Descriptive analyses of mortality rates attributed to behavioural health conditions (see Figure 5.6) indicate increases in mortality rate, associated with behavioural health across many of the OECD comparison countries, including striking increases in Canada, Ireland, Germany, and Australia. A subset of the OECD comparison countries maintained stable levels of mortality rates attributed to behavioural health, including Japan, France, Finland, and Denmark. In the UK, in contrast to other OECD countries, the figure shows a striking increase in mortality rate associated with behavioural health. At the beginning of the period in 2010, mortality rates in the UK are like many other OECD countries. However, by 2012, the UK was leading within this comparison group, and by 2020, the mortality rate associated with behavioural health increased by 90%, from 35 deaths per 100,000 to 67 deaths

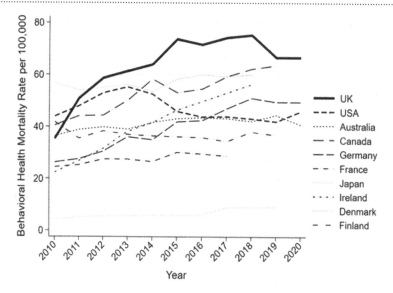

FIGURE 5.6 Behavioural Health Associated Mortality Rate by Country

per 100,000. In addition to the growing burden of behavioural health conditions, that greater burden appears to be translating to increases in related mortality rates in the UK and several other OECD countries.

COMPARISON ACROSS OECD COUNTRIES

This chapter describes a set of health indicators, across a subset of OECD countries, using all available data between 2010 and 2022. OECD countries were selected into the comparison countries, primarily to serve as particularly similar or contrasting to the UK. This analysis included several countries that provide automatic health coverage from the entire population, financed by taxation, much like in the UK (i.e., Australia, Canada, Denmark, Finland, Ireland, and Norway) (Devaux, 2010). Further, the analysis also included countries with notable, well-documented trends in life expectancy, to contrast and anchor life expectancy trends in the UK (e.g., US and Japan). The US also serves as an indicator for health inequalities within the context of privatised healthcare. The policy questions surrounding privatisation of the National Health Service (NHS) is likely to be a focal point of discussions on the future of the NHS in the coming years in the UK (Abbasi, 2023). The UK is a unique country among many OECD countries because its health system, the NHS, is a publicly funded system. However, its welfare state regime is increasingly classified as liberal, characterised by limited state provision of welfare, and modest social protection benefits, which are often tied to entitlement criteria and means-tested (Forster et al., 2018).

One of the key advantages of this descriptive analysis is the examination of the effects of COVID-19 on several indicators of health inequalities. Previous studies have suggested that COVID-19 is syndemic, that is, a synergistic pandemic that compounds the effects of existing non-communicable diseases and the inequalities in the social determinants of health (Bambra et al., 2020). The key limitation of this approach is the descriptive examination of health distributions as a measure of health inequalities. Experts on health inequality and inequity have pointed to the difficulty of comparing across countries, especially international comparisons stratified by social groups, because of cultural differences across countries in the definitions and impacts of those social groups (Kawachi et al., 2002).

UK LEARNING POINTS

These analyses of OECD life expectancy data demonstrate the diminishing gains in UK life expectancy followed by a decline in the past several years. Though the focus of these descriptive analyses was on differences in life expectancy between countries, there are other indications that the life expectancy gap within the UK is widening (Corris et al., 2020). In terms of preventable mortality, the UK follows the general trend of OECD countries within the EU, but during the most recent years of available data (coinciding with the COVID-19 pandemic), the strong increase in preventable mortality mirrors the preventable mortality rates of the US. Treatable mortality, though the UK is comparatively on the higher end of the trend over time, appears to be decreasing, though the impact of the COVID-19 pandemic on treatable mortality may lag behind the pandemic's effect on preventable mortality. Analyses of privatisation of the NHS and treatable mortality have found that private sector outsourcing corresponded to a significant increase in the rate of treatable mortality, pointing to a decline in quality of healthcare services, associated with privatisation (Goodair and Reeves, 2022).

Other analyses of self-reported mental health in the UK indicate that population mental health has worsened since the 2008 financial crisis, and compounded significantly more between 2009 and 2013, compared to previous periods (Barr et al., 2015). The same study also indicated a widening gap between higher and lower educational groups. Those shifts in trend were partially attributed to welfare policies and austerity measures which were implemented following the 2008 financial crisis. The current descriptive analyses mirror that pattern by indicating a pronounced increase in mortality rates, associated with behavioural health conditions.

UK POLICY IMPLICATIONS

Reducing health inequalities is an established policy priority for many countries, with several European countries setting national targets for reducing inequalities in mortality. Target setting has been identified as a key requirement for creating (and measuring) successful health policy (Dahlgren and Whitehead, 2006). Of the EU countries, the UK is at the forefront of advanced, quantitative targets and data collection related to health inequalities (Bauld et al., 2008). While policy is often the focal point of strategies to reduce health inequalities, it is also worth considering non-health policies, which can exacerbate those inequalities. For example, the UK's Work Capability Assessment (WCA) scheme is one such policy implementation, introduced in 2008 (Baumberg et al., 2015). The scheme's result was that individuals claiming Employment and Support Allowance had to undergo fitness to work assessments. An analysis of the policy's implementation in England between 2010 and 2013 showed that areas of higher reassessment were linked to increases in adverse mental health outcomes (Barr et al., 2016a) including an increase in suicides (Barr et al., 2016b) rather than improvement in the probability of transitioning to employment, as intended.

Even effective public health interventions may increase health inequalities if that intervention disproportionately benefits, for example, individuals belonging to higher socio-economic status (SES) groups more than lower SES groups. A systematic review of intervention types found that specific types of interventions were more likely to reduce health inequalities (Lorenc et al., 2013), specifically interventions, focused upon resource provision/fiscal interventions, such as free fruit provision in schools and free folic acid supplements have been shown to reduce inequalities by SES in healthy eating behaviours and folic acid intake, respectively (de Sa and Lock, 2008; Stockley and Lund, 2008). Structural workplace interventions were also indicated as reducing health inequalities. By contrast, interventions that were more downstream, such as mass media campaigns, were found to increase health inequalities and should be implemented with caution (Niederdeppe et al., 2008).

CONCLUSION

This chapter has explored several measures of health inequalities across a range of OECD countries. Across measures, there were strong health inequalities across countries, which were maintained or increased over time. Trends in life expectancy, in these analyses and previous research, showed that life expectancy is malleable to events, such as influenza outbreaks, and was especially affected by the COVID-19 pandemic beginning in 2020. The combination of trends in health indicators in OECD data and other analyses points to increasing health inequalities in the UK, the US, and in some European countries, beginning before the COVID-19 pandemic. As the UK shifts towards accomplishing its policy goals of reducing health inequalities, it will be necessary to evaluate interventions to ensure that their intended effect is met, and they primarily benefit the most disadvantaged groups.

RESEARCH POINTS AND REFLECTIVE EXERCISES

- Research the impact of COVID-19 on countries across the OECD. Which groups were impacted the most by the pandemic across countries?
- Variation in life expectancy across countries can be highly informative and provide policy makers with points of comparison that may lead to translational policy, where one country develops health policies based on the existing health policies of another country. However, within-country comparisons can yield similar lessons. For example, much like the variation in life expectancy across countries, there is strong variation in life expectancy across the UK. Explore the range of life expectancies across Northern Ireland, England, Wales, Scotland. What kinds of pattern do you see within the UK? Reflect upon reasons for these differences.

REFERENCES

Abbasi, K. (2023). The BMJ's Commission on the Future of the NHS. *BMJ*, 381: 1379. https://doi.org/10.1136/bmj.p1000

Arcaya, M. C., Arcaya, A. L. and Subramanian, S. V. (2015). Inequalities in Health: Definitions, Concepts, and Theories. *Global Health Action*, 24 (8): 27106. https://doi.org/10.3402/gha.v8.27106

Avendano, M. and Kawachi, I. (2014). Why Do Americans Have Shorter Life Expectancy and Worse Health than Do People in Other High-Income Countries? *Annual Review of Public Health*, 35: 307–25. https://doi.org/10.1146/annurev-publhealth-032013-182411

Bambra, C., Riordan, R., Ford, J. and Matthews, F. (2020). The COVID-19 Pandemic and Health Inequalities. *Journal of Epidemiology and Community Health*, 74 (11): 964–968. https://doi.org/10.1136/jech-2020-214401

Barr, B., Kinderman, P. and Whitehead, M. (2015). Trends in Mental Health Inequalities in England During a Period of Recession, Austerity and Welfare Reform 2004 to 2013. *Social Science and Medicine*, 147: 324–331. https://doi.org/10.1016/j.socscimed.2015.11.009

Barr, B., Taylor-Robinson, D., Stuckler, D., Loopstra, R., Reeves, A., et al. (2016a). 'First, Do No Harm': Are Disability Assessments Associated with Adverse Trends in Mental Health? A Longitudinal Ecological Study. *Journal of Epidemiology and Community Health*, 70 (4): 339–345. https://doi.org/10.1136/jech-2015-206209

Barr, B., Taylor-Robinson, D., Stuckler, D., Loopstra, R., Reeves, A., et al. (2016b). Fit-for-Work or Fit-for-Unemployment? Does the Reassessment of Disability Benefit Claimants Using a Tougher Work Capability Assessment Help People into Work? *Journal of Epidemiology and Community Health*, 70 (5): 452–458. https://doi.org/10.1136/jech-2015-206333

Bauld, L., Day, P. and Judge, K. (2008). Off Target: A Critical Review of Setting Goals for Reducing Health Inequalities in the United Kingdom. *International Journal of Health Services: Planning, Administration, Evaluation*, 38 (3): 439–454. https://doi.org/10.2190/HS.38.3.d

Baumberg, B., Warren, J., Garthwaite, K. and Bambra, C. (2015). Rethinking the Work Capability Assessment. Available at: https://eprints.ncl.ac.uk/231970. (Accessed: 15 August 2023)

Corris, V., Dormer, E., Brown, A., Whitty, P., Collingwood, P., et al. (2020). Health Inequalities Are Worsening in the North East of England. *British Medical Bulletin*, 134 (1): 63–72. https://doi.org/10.1093/bmb/ldaa008

Dahlgren, G. and Whitehead, M., (2006). European Strategies for Tackling Social Inequities in Health: Levelling up Part 2 European Strategies for Tackling Social Inequities in Health: Levelling up Part 2. apps.who.int. 2006. Available at: https://apps.who.int/iris/bitstream/handle/10665/107791/E89384.pdf. (Accessed: 20 August 2023).

De Sa, J. and Lock, K. (2008). Will European Agricultural Policy for School Fruit and Vegetables Improve Public Health? A Review of School Fruit and Vegetable Programmes. *European Journal of Public Health*, 18 (6): 558–568. https://doi.org/10.1093/eurpub/ckn061

Desai, M., Nolte, E., Karanikolos, M., Khoshaba, B. and McKee, M. (2011). Measuring NHS Performance 1990–2009 Using Amenable Mortality: Interpret with Care. *Journal of the Royal Society of Medicine*, 104 (9): 370–379. doi 10.1258/jrsm.2011.110120

Devaux, M. (2010). Health Systems Institutional Characteristics, OECD Health Working Papers. Organisation for Economic Co-Operation and Development. Available at: https://doi.org/10.1787/5kmfxfq9qbnr-en. (Accessed: 20 August 2023).

DiMatteo, M. R., Lepper, H. S. and Croghan, T. W. (2000). Depression Is a Risk Factor for Noncompliance with Medical Treatment: Meta-Analysis of the Effects of Anxiety and Depression on Patient Adherence. *Archives of Internal Medicine*, 160 (14): 2101–2107. https://doi.org/10.1001/archinte.160.14.2101

Forster, T., Kentikelenis, A. and Bambra, C. (2018). *Health Inequalities in Europe: Setting the Stage for Progressive Policy Action*. Freie Universität Berlin. Available at: https://doi.org/10.17169/REFUBIUM-1014. (Accessed: 20 August 2023).

Goodair, B. and Reeves, A. (2022). Outsourcing Health-Care Services to the Private Sector and Treatable Mortality Rates in England, 2013–20: An Observational Study of NHS Privatisation. *The Lancet Public Health,* 7 (7): e638–e646. https://doi.org/10.1016/S2468-2667(22)00133-5

Harris, K. H., Majmundar, M. K. and Becker, T. (2021). High and Rising Mortality Rates Among Working-Age Adults. Available at: https://nap.nationalacademies.org/read/25976/chapter/1 (Accessed: 2 August 2023).

Ho, J. Y. and Hendi, A. S. (2018). Recent Trends in Life Expectancy Across High Income Countries: Retrospective Observational Study. *BMJ,* 362: k3622. https://doi.org/10.1136/bmj.k2562

Kawachi, I., Subramanian, S. V. and Almeida-Filho, N. (2002). A Glossary for Health Inequalities. *Journal of Epidemiology and Community Health,* 56 (9): 647–652. https://doi.org/10.1136/jech.56.9.647

König, H., König, H- H. and Konnopka, A. (2019). The Excess Costs of De pression: A Systematic Review and Meta-Analysis. *Epidemiology and Psychiatric Sciences,* 5: (29): e30. https://doi.org/10.1017/S2045796019000180

Kroll, L.E., Schumann, M., Hoebel, J. and Lampert, T. (2017). Regional Health Differences: Developing a Socioeconomic Deprivation Index for Germany. *Journal of Health Monitoring,* 2 (2): 98–114. Available at: https://edoc.rki.de/handle/176904/2657.2

La Placa, V. and Morgan, J. (2023). *Social Science Perspectives on Global Public Health.* London: Routledge.

Lorenc, T., Petticrew, M., Welch, V. and Tugwell, P. (2013). What Types of Interventions Generate Inequalities? Evidence from Systematic Reviews. *Journal of Epidemiology and Community Health,* 67 (2): 190–193. https://doi.org/10.1136/jech-2012-201257

Mackenbach, J. P., Hoffmann, R., Khoshaba, B., Plug, I., Rey, G., et al. (2013). Using 'Amenable Mortality' as Indicator of Healthcare Effectiveness in International Comparisons: Results of a Validation Study. *Journal of Epidemiology and Community Health,* 67 (2): 139–146. https://doi.org/10.1136/jech-2012-201471

Molbak, K., Espenhain, L., Nielsen, J., Tersago, K., Bossuyt, N., et al. (2015). Excess Mortality among the Elderly in European Countries, December 2014 to February 2015. *Euro Surveillance: Bulletin Europeen Sur Les Maladies Transmissibles = European Communicable Disease Bulletin,* 20 (11). https://doi.org/10.2807/1560-7917.es2015.20.11.21065.

Murtin, F., Mackenbach, J., Jasilionis, D. and Mira d'Ercole, M. (2017). Inequalities in Longevity by Education in OECD Countries. OECD Statistics Working Papers. Organisation for Economic Co-Operation and Development. Available at: https://doi.org/10.1787/6b64d9cf-en (Accessed: 20 August 2023).

Naylor, C., Parsonage, M., McDaid, D., Knapp, M., Fossey, M., et al. (2012). *Long-Term Conditions and Mental Health: The Cost of Co-Morbidities.* London: King's Fund.

Niederdeppe, J., Kuang, X., Crock, B. and Skelton, A. (2008). Media Campaigns to Promote Smoking Cessation among Socioeconomically Disadvantaged Populations: What Do We Know, What Do We Need to Learn, and What Should We Do Now? *Social Science and Medicine,* 67 (9): 1343–1355. https://doi.org/10.1016/j.socscimed.2008.06.037

Nolte, E. and McKee, M. (2011). Variations in Amenable Mortality—Trends in 16 High-Income Nations. *Health Policy,* 103 (1): 47–52. https://doi.org/10.1016/j.healthpol.2011.08.002

OECD. (2014). Data Warehouse. Available at: https://doi.org/10.1787/data-00900-en (Accessed: 3 August 2023).

OECD. (2021). *Health at a Glance 2021: OECD Indicators.* Paris: OECD.

OECD. (2022). Avoidable Mortality: OECD/Eurostat Lists of Preventable and Treatable Causes of Death, January. Available at: www.oecd.org/health/health-systems/Avoidable-mortality-2019-Joint-OECD-Eurostat-List-preventable-treatable-causes-of-death.pdf. (Accessed: 21 August 2023)

Palladino, R., Lee, J. T., Ashworth, M., Triassi, M. and Millett, C. (2016). Associations Between Multimorbidity, Healthcare Utilisation and Health Status: Evidence from 16 European Countries. *Age and Ageing,* 45 (3): 431–435. https://doi.org/10.1093/ageing/afw044

Papanicolas, I., Woskie, L. R. and Jha, A. K. (2018). Health Care Spending in the United States and Other High-Income Countries. *JAMA: The Journal of the American Medical Association*, 319 (10): 1024–1039. https://doi.org/10.1001/jama.2018.1150

Parker, M., Bucknall, M., Jagger, C. and Wilkie, R. (2020). Population-Based Estimates of Healthy Working Life Expectancy in England at Age 50 Years: Analysis of Data from the English Longitudinal Study of Ageing. *The Lancet. Public Health*, 5 (7): e395–e403. https://doi.org/10.1016/S2468-2667(20)30114-6

Pebody, R. G., Green, H. K., Warburton, F., Sinnathamby, M., Ellis, J., et al. (2018). Significant Spike in Excess Mortality in England in Winter 2014/15–Influenza the Likely Culprit. *Epidemiology and Infection*, 146 (9): 1106–1113. https://doi.org/10.1017/S0950268818001152

Proksch, D., Busch-Casler, J., Haberstroh, M. M. and Pinkwart, A. (2019). National Health Innovation Systems: Clustering the OECD Countries by Innovative Output in Healthcare Using a Multi Indicator Approach. *Research Policy*, 48 (1): 169–179. https://doi.org/10.1016/j.respol.2018.08.004

Raleigh, V. S. (2019). Trends in Life Expectancy in EU and Other OECD Countries. OECD Health Working Papers. Organisation for Economic Co-Operation and Development. Available at: https://doi.org/10.1787/223159ab-en (Accessed 5 August 2023).

Singh, G. K. and Siahpush, M. (2006). Widening Socioeconomic Inequalities in US Life Expectancy, 1980–2000. *International Journal of Epidemiology*, 35 (4): 969–979. https://doi.org/10.1093/ije/dyl083

Stockley, L. and Lund, V. (2008). Use of Folic Acid Supplements, Particularly by Low-Income and Young Women: A Series of Systematic Reviews to Inform Public Health Policy in the UK. *Public Health Nutrition*, 11 (8): 807–821. https://doi.org/10.1017/S1368980008002346

Tobias, M. I. and Cheung, J. (2003). Monitoring Health Inequalities: Life Expectancy and Small Area Deprivation in New Zealand. *Population Health Metrics*, 1 (1): 2. https://doi.org/10.1186/1478-7954-1-2

Tobias, M. and Jackson, G. (2001). Avoidable Mortality in New Zealand, 1981-97. *Australian and New Zealand Journal of Public Health*, 25 (1): 12–20. https://doi.org/10.1111/j.1467-842x.2001.tb00543.x

Venkataramani, A. S., O'Brien, R. and Tsai, A. C. (2021). Declining Life Expectancy in the United States: The Need for Social Policy as Health Policy. *JAMA: The Journal of the American Medical Association*, 325 (7): 621–622. https://doi.org/10.1001/jama.2020.26339

Whiteford, H. A., Degenhardt, L., Rehm, J., Baxter, A. J., Ferrari, A. J., et al. (2013). Global Burden of Disease Attributable to Mental and Substance Use Disorders: Findings from the Global Burden of Disease Study 2010. *The Lancet*, 382 (9904): 1575–1586. https://doi.org/10.1016/S0140-6736(13)61611-6

Woolf, S. H., Masters, R. K. and Aron, L. Y. (2022). Changes in Life Expectancy Between 2019 and 2020 in the US and 21 Peer Countries. *JAMA Network Open*, 5 (4): e227067. https://doi.org/10.1001/jamanetworkopen.2022.7067

CHAPTER 6

Partnership Working in Health and Social Care

....

Julia Morgan and Jackie Yaskey

INTRODUCTION

Partnership working has been the focus of government policy across the OECD for many years, resulting in the introduction of a range of policies and legislation which has led to the reorganisation of health and social care services. The aim is to foster partnership working within and between health and social care sectors as well as with the public, service users, voluntary sector, and private sector. This focus on policy reform and partnership working, however, is often uncritical; taking for granted that partnership working is beneficial without compelling and robust evidence to support these claims. Coupled with this, partnership working can be challenging due to the complexity of health and social care systems and the complexity of service user needs with numerous barriers to partnership working being evident. This chapter will explore the meaning of partnership working, focusing on partnership working between professionals and between organisations or agencies, and outline the benefits and challenges of this way of working. It continues by focusing on two examples of partnership working across the four devolved nations of the UK: the integration of health and social care services, and integrated partnership working to safeguard children.

WHAT IS PARTNERSHIP WORKING?

Partnership working in health and social care is complex and there is variation in the types of partnership working that exist. This means that the term can be difficult to define often relating to a wide range of differing activities. Numerous other terms such as joint or joined up working, multiagency working, multi-disciplinary teams, collaboration, coordinated working, inter-professional or interdisciplinary working, integration, and integrated care may also be used to refer to partnership working

DOI: 10.4324/9781003343608-7

(Atkinson et al., 2007). Partnership working can assume several forms ranging from informal collaborations between practitioners and organisations (for example, one off multiagency panels, information exchange or training courses offered by one discipline/agency to another) through to more formalised structures within and between organisations, for example, in England and Wales, multi-disciplinary teams such as multi-agency safeguarding hubs (MASH), multi-agency risk assessment co-ordination (MARAC), and multi-agency public protection arrangements (MAPPA).

BOX 6.1 MARACs, MAPPAs, AND MASH

MARACs in England and Wales include a range of different partners from police, social services, health, voluntary sector, education, and housing working, in an integrated way, to coordinate responses to address high-risk cases of domestic abuse. By working together across agencies, MARACs are perceived as best placed to safeguard adult survivors of domestic abuse through sharing of information and shared risk assessment and to work with perpetuators of abuse.

MAPPAs in England and Wales focus on the risk management of individuals, convicted of sexual and violent crimes, and include agencies such as the police, prison service, probation service, and other agencies who have a 'duty to co-operate'.

MASHs aim to improve the coordination of child protection investigations, improve communication between agencies, bring thresholds into line, and improve decision making in child protection. MASH teams are comprised of representatives from police child protection teams, local authority social workers, and other key professionals, such as education and health. The development of MASH was designed to lead to efficient and effective information sharing, faster completion of assessments and decision making and increased collaboration between agencies.

Integration is the current focus of much partnership working across the countries of the UK and OECD. The term integration is an umbrella term, which often describes a range of partnership initiatives, whose aim is to bring together organisations, professionals, and services, to avoid fragmentation of care between and within public services which can result in service users 'falling through the gaps' between services and not receiving the care that they need. Tackling unmet need through partnership working is seen as key to reducing health inequalities, improving wellbeing, and managing risk and vulnerability. Integration can relate to a range of activities including organisations pooling funding; joint planning, delivery, and commissioning of services; co-location of services; joint training; joint staffing using multi-disciplinary teams; centralised information systems; joint risk assessments, and joint monitoring, needs assessments, and protocols (Heenan and Birrell, 2018). At the centre of integrative models is the patient or service user with their lived experiences and expertise meaning that they are important partners in decisions about, and co-production of, future health and social care provision (please see chapter seven for more discussion).

Integration has been understood in several ways, and one such model focuses on three levels, which are often interconnecting. First, the macro level, where integration is focused at the population or policy or sector level. Second, the meso level, where integrated care is focused on the organisation level or on a particular care pathway, for example, services for diabetes or services for older people. Lastly there is the micro level, where delivery of integrated care is focused on the individual service user level (Curry and Ham, 2010; Valentijn et al., 2013). Complexity is at the heart of integrated working and managing complexity, uncertainty and risk are key components of integration (Hood, 2014). For example, services which are integrated normally focus on managing complex service user needs which require multiple interventions from many different agencies. Complexity therefore arises both in relation to the complexity of the service users' needs but also in relation to managing the co-ordination of different systems, agencies, and practitioners at various levels (macro, meso, micro) to offer person-centred integrated services. Table 6.1 depicts some of the current focuses of integrated partnership working.

TABLE 6.1 Focuses of Integrated Working

Focus of integrated working	Characteristics
Integration of primary and secondary healthcare services	Consists of vertical integration and collaboration between health services in the community (for example primary health services such as general practitioners (GPs) and other community health services) and secondary health services such as hospitals. This could include joined up information technology (IT) systems, information sharing, shared funding, and joint working. An example of integrated care could include primary care and secondary care professionals working together in the community to reduce the risk of hospital admissions for older people by increasing home-based care or care in the community.
Integration of mental and physical health	A service user may experience input from both mental and physical health services but experience a lack of joined up working between these services, with information not being shared and fragmented service delivery. The fragmented nature of service delivery may often mean that the mental health of service users with physical illnesses may not be a priority and vice versa. This is problematic as people with schizophrenia are three times more likely to die from untreated physical illnesses than the general population (Naylor et al., 2016). The importance of a 'whole person approach' to health, therefore, through integrated working across mental and physical health services is perceived as key to improving outcomes.

(Continued)

TABLE 6.1 Focuses of Integrated Working (Continued)

Focus of integrated working	Characteristics
Integration of health and social care	This focuses on increasing alignment between health services and social care services to provide holistic person-centred care which improves outcomes for service users who may have multiple and complex health and social care needs. A case study of multi-organisational integrated partnership working in Birmingham, UK, between the local authority, NHS, and a range of partners, focused on early intervention to prevent people from being unnecessarily admitted into hospital. Other aims of this intervention were to reduce delays in discharge from hospital; to reduce hospital re-admission; and to support people to stay in their own home rather than be admitted into long term care. The COVID 19 pandemic highlighted, in England for example, the divide between health and social care systems with health systems prioritised over social care, and in some cases, especially at the early stages of COVID 19, a lack of joined up working between health and social care systems (Miller et al., 2021). However, COVID 19 also led to some examples of increased partnership working between health and social care (Bell et al., 2022).
Integration of child and adult services	This could refer to enhanced joint working in transitioning children from child and adolescent mental health services (CAMHS) to adult mental health services. It could also refer to the transitioning from child social care to adult social care to ensure a continuum of care, so that young people do not fall between the gaps because of fragmentation between child and adult service provision. Integrated joint working across child and adult services is also required as adult safeguarding concerns could impact on children's safeguarding within the family and vice versa.
Sectoral integration and integrated care pathways	This could include sectoral integration for example, integrated children's services where a range of professionals and agencies work together to improve outcomes for children (for example, through multi agency safeguarding hubs). It could include horizontal integration in terms of primary care networks, where primary care providers work together to offer services to their community including a joined-up appointment system so that more appointments are available. Alternatively, acute hospitals could join up with other acute hospitals to work more effectively and efficiently. Some examples of integrated care pathways could be a range of professionals and agencies working together in diabetes care or cancer care, or autism support, or cerebral palsy care.

Although, there may be difficulties defining partnership working, what partnership working has at its core is a focus on cooperation, collaboration and coordination between practitioners, agencies, disciplines, organisations (both public and private including public–private partnerships), and services to improve outcomes for service users and improve efficiency in delivering public services. Partnership working, therefore, is said to be about 'adding value'; it is relational (between people and organisations); it is holistic; it is about reducing costs and duplication of services including conflicting advice from multiple providers; and aims to locate the service user at the centre of the partnership. Partnership working proceeds beyond silo working and aims to overcome the inflexibilities of professional and organisational boundaries, and is said to respond more effectively, more holistically, and more efficiently to the complexity of service user needs (Glasby and Dickinson, 2014).

CHALLENGES OF PARTNERSHIP WORKING WITH OTHER PROFESSIONALS

Despite the emphasis on public sector partnership working in policy and legislation, partnership working is often difficult to achieve (Perkins et al., 2020), with previous poor experiences of partnership working influencing present day attempts. Differences between the cultures of organisations, including private and public providers, can also make partnership working challenging. Moreover, even though partnership working is often mandated by legislation, for example, the recent Health and Care Act (2022) in England and the introduction of Integrated Care Systems, there are wide variations in the implementation and outcomes of partnership working initiatives (Joseph et al., 2019); with some questioning whether partnership working precipitates benefits (National Audit Office, 2017; Reed et al., 2021). For example, in relation to integrated care, some research has found that integration of care did not reduce hospital admissions, and in some cases, increased admissions (Georghiou and Keeble, 2019; Parry et al., 2019). In addition, the evidence base evaluating the implementation of partnership working is often underdeveloped with Cameron et al. (2014) stating that most evaluations are small scale and of poor quality. Coupled with this, many evaluations have been found to focus on process, for example, the process of implementation of working in partnership, rather than on the outcomes for service users (Petch et al., 2013; Glasby and Dickinson, 2014). This makes it difficult to assess, in a rigorous way, how beneficial partnership working is in improving a range of outcomes (for more discussion, see Heenan and Birrell, 2018).

Several challenges to achieving effective partnership working have been identified and Table 6.2 explores some of these barriers.

TABLE 6.2 Barriers to Implementing Partnership Working

Types of Barriers	Examples
Structural and Process Barriers	The history of working separately can create obstacles to partnership working. These complex barriers could include separation in terms of diverse ways of working; different priorities, eligibility criteria and concepts of risk; separation in where services are located, and a lack of a shared vision or mission statement across organisations (including differing legal, assessment, regulatory, and policy frameworks). Non-integrated management and information systems with different IT systems and assessments can result in a lack of sharing of information and poor communication across professional boundaries. Moreover, the structural privileging of the biomedical model may mean that the health sector assumes a more dominant role in partnership working, which can result in social care being viewed as 'junior partners' (Heenan and Birrell, 2018: 144).
Financial Barriers	Overall, across the countries of the UK, health services receive more funding than social care services which can lead to greater infrastructure and resources for health services; this may have implications for who leads integration projects (Eastwood and Miller, 2021). Market forces which promote competition between organisations can also mean that collaboration across agencies can be difficult. Moreover, within the UK, health services tend to be free at the point of contact while social care services are often means tested (with greater private provision) creating complex barriers to partnership working in relation to the pooling of finances and the commissioning of services across the health and social care sector. There may also be different funding cycles between agencies which makes it difficult to plan and collaborate. Where budgets are pooled between services, this may lead to disagreement on what services should be commissioned. A lack of investment and adequate funding to plan and implement integration and partnership working is evident.
Professional and Staffing Barriers	Differences in professional values, philosophies and attitudes may lead to potential clashes and rivalries which can reduce trust between professional groups and impact on partnership working. Status and equity issues can arise with a particular agency often taking the lead. There may be status and power barriers relating to qualifications and professional bodies which can disempower social care workers, for example, who are more likely to have less recognised qualifications than those who are registered professionals such as doctors, nurses, and social workers. This can result in some views assigned less weight in decision making regardless of their knowledge of the service user. Moreover, insufficient joint training and knowledge of the roles of other professionals and a lack of clarity on why partnership working, and integration is needed, may cause challenges. Time may also be a barrier to developing this knowledge as time for training, critical thinking, and developing partnership skills and relationships, may not be allocated. There may also be differences in the pay of professionals, for example health and social care workers, which may act as a barrier to effective partnership working.

(Continued)

TABLE 6.2 Barriers to Implementing Partnership Working (Continued)

Types of Barriers	Examples
Complex Systems as a Barrier	Partnership working is complex, both in terms of service users' needs as well as the complexity of integrated working in health and social care. Complexity may be a barrier to partnership working because it may be experienced, by practitioners, as overwhelming and stressful impacting their judgements, critical thinking, and behaviours; creating divisions within integrated teams (Hood, 2014). The complex nature of partnership working can lead to confusion, a lack of accountability, increased bureaucracy, and inefficiency (Reed et al., 2021). For example, partnerships may be fluid and constantly changing, with a range of different stakeholders being involved outside of the core group leading to different perspectives, relationship dynamics and values. Moreover, repeated reorganisations of health and social care with new systems and ways of working as well as financial uncertainty in terms of funding of integrated care can increase complexity. While both new perspectives and re-organisations can be positive if managed well through a complexity lens, they can also lead to unpredictability, a lack of clarity and uncertainty impacting on the success of partnership working.

BOX 6.2 THE CASE OF STEVEN HOSKIN

Some barriers to partnership working can be seen in the case study of Steven Hoskin. Steven Hoskin was a vulnerable man with learning disabilities who was murdered by people who had befriended him. The serious case review (Flynn, 2007) identified several failings across agencies who were responsible for working together to safeguard him (SCIE, 2020). These failings included:

- A lack of sharing of information, which meant that the full picture was not available to agencies who were assessing the risk that Steven faced. Each agency had a small part of the jigsaw, and this was not shared with one another.
- Agencies worked in parallel (silos) rather than in a joined-up integrated way. This may have been a result of historical structural barriers between agencies.
- A lack of communication between agencies about Steven.
- A lack of understanding and agreement around risk. For example, people who do not meet the thresholds of social care eligibility may repeatedly contact emergency services such as the police and Accident and Emergency services for help and this should be an indicator of concern. The need for ambulance, health, and police services to have a shared understanding of risk was key as was working together in an integrated fashion to share information about repeated call outs from vulnerable people.
- A need for training for staff on working together including the limits to data protection and confidentiality which is embedded within a culture of partnership working and strong effective leadership was required.

See SCIE (2020) for a video examining this case in more detail.

INTEGRATING HEALTH AND SOCIAL CARE

The integration of health and social care has been a prime policy objective for many years in the devolved nations of the United Kingdom as well as across OECD countries. Integration of health and social care is a policy priority for many countries because of the changing needs of populations which requires more focus on long-term care and complex health needs rather than a focus on acute services (the latter, for example, being primarily and historically the focus of the NHS). Aging populations, and increases in the number of service users, with multiple long-term conditions, who require care from numerous providers, who may have limited contact with one another, calls for health and social care organisations (including informal carers) to work together to ensure co-ordinated person-centred services across a person's lifespan (OECD, 2021). Integration of health and social care, it is hoped, will result in several benefits, including a reduction of health inequalities, and a prioritising of population health; a reduction in duplication and fragmentation of services; finances spent more efficiently to ensure more sustainable health and social care systems; an increase in continuity of care; and improvements in the quality of services and improved outcomes for service users (Department of Health and Social Care, 2022).

In England, over the past decade, while there has been some partnership working between health and social care organisations, progress towards integrated care has been slow (King's Fund, 2022). The recent Health and Care Act (Department of Health and Social Care, 2022), which builds on the NHS Long Term Plan (NHS, 2019), has, however, made integrated working a statutory duty, requiring the setting up of formal geographically based integrated care systems (ICS) to bring together public health, NHS, and social care organisations including the voluntary sector and local authorities in what are now called integrated care partnerships. Integrated care partnerships are responsible for producing an integrated care strategy on how the jointly assessed needs of the local population will be met at both 'place' level (for example, at borough or county level) and 'neighbourhood' level (for example, primary care localities with populations of between 30,000 and 50,000 with multi-disciplinary teams across health and social care being the driver at this level for integrated care). In addition, integrated care boards (ICBs) have been introduced, replacing clinical commissioning groups, with the requirement to design a five-year forward plan focusing on collaborative, rather than competitive, commissioning and delivery of NHS services. However, as stated by the King's Fund (2022), although legislation and policy are important to compel organisations to work together, so too is effective implementation of ICS, including a focus and commitment to long term change (including taking on board existing partnerships) and listening to the needs of communities and service users. Moreover, concerted effort is needed to ensure that social care is not side-lined as previous attempts at integration have focused primarily on integration across health services with minimal integration with social care (Eastwood and Millar, 2021).

Comparing countries across the devolved nations of the UK in relation to integrated care shows that only small improvements have been evidenced in service user outcomes given the amount of focus on integrated care over the past decades (Reed et al., 2021). Although, England has only recently legislated for statutory integrated care systems, this is not the case in Northern Ireland, Scotland, and Wales, where legislation already exists. For example, Scotland legislated in 2014 to integrate adult health and social care services resulting in the formation of health and social care partnerships (HSCPs). It is, thus, surprising that Reed et al. (2021) found little difference across all four countries in relation to integrated care and outcomes for service users and little evidence from any of the four countries that pooling of resources saved money. This raised questions about 'what integrated care can realistically deliver' (Reed et al., 2021: 2), and whether too much is being asked of integrated care.

Thinking back to the challenges that were identified in Table 6.2, it is unlikely that legislation, or a policy focus on integrated care at the macro level will, on its own, result in barriers to integrated working being overcome on the ground. For example, restructuring health and social care systems through top-down legislation does not necessarily result in organisational cultures and priorities, unequal power relationships, and professional commitment to collaboration changing to facilitate partnership working and, in many cases, can be disruptive impacting on service development. Of importance to effective partnership working is the availability of appropriate resources and time to develop local-level relationships which focus on reducing power dynamics, support understandings of each other's work and enable a consensus to be reached on a shared vision of partnership working including how partnerships can be facilitated locally. A need for specialist 'systems-focused' training for leaders and managers on how to manage complex partnerships across health and social care systems is key including an understanding of complex adaptive systems (Plsek and Greenhalgh, 2001; Holland, 2014).

Integrated systems are complex systems which are dynamic, non-linear, multi-faceted, include a range of diverse stakeholders and can be unpredictable with changes in one part of the system, for example in social care, having unintended consequences in another part of the system, for example healthcare. Complex adaptive systems, such as integrated systems, are highly dependent on co-operation and relationships between all parts of the system to work effectively and to adapt to local concerns and complexity. As a result, time and resources are not only needed to equip managers with skills to support the complexity of partnership working but also to enable members of the system/s to come together to network and to build relationships of trust (Huxham and Vangen, 2005) facilitating the development of 'boundary spanning' practitioners (Crosby and Bryson, 2010). This can be difficult to achieve without extra resourcing; especially in areas where there are high vacancies rates which allow little time to focus of developing boundary spanning skills and relationships between partners.

WORKING IN PARTNERSHIP TO SAFEGUARD AND PROTECT CHILDREN

Across the four devolved nations of the UK, there are a range of laws and child protection systems to safeguard children. Integration and partnership working are key components of the child protection systems in these countries as can be seen from Table 6.3. In all the four countries, there are a range of complex local level partnerships who lead child safeguarding initiatives: in England, local safeguarding

TABLE 6.3 Children's Safeguarding across Devolved Nations of the UK

Children's safeguarding	England	Wales	Scotland	Northern Ireland
Selected legislation	Children Act 1989, 2004, Children and Social Work Act 2017.	Children Act 1989, 2004; Social Services and Well-being Act 2014; The Safeguarding Boards (General) (Wales) Regulations 2015; Wellbeing of Future Generations Act, 2015.	The Children (Scotland) Act 1995; Children's Hearings (Scotland) Act, 2011; Children and Young People (Scotland) Act 2014; Public Bodies (Joint Working) (Scotland) Act 2014.	The Children (Northern Ireland) Order 1995; Safeguarding Board Act (Northern Ireland) 2011; Children's Services Co-operation Act (Northern Ireland) 2015.
Selected policy/ guidance on partnership working	Working Together to Safeguard Children (HM Government, 2018; 2023).	Working Together to Safeguard People Volume 5, 2018; Working Together to Safeguard People Volume 2, 2016; Codes and guidance: Part 9 Statutory Guidance 2020.	Getting it Right for Every Child, 2022; National Guidance for Child Protection in Scotland 2021 (updated 2023).	Co-operating to Safeguard Children and young people in Northern Ireland 2017; Children and Young People's Strategy 2020–2030; Regional core child protection policies and procedures for Northern Ireland, 2018.
Who takes strategic lead on children's safeguarding	Department of Education responsible for child protection. Local level: Local safeguarding partners led by the local authority; the integrated care board (ICB) (health) and Chief Officers of the police.	Responsibility evolved to Senedd Cymru. Local authorities responsible for establishing Safeguarding Children Boards including local representatives from local authorities, police health board, NHS Trust, probation board, youth offending team and other organisations.	Scottish government takes the lead on child protection. Child Protection Committees (CPCs) at the local authority level are responsible for multi-agency children's safeguarding, working with health, children's social work, police, and other agencies.	The Northern Ireland Executive, through the Department of Health (DoH), takes lead for child protection. The Safeguarding Board for Northern Ireland (SBNI) develops policies on how agencies work together. Five local Safeguarding Panels, aligned with five Health and Social Care Trusts, support the work of the SBNI at the local level and include members from a range of organisations.

partnerships; in Wales, safeguarding children boards; in Scotland, child protection committees; and in Northern Ireland, local safeguarding panels. All these partnerships have a core membership including the local authority, health, and police, as well as a range of other partners including education, voluntary organisations, probation, and youth offending. Across the four nations there is a duty to co-operate in relation to partnership working around child protection, which is supported by legislation with relevant policy and guidance available on partnership working and managing risk.

However, serious case reviews in the United Kingdom (now called child safeguarding practice reviews (CSPRs) in England; case management reviews (CMRs) in Northern Ireland; learning reviews in Scotland; child practice reviews (CPRs) in Wales) have all highlighted challenges in partnership working which may have contributed to the ineffective safeguarding of children. In England, this included issues around information sharing with a lack of dialogue and critical thinking between professionals and agencies leading to shared information being misinterpreted or misunderstood (Dickens et al., 2022). This lack of dialogue and critical thinking may be a result of workload and time pressures with a lack of sufficient resourcing of time being a barrier to effective partnership working (Porter et al., 2023). Moreover, the review into the murders of Arthur Labinjo-Hughes and Star Hobson (Hudson and Child Safeguarding Review Panel, 2022), both who lived in areas of England with MASH initiatives, highlighted poor joint working and an 'over-reliance on single agency processes' (in the case of Labinjo-Hughes), and 'superficial assessments' (in the case of Star Hobson) with the latter potentially being exacerbated by high workloads, unfilled vacancies and the large numbers of agency staff working within the local authority at the time.

The review stated that 'multi-agency safeguarding arrangements are not yet fit for purpose everywhere' (p. 5) and recommends restructuring with the introduction of new multi-agency child protection units (MACPUs) which are co-located and fully integrated in every local authority area. In Scotland, a review highlighted issues concerning information sharing, communication, and knowing who the lead professional was which resulted in a lack of co-ordinated action (NSPCC Learning, 2021). While in Northern Ireland challenges included fragmentation of services especially between health and social care, lack of joined up working, and different information systems across health and social care trusts (Jones et al., 2023). Similar issues are evident in Wales (Rees et al., 2021) including a lack of representation from all agencies at meetings and more clarity needed around which models and frameworks are currently being used to inform child protection responses (Care Inspectorate Wales, 2023).

Child protection is complex characterised by uncertainty and the difficulty of predicting risk with 'technical' top-down approaches (Munro, 2010) such as the introduction of tools to support partnership working and procedures for information sharing not necessarily leading to significant increases in collaboration between partners (Dickens et al., 2022). Moreover, child protection is complex because of the wide number of agencies and professionals involved in safeguarding children. For complex systems to effectively work it is important to support opportunities for face-to-face dialogue and learning so that practitioners develop 'interprofessional expertise' (Hood et al., 2017: 705). This interprofessional expertise arises through regularly interacting with other professionals and is not necessarily something that can be learnt through guidelines on how to do partnership working. Moreover, engaging, face to face, with other practitioners has been shown to build trusting relationships, and to support critical thinking, the exchange of information and communication between practitioners (Feinstein et al., 2023). Again, appropriate resourcing including time to enable practitioners to develop relationships is key to strengthening partnership working.

CONCLUSION

This chapter has given an overview of partnership working between professionals, organisations, and agencies. It briefly explored partnership working in health and social care and in the safeguarding of children across the four devolved nations of the UK. Although, partnership working, and the integrating of services are said to be critical components in improving outcomes for service users, there is often a lack of clarity over what these terms mean as well as a lack of evidence on how partnership working can lead to improved outcomes for service users. Numerous challenges exist to successful partnership working which have been regularly highlighted in reports and serious case reviews across all four countries of the UK. A key factor in supporting long term change is managing the complexity of partnership working; this requires the development of specific knowledge and skills to work within complex systems. Significant resourcing is needed to support time pressurised staff not only to develop trusting relationships with one another to overcome operational, cultural, and territorial barriers but also to support the extra work that is required to facilitate successful partnership working.

RESEARCH POINTS AND REFLECTIVE EXERCISES

- 'Complexity is inherent in partnership working'. Research complexity theory, including complex adaptive systems, and outline why an understanding of these theories may offer insight for those working within and across complex systems.
- Explore how COVID 19 impacted on partnership working and reflect upon the lessons that can be learnt from COVID 19 to support partnership working (for example Bell et al., 2022; NHS Confederation, 2022).

REFERENCES

Atkinson, M., Jones, M. and Lamon, E. (2007). Multi-Agency Working and its Implications for Practice: A Review of the Literature. Available at: www.nfer.ac.uk/publications/MAD01/MAD01.pdf (Accessed: 15 February 2023).

Bell, L., Whelan, M., & Lycett, D. (2022). Role of an Integrated Care System during COVID-19 and beyond: a qualitative study with recommendations to inform future development. *Integrated Healthcare Journal*, 4 (1), e000112. https://doi.org/10.1136/ihj-2021-000112

Cameron, A., Lart, R., Bostock, L. and Coomber, C. (2014). Factors that Promote and Hinder Joint and Integrated Working between Health and Social Care Services: A Review of Research Literature. *Health and Social Care in the Community*, 22 (3): 225–233. https://doi.org/10.1111/hsc.12057

Care Inspectorate Wales. (2023). *Rapid Review of Child Protection Arrangements*. Wales: Care Inspectorate Wales.

Crosby, B. C. and Bryson, J. M. (2010). Integrative leadership and the creation and maintenance of cross-sector collaborations. *Leadership Quarterly*, 21 (2): 211–230. https://doi.org/10.1016/j.leaqua.2010.01.003

Curry, N. and Ham, C. (2010). *Clinical and Service Integration: The Route to Improved Outcomes*. London: King's Fund.

Department of Health and Social Care. (2022). Health and Care Act. Available at: www. legislation.gov.uk/ukpga/2022/31/contents/enacted (Accessed: 27 February 2023).

Dickens, J., Cook, L., Cossar, J., Rennolds, N., Rimme, J., et al. (2022). Learning for the Future: Final Analysis of Serious Case Reviews, 2017 to 2019. Available at: https://assets.publishing. service.gov.uk/government/uploads/system/uploads/attachment_data/file/1123286/Learning_ for_the_future_-_final_analysis_of_serious_case_reviews__2017_to_2019.pdf (Accessed: 18 October 2023)

Eastwood, J. and Miller, R. (2021). Integrating Health and Social Care Systems. In V. Amelung, V. Stein, E. Suter, N., Goodwin, E. Nolte and R. Balicer (eds), *Handbook of Integrated Care*. Springer: Cham, 81–103.

Feinstein, L., Hyde-Dryden, G., Baginsky, M. and Hood, R. (2023). *Overcoming Behavioural and Cultural Barriers to Multi-agency Information: Sharing in Children's Social Care: A Rapid Review to Inform the Newham-Led Project for the DfE Data and Digital Fund*. Oxford: Rees Centre, Department of Education and University of Oxford.

Flynn, M. C. (2007). The Murder of Steven Hoskin. A Serious Case Review. Available at: www.hampshiresab.org.uk/wp-content/uploads/2007-December-Serious-Case-Review- regarding-Steven-Hoskin-Cornwall.pdf (Accessed: 10 February 2023).

Georghiou, T. and Keeble, E. (2019). *Age UK's Personalised Integrated Care Programme: Evaluation of Impact on Hospital Activity*. London: Nuffield Trust.

Glasby, J. and Dickenson, H. (2014). *Partnership Working in Health and Social Care: What is Integrated Care and How Can we Deliver it?* Bristol: Policy Press.

Heenan, D. and Birrell, D. (2018). *The Integration of Health and Social Care in the UK*. London: Palgrave.

HM Government. (2015). *Working Together to Safeguard Children*. London: Department for Education.

HM Government. (2023). Draft: Working Together to Safeguard Children 2023. A Guide to Multi-Agency Working to Help, Safeguard, Protect and Promote the Welfare of Children. Available at: https://consult.education.gov.uk/child-protection-safeguarding- division/working-together-to-safeguard-children-changes-to/supporting_documents/ Working%20Together%20to%20Safeguard%20Children%202023%20%20draft%20 for%20consultation.pdf (Accessed: 19 October 2023).

Holland, J. H. (2014). *Complexity: A Very Short Introduction*. Oxford: Oxford University Press.

Hood, R. (2014). Complexity and Integrated Working in Children's Services. *The British Journal of Social Work*, 44 (1): 27–43. https://doi.org/10.1093/bjsw/bcs091

Hood, R., Price, J., Sartori, D., Maisey, D., Johnson, J., et al. (2017). Collaborating Across the Threshold: The Development of Interprofessional Expertise in Child Safeguarding. *Journal of Interprofessional Care*, 31 (6): 705–713. https://doi.org/10.1080/13561820. 2017.1329199

Hudson, A. and Child Safeguarding Review Panel. (2022). National Review into the Murders of Arthur Labinjo-Hughes and Star Hobson. Available at: https://assets.publishing.

service.gov.uk/media/628e262d8fa8f556203eb4f8/ALH_SH_National_Review_26-5-22.pdf (Accessed: 19 October 2023).

Huxham, C. and Vangen, S. (2005). *Managing to Collaborate: The Theory and Practice of Collaborate Advantage.* London: Routledge.

Jones, R., et al. (2023), The Northern Ireland Review of Children's Social Care Services Report. Available at: www.cscsreviewni.net/ (Accessed: 18 January 2024).

Joseph, S., Klein, S., McCluskey, S., Woolnough, P. and Diack, L. (2019). Inter-Agency Adult Support and Protection Practice: A Realistic Evaluation with Police, Health and Social Care Professionals. *Journal of Integrated Care*, 27 (1): 50–63. https://doi.org/10.1108/JICA-06-2018-0041

King's Fund. (2022). Integrated Care: Our Position. Available at: www.kingsfund.org.uk/projects/positions/integrated-care (Accessed: 28 February 2023).

Miller, R., Glasby, J., and Dickinson, H. (2021). Integrated Health and Social Care in England: Ten Years On. *International Journal of Integrated Care*, 21 (4), 6: 1–9 https://doi.org/10.5334/ijic.5666

Munro, E. (2010). *The Munro Review of Child Protection Part One: A Systems Analysis.* London: Department for Education.

National Audit Office. (2017). Health and Social Care Integration: HC 1011 Session 2016–2017. Available at: www.nao.org.uk/wp-content/uploads/2017/02/Health-and-social-care-integration.pdf (Accessed: 20 February 2023).

Naylor, C., Das, P., Ross, S., Honeyman, M., Thompson, J., et al. (2016). *Bringing Together Physical and Mental Health: A New Frontier for Integrated Care.* London: The King's Fund.

NHS. (2019). The NHS Long Term Plan. Available at: www.longtermplan.nhs.uk/ (Accessed: 27 February 2023).

NHS Confederation. (2022). *The COVID-19 Inquiry Learning the Lessons.* Available at: www.nhsconfed.org/system/files/2022-07/The-COVID-19-inquiry-learning%20the-lessons.pdf (Accessed: 22 February 2024).

NSPCC Learning. (2021). A Summary of the Care Inspectorate's Triennial Review of Initial Case Reviews and Significant Case Reviews in Scotland, CASPAR *Briefing*. Available at: https://learning.nspcc.org.uk/media/2609/caspar-briefing-scotland-triennial-review-scrs.pdf (Accessed: 20 October 2023).

OECD. (2021). Safe Long-Term Care. In *Health at a Glance 2021: OECD Indicators.* Paris: OECD Publishing. https://doi.org/10.1787/d70b7f79-en.

Parry, W., Wolters, A. T., Brine, R. J., and Steventon, A. (2019). Effect of an Integrated Care Pathway on Use of Primary and Secondary Healthcare by Patients at High Risk of Emergency Inpatient Admission: A Matched Control Cohort Study in Tower Hamlet. *BMJ Open 9*: e026470. https://doi.org/10.1136/bmjopen-2018-026470

Perkins, N., Hunter, D. J., Vistram, S., Finn, R., Gosling, J., et al. Partnership or Insanity: Why do Health Partnerships do the Same Thing Over and Over Again and Expect a Different Result? *Journal of Health Services Research and Policy*, 25 (1): 41–48. https://doi.org/10.1177/1355819619858374

Petch, A., Cook, A. and Miller, E. (2013). Partnership Working and Outcomes: Do Health and Social Care Partnerships Deliver for Users and Carers? *Health Soc Care Community*, 21: 623–633. https://doi.org/10.1111/hsc.12050

Plsek, P. E. and Greenhalgh, T. (2001). The Challenge of Complexity in Health Care. *BMJ*, 323 (7313): 625–628. https://doi.org/10.1136/bmj.323.7313.625.

Porter, R., Young, E., Scott, J., McIver, L., Mackinnon, K., et al. (2023). *Children's Services Reform Research: Rapid Evidence Review.* Scotland: Centre for Excellence for Children's Care and Protection.

Reed, S., Oung, C., Davies, J., Dayan, M. and Scobie, S. (2021). Integrating Health and Social Care: A Comparison of Policy and Progress Across the Four Countries of the UK. Available at: www.nuffieldtrust.org.uk/files/2021-12/integrated-care-web.pdf (Accessed: 1 March 2023).

Rees, A. M., Fatemi-Dehaghani, R., Slater, T., Swann, R. and Robinson, A. L. (2021). Findings from a Thematic Multidisciplinary Analysis of Child Practice Reviews in Wales. *Child Abuse Review*, 30: 141–154. https://doi.org/10.1002/car.2679

SCIE. (2020). Have We Learned from Steven Hoskin's Murder?. Available at: www.scie.org.uk/safeguarding/adults/practice/lessons-learnt/steven-hoskin-ten-years-on (Accessed: 20 February 2023).

Valentijn, P. P., Schepman, S. M., Opheij, W. and Bruijnzeels M. A. (2013). Understanding Integrated Care: A Comprehensive Conceptual Framework Based on the Integrative Functions of Primary Care. *Int J Integr Care*, 13 (1): e010. https://doi.org/10.5334/ijic.886

CHAPTER 7

Service User Involvement in Health and Social Care

Understanding Power Relations and the Political Nature of Participation

....

Julia Morgan

INTRODUCTION

Service user involvement is seen as key to the development of health and social care systems across many OECD countries with service user involvement being the focus of much international and national health and social care legislation and policy. There are several terms used to refer to service user involvement which can cause confusion including terms such as public and patient involvement (PPI); patient involvement, engagement, and experience; shared decision making; patient participation; citizen participation and working with people and communities. All these terms comprise a focus on putting people who use health and social care services at the centre of care to involve them in how care is realised, to listen to their voices, understand their experiences of services, and empower them as active agents to make decisions which relate both to themselves and to the services they currently use or may use in the future. This chapter explores key concepts in service user involvement including participation, and empowerment before discussing how an understanding of power relations and the political nature of participation is needed when planning service user involvement initiatives.

SERVICE USER INVOLVEMENT

Service users possess important knowledge because of their agency, individual and collective lived experiences of illnesses conditions or situations, use of services, and because they experience social policies (Beresford, 2000; McLaughlin et al., 2020). Service user involvement in health and social care may refer to the participation

DOI: 10.4324/9781003343608-8

of patients and/or service users as well as carers and the public at four main levels (Tambuyzer et al., 2014). First, there is the individual or micro level where service users are involved directly in their own care, for example, through use of direct payments where personal budgets are transferred to individuals to make choices about control over care. This includes shared decision making in relation to care plans and self-management, with service user involvement an important part of personalised or person-centred care. The setting up of self-help groups, advocacy groups, and peer support groups is also important in self-management and service user involvement. Second, service users may be involved in health and social care at the meso level through participating in the co-production of services including the planning, commissioning, delivery, and evaluation of services. Service users may also be involved in recruitment of staff, and strategic management boards. Third, they may be involved at the macro level in the creation of health and social care legislation and policy. Lastly, they may be involved at the meta level in the design and production of research and knowledge, and in the education of health and social care professionals. Table 7.1 outlines some key concepts, that arise in relation to service user involvement.

TABLE 7.1 Glossary of Key Concepts

Key concepts	Definitions
Co-production	Co-production is defined as delivering public services in an equal and reciprocal relationship between professionals, people using services, their families, and neighbours. Where activities are co-produced in this way, both services and neighbourhoods become effective agents of change (Boyle et al., 2010: 11). Coproduction is about reducing power imbalances between service users and professionals with a focus on recognising the skills and knowledge service users bring to partnership working through their lived experiences. It moves beyond listening to service users and engages them as active agents in the design and delivery of services, strategic decision-making and the production of policy and knowledge. See SCIE (2022) for further discussion. Coproduction is often used interchangeably with the words co-design or co-create, although they often relate to different activities.
Personalised care/ person centred care	Focus is on partnership working between professionals, the service user and their families, to co-create or co-produce individual care plans. Users have control and choice over their lives with professionals listening to them. The OECD has introduced a People-Centred Health Systems Framework which focuses on, ensuring voice, choice, co-production, and respectfulness, including the introduction of benchmarks to support countries to measure how people-centred health systems are (OECD, 2021).

(Continued)

TABLE 7.1 Glossary of Key Concepts (Continued)

Key concepts	Definitions
Agency	Humans are active knowledgeable social actors who have agency. Agency refers to self-determination, meaning humans are not passive by-standers but respond, understand and engage with the world, and make choices as a result. Individual, and collective agency, however, may be constrained through structures such as social class, ethnicity, gender, disability, and social norms.
Advocacy	Advocacy is about speaking up to precipitate change and is about addressing issues of power within the health and social care system. Often, we view advocacy as speaking on behalf of someone else by finding out their views and needs, and then representing them (sometimes known as proxy agency). However, this is not always the case, and individuals may be their own advocate. People may also collectively advocate for a group of people through self-help groups or formal advocacy groups. Morgan (2023), for example found that many women diagnosed as adults with ADHD in England received support from online ADHD forums, which were set up by women diagnosed with ADHD as adults. This peer-to-peer support was transformational and empowered some to seek diagnosis.

Service user involvement is said to bring about many benefits (see box 7.1 for an example of integrated care in England). These benefits include increased patient knowledge about their condition including treatments, compliance with treatments, and self-management of care; reductions in lengths of stay in hospital and readmission rates as a result of a deeper understanding of their condition leading to potential cost savings; improved health and social care satisfaction ratings; more independence and feeling in control of their care; and increases in self-esteem through involvement in decision making (Coulter, 2011; Da Silva, 2011; Nesta, 2013; NEF, 2013; Foot et al., 2014; National Voices, 2014; CQC, 2016). Moreover, service user expertise and lived experiences, are a crucial component of evidence-based practice and enables professional practice and services to be responsive to and informed by service user preferences and values (Davies and Gray, 2017). In relation to service user involvement in service delivery and commissioning, benefits include reductions in health inequalities by responding to the needs of communities; better use of public funds as services reflect need; increased transparency and accountability of service providers to communities; and improved quality of services (NHS England and Department of Health and Social Care, 2022). Involving service users in the education of professionals, such as social workers, can bring benefits including greater understanding of experiences from the service users' point of view, enhanced compassion among professionals, reductions in stigmatising attitudes from social workers and increased partnership working in decision making (Waterson and Morris, 2005; Beresford and Boxall, 2012; Duffy et al., 2013). Service user participation is also seen as beneficial as it can direct transformative change in services, provision and knowledge, empowering service users (Freire, 1970).

BOX 7.1 INTEGRATED CARE SYSTEMS AND SERVICE USER INVOLVEMENT: ENGLAND

Service user involvement and person-centredness underpins integrated care and is key to the successful implementation of integration both in England and across European countries (Czypionka et al., 2020). Integrated Care Systems (ICSs) in England situate service users, their carers, and the local community at the heart of partnership working. ICSs are partnerships of health and social care organisations that work together to plan and deliver joined up services to improve the health and wellbeing of local communities. ICSs have a Public Involvement Duty under the NHS Act 2006 amended by the Health and Care Act 2022 to ensure that 'people are appropriately 'involved' in planning, proposals, and decisions regarding NHS services' (NHS England and Department of Health and Social Care, 2022: 16). Co-production is critical to the effective working of ICSs, bringing about increases in community trust and community relationships as well as cost-effective and safe services which respond to local need and lived experiences. Guidance on the involvement of services users and communities in integrated care initiatives (NHS, 2021) identifies a spectrum of involvement of service users and communities including being informed through the use of newsletters and events; to obtaining feedback about services through surveys; to discussions about services through focus groups; to collaboration on decision making through working in partnership with the public and to empowerment where the final decision making is in the hands of the public.

Each ICS consists of an:

- **Integrated care board:** which develop health plans with communities and service users.
- **Integrated care partnerships** which include representatives and community leaders in planning and develop integrated care strategies with communities and service users.
- **Place-based partnerships:** which fully engage people who are impacted by their decisions and involve people in decision making.
- **Provider collaboratives:** which need to build on co-production and links to local communities.

KEY CONCEPTS IN SERVICE USER INVOLVEMENT: PARTICIPATION

Participation is a key element of service user involvement. Participation is viewed, by many, as a political act which supports people to exercise their agency and own their destinies (Freire, 1970; Fals-Borda and Rahman, 1991). Cornwall (2002; 2003) differentiates between invited and claimed spaces of participation with the former (invited) being more formal events where organisations create forums for stakeholders or service users to contribute and reach consensus. However, these invited spaces

TABLE 7.2 Arnstein's Ladder of Participation

Rungs		
8	Service user control	Degrees of service user power
7	Delegated power	
6	Partnership	
5	Placation	Degrees of tokenism
4	Consultation	
3	Informing	
2	Therapy	Nonparticipation
1	Manipulation	

Source: adapted from Arnstein (1969)

for participation do not necessarily result in political transformation in the operation of services. Claimed participation, however, according to Cornwall, is more organic and involves service users taking control of the political processes without necessarily being invited in by service providers. Social movements such as the disability movement are a good example of claimed participation, challenging societal perspectives on disability and oppression, while advocating for change for disabled people. Similarly, Parfitt (2004) distinguishes between 'participation as an end' (for example claimed participation as envisaged by Cornwall) and 'participation as a means' (for example as an apolitical way to improve service delivery through listening to the voices of service users).

Arnstein's ladder of participation develops understanding of participation. Table 7.2 shows that rungs six to eight, service user control, delegated power and partnership, are at the top of the ladder of participation with differing degrees of service user power. For example, if we think about a project that was being developed, rung eight would result in service users exercising complete control over the project including the initial idea and power to make decisions. While in rung seven, a professional may have originally thought of the project idea, but decision making about the project is then delegated to service users. Rung six, on the other hand, is about equal partnership between service users and professionals in decision making. Rungs three-five, however, involve little or no real transfer of power to service users over the decisions that will made about the project. For example, service users may be consulted about a particular project (rung four), but this does not mean their views will influence decisions about the project. Rungs three to five are, therefore, often seen as tokenistic and have been critiqued as a tick box participatory exercise, which gives the appearance of participation with no transfer of power to make decisions, to service users. Rungs one to two do not constitute participation. For a critique of Arnstein's model, please see Tritter and McCallum (2006).

Beresford (2002) identifies two contrasting approaches to service user involvement. First there is the consumerist approach which is influenced by neoliberalism and New Public Management (NPM) and emphasises choice, viewing service users as consumers or customers of health and social care. By virtue of being a customer, service users have important information that they can share to service providers and policy makers about how to make services more effective and efficient. The aim of the consumerist approach is not necessarily to increase service user participation in decision making but is more about consultation and feedback. This could be seen to correspond to Arnstein's ladder rungs three to five above and notions of invited participation (Cornwall, 2002; 2003) or participation as a means (Parfitt, 2004). Second, there is the democratic approach which focuses more on the re-distribution of power and empowerment of service users to direct change. Service user involvement in the democratic approach, therefore, focuses on their active participation to ensure activities are undertaken 'with' or 'by' service users as opposed to 'on', 'to', 'about' or 'for' service users. Service user involvement, as constructed by the democratic approach, is linked to citizenship, democracy, and human rights (Newman, 2001) and focuses on empowering service users as decision makers in the co-production of services, research and policy. Participation, in the democratic approach therefore, is 'not simply [about] 'taking part' or 'being present' but [is about] having some influence over decisions and action' (Kirby et al., 2003: 5).

Exploring the statutory guidance for integrated services in England (NHS England and Department of Health and Social Care, 2022) shows that both approaches to service user involvement are evident including a focus on the collection of information from service users to inform decision-making and service provision (consumerist approach) and the sharing of power in decision making (democratic approach). A comparison of service user involvement policies for older people, who use social care, in England and Norway, indicates that although both countries are influenced by similar discourses about service user participation, these discourses are interpreted differently due to variation in welfare philosophies, and historical, political and cultural contexts, with consumerist perspectives stronger in England but democratic approaches also evident across both countries (Christensen and Pilling, 2019).

KEY CONCEPTS IN SERVICE USER INVOLVEMENT: EMPOWERMENT AND POWER

Underpinning participation and service user involvement is the term empowerment. Empowerment has been defined as 'a process through which people gain greater control over decisions and actions' which affect their health and quality of life (World Health Organization, 2020). Freire (1970) emphasises 'conscientisation' whereby individuals and communities are empowered through participatory dialogue to critically engage with factors which impact their lives. Empowerment, therefore, is political, transformational, and emancipatory. To fully understand empowerment, however, we must firstly reflect upon the word 'power' as reflections on meanings of power are often missing in initiatives aiming to empower service users and communities (Morgan, 2016), often leading to tokenistic attempts at participation with little change in decision making opportunities.

Power is often difficult to define (Lukes, 2005). Foucault (1972) emphasises power as exercised through social relationships, the production of knowledge, and discourses. By way of illustration, power exercised by medical practitioners has led to hegemonic biomedical bodies of knowledge, constructing discourses around autism as pathological, a condition outside of the norm, which requires cure (Waltz, 2020). The construction of biomedical knowledge is a form of 'biopower' which acts on 'bodies'(people) through a process of self-control, self-discipline, and self-evaluation in response to accepted 'regimes of truth' or social norms. As a result, the construction of knowledge, and thus the exercising of power, by autistic people themselves through, for example, Participatory Autism Research (Chown et al., 2017) can be empowering and emancipatory, offering a counter-narrative or critical resistance to biomedical research undertaken 'on' autistic people. This challenge to biomedical models of autism is apparent within the Neurodiversity Movement which offers alternative conceptualisations to neurotypical discourses which position autistic subjects as 'deviant' in relation to the 'norm' (Bertilsdotter et al., 2020). Power, therefore, is not just about top-down power (for example, coercion) such as the power of the State over its citizens, which tends to be the Structuralist Marxist standpoint, but about power relationships which also exist at the micro level (Foucault, 1975). Power is, therefore, exercised in everyday life and within taken for granted knowledge, social norms, and regimes of truths (Foucault, 1975). For Foucault, power 'is everywhere, not because it embraces everything, but because it comes from everywhere' (Foucault, 1976: 93). Foucault's theory of power can be located within the postmodernist approach to power and its construction, as outlined in chapter two. Power and authority emerge through a complex process of creation and contingencies and cannot be reduced to stabilised social structures and pre-determined stages of historical development.

Others have outlined four types of power relations: power within (relates to self-worth), power to (an individual's ability to act including increasing capacity, knowledge, and skills), power with (collective action) and power over (obedience or force) (Rowlands, 1995).'Power over' (Rowland, 1995) is often how power is conceptualised, for example violence against women and girls by men in a patriarchal society (Morgan and Choak, 2023) or health professional power over service users. 'Power to', on the other hand, emphasises individuals' productive and generative power and links to the potential of all people to control their lives. Empowerment based on 'power to' recognises that service users possess the potential to make decisions about their life and the services they receive because they not only have agency but are experts by experience. 'Power within' refers to confidence, self-awareness, consciousness raising and self-esteem which are important in building the capacities of service users to advocate for themselves. While 'power with' can empower service users through collective action to challenge hegemonic biomedical discourses to ensure needs are met. Understanding power, and the multiple ways that power plays out, including through social relationships and the production of knowledge, is key to ensuring ways of working that focus on empowerment as opposed to tokenistic attempts at participation which reinforce existing power relationships.

POWER IMBALANCES AND SERVICE USER INVOLVEMENT

Reflections on how power or a lack of power-sharing can be barrier to service user involvement are needed to support participatory initiatives. Power can be exercised in service user involvement initiatives variously and can be seen, for example, in expectations that service users will volunteer and give their time and knowledge freely, while professionals participate as part of their paid role. This can be reflective of a lack of value placed on service user experience. Power over can also play out over which service users participate in participatory processes and knowledge exchange. Service users are not a homogenous group and research indicates that some service users are under-represented in service user involvement initiatives. For example, evidence shows that that those involved in patient participation initiatives within the NHS in England tend to be 'white, middle class, educated and older people' (Ocloo, 2018:1); are of high socio-economic status in Canada (Boutilier et al., 2001) with barriers for women and those with English as a second language identified in Australia (Lee et al., 2009). While the CQC (2016) in England report that those with long term physical and mental health conditions and people over the age of 75 years old are less likely to feel that they were involved in making decisions about their care. Beresford (2020; 2013) identified groups who tend to be excluded from service user involvement initiatives including those individuals excluded, due to, for instance, class and ethnicity, groups within particularly marginalised settings such as the homeless and Gypsies and Travellers to those marginalised individually, for instance, people who communicate outside of the dominant rules of expression such as sign language. Moreover, those with severe and complex conditions or disabilities (Cameron et al., 2019) are often excluded as well as people viewed as 'unwanted' voices, offering alternative viewpoints, which do not automatically fit current agendas (Beresford, 2013; Ocloo and Matthews, 2016; Beresford, 2019). The exercising of top-down 'power over' in terms of who is invited to participate can, therefore, reinforce hegemonic narratives and reduce emancipatory change and enhance discrimination.

A lack of reflection on power dynamics can also result in tokenistic participatory initiatives. Although many service users participate in participatory processes because they want to bring about change (Beresford and Croft, 1993), the reality may be that opportunities to bring about change may be curbed leading to 'participation fatigue', and a perception that their knowledge and life experiences are not valued. In Sweden, for example, which is often heralded as a civic minded society, research has indicated that around 42–50% of people felt that their participation in initiatives had very little impact (or they were not aware of any impact) (Fredriksson and Tritter, 2020). While in Chile, service users reported being asked to comment on draft mental health plans, which had already been decided upon by service providers resulting in tensions around whose voices were heard and who had decided what to focus upon in the plans (Montenegro, 2018). Beresford (2019; 2020) has argued that often patient involvement initiatives ignore the political nature of participation and give the illusion of participation by using the language of rights, democracy, empowerment and participation but instead offer up tokenistic and restricted opportunities for power-sharing (Beresford, 2020; Tritter, 2009).

What is also evident is that service user involvement may be more likely at the micro level (individual) than at other levels, with research undertaken in New Zealand, and Norway indicating that service users are less likely to be involved at the service provision and organisational level, and more likely to be involved in decisions about their own care (Kent and Read, 1998; Storm et al., 2011). This was also found across OECD countries with higher levels of service user involvement in choices around their own care but less formal opportunities for participation in health policy decision making, with only three out of twenty-seven countries across the OECD, Portugal, Australia, and Germany, systematically including patients in at least four areas of health policy decision-making (OECD, 2021). This appears to be indicative of a consumerist approach to service user involvement (for example, choice of care at the individual level) as well as indicative of narratives that service users are experts only in their own condition (Cameron et al., 2019).

CONCLUSION

Service user involvement in health and social care is seen to bring direct benefits including the empowerment of service users. While participation in initiatives may take many forms from feedback to direct involvement in decision making, it is not always that service users feel listened to, respected, or involved in decision making, with power asymmetries often characterising participatory processes. These power asymmetries may be evident regardless of the presence of participatory language or policy, which supports democratic participation, giving the appearance that organisations are doing something differently, while doing very little to change the way that services operate. It is, therefore, important that those who plan participatory initiatives in health and social care go beyond 'speech acts' (Ahmed, 2012) to authentically engage with the political nature of participation and how services and the production of knowledge can be transformed through the direct involvement of service users. While hearing the views of service users is important and may be what some service users prefer as opposed to being directly involved in decision making processes, it is important to recognise that participation is about more than just having voices heard. It is also about challenging oppression and discrimination and is emancipatory and driven by service users. The political nature of participation, however, is often forgotten in service user involvement initiatives with a focus on more consumerist approaches to participation usually being the norm. Reflection is thus required on how power is implicated in service user involvement initiatives including reflection on how diverse groups can be supported to participate. The latter would involve building trust with communities, working with communities to enable opportunities to participate as decision makers and the use of a range of inclusive participatory methods to facilitate active engagement.

RESEARCH POINTS AND REFLECTIVE EXERCISES

- Research the barriers to service user involvement and discuss how they can be overcome (for example, Bee et al., 2015; Amann and Sleigh, 2021; Ocloo, et al., 2021). Then research the barriers for participation for children (for example Morgan and Sengedorj, 2015; Kiili at al., 2021).
- Read the paper by Duffy et al. (2022) and explore how COVID-19 has impacted on service user involvement. Do you agree that service user involvement is an afterthought?
- Discuss whether more of a focus on 'power' and the 'political' is needed in service user involvement initiatives across OECD countries. What issues do you think may arise from such a focus?

REFERENCES

Ahmed, S. (2012). *On Being Included: Racism and Diversity in Institutional Life*. Durham, NC: Duke University Press.

Amann, J. and Sleigh, J. (2021). Too Vulnerable to Involve? Challenges of Engaging Vulnerable Groups in the Co-Production of Public Services through Research. *International Journal of Public Administration*, 44 (9): 715–727. https://doi.org/10.1080/01900692.2021.1912089

Arnstein, S. (1969). A Ladder of Citizen Participation. *Journal of the American Institute of Planners*, 35 (4): 216–224. https://doi.org/10.1080/01944366908977225

Bee, P., Price, O., Baker, J. and Lovell, K. (2015). Systematic Synthesis of Barriers and Facilitators to Service User-Led Care Planning. *The British Journal of Psychiatry*, 207 (2): 104–114. https://doi.org/10.1192/bjp.bp.114.152447

Beresford, P. (2000). Service Users' Knowledges and Social Work Theory: Conflict or Collaboration? *The British Journal of Social Work*, 30 (4): 489–503. http://www.jstor.org/stable/23716149

Beresford, P. (2002). User Involvement in Research and Evaluation: Liberation or Regulation? *Social Policy and Society*, 1 (2): 95–105. doi:10.1017/S1474746402000222

Beresford, P. (2013). *Beyond the Usual Suspects*. London: Shaping Our Lives.

Beresford, P. (2019). Public Participation in Health and Social Care: Exploring the Co-production of Knowledge. *Front. Sociol*, 3 (41). https://doi.org/10.3389/fsoc.2018.00041

Beresford, P. (2020). PPI Or User Involvement: Taking Stock from a Service User Perspective in the Twenty First Century. *Res Involv Engagem*, 6 (36). https://doi.org/10.1186/s40900-020-00211-8

Beresford, P. and Boxall, K. (2012). Service Users, Social Work Education and Knowledge for Social Work Practice. *Social Work Education*, 31 (2): 155–167. https://doi.org/10.1080/02615479.2012.644944

Beresford, P. and Croft, S. (1993). *Citizen Involvement: A Practical Guide for Change*. Basingstoke: Macmillan.

Bertilsdotter Rosqvist, H., Chown, N. and Stenning. A. (2020). *Neurodiversity Studies: A New Critical Paradigm*. London: Routledge.

Boutilier, M. A., Rajkumar, E., Poland, B. D., Tobin, S. and Badgley, R. F. (2001). Community Action Success in Public Health: Are We Using a Ruler to Measure a Sphere? *Can J Public Health*, 92 (2): 90–94. https://doi.org/10.1007/BF03404937

Boyle, D., Coote, A., Sherwood, C. and Slay, J. (2010). *Right Here, Right Now: Taking Co-production into the Mainstream*. London: NESTA.

Cameron, C., Moore, M., Nutt, A. and Chambers, E. (2019). Improving Understanding of Service-User Involvement and Identity: Collaborative Research Traversing Disability, Activism and the Academy. *Disability and Society*, 34 (7-8): 1312–1331. https://doi.org/10.1080/09687599.2019.1632693

Chown N., Robinson J., Beardon L., Downing J., Hughes L., et al. (2017). Improving Research About Us, With Us: A Draft Framework for Inclusive Autism Research. *Disability and Society*, 32 (5): 720–734. https://doi.org/10.1080/09687599.2017.1320273

Christensen, K. and Pilling, D. (2019). User Participation Policies in Norway and England – the Case of Older People and Social Care. *Journal of Social Policy*, 48 (1): 43–61. doi:10.1017/S0047279418000272

Cornwall, A. (2002). *Making Spaces, Changing Places: Situating Participation in Development, IDS Working Paper 170*. Brighton: Institute of Development Studies.

Cornwall, A. (2003). *Beneficiary, Consumer, Citizen: Perspectives on Participation for Poverty Reduction, SIDA Studies No 2*. Stockholm: Swedish International Development Cooperation Agency.

Coulter, A. (2011). *Engaging Patients in Healthcare*. Milton Keynes: Open University Press.

CQC. (2016). *Better Care in My Hands: A Review of How People are Involved in Their Care*. Newcastle upon Tyne: CQC.

Czypionka, T., Kraus, M., Reiss, M. Baltaxe, E., Roca, J., et al. (2020). The Patient at the Centre: Evidence From 17 European Integrated Care Programmes for Persons with Complex Needs. *BMC Health Serv Res*, 20: 1102. https://doi.org/10.1186/s12913-020-05917-9

Da Silva, D. (2011). *Helping People Help Themselves, A Review of the Evidence Considering Whether it is Worthwhile to Support Self-Management*. London: The Health Foundation.

Davies, K. and Gray, M. (2017). The Place of Service-User Expertise in Evidence-Based Practice. *Journal of Social Work*, 17 (1): 3–20. https://doi.org/10.1177/1468017316637222

Duffy, J., Cameron, C., Casey, H., Beresford, P. and McLaughlin, H. (2022). Service User Involvement and COVID-19—An Afterthought? *The British Journal of Social Work*, 52 (4): 2384–2402. https://doi.org/10.1093/bjsw/bcac007

Duffy, J., Das, C. and Davidson, G. (2013). Service User and Carer Involvement in Role-Plays to Assess Readiness for Practice. *Social Work Education*, 32 (1): 39–54. https://doi.org/10.1080/02615479.2011.639066

Fals-Borda, O. and Rahman, M. A. (1991). *Action and Knowledge: Breaking the Monopoly with Participatory Action-Research*, 1st edn. New York: Apex Press.

Foot, C., Gilburt, H., Dunn, P., Jabbal, J., Seale, B., et al. (2014). *People in Control of Their Own Health and Social Care, the State of Involvement*: London: The King's Fund and National Voices.

Foucault, M. (1972). *Power/Knowledge, Selected Interviews and Other Writings*. New York: Pantheon Books.

Foucault, M. (1975). *Discipline and Punish: The Birth of the Prison*. New York: Random House.

Foucault, M. (1976). *The History of Sexuality. Vol. 1, The Will to Knowledge*. London: Penguin.

Fredriksson, M. and Tritter, J. (2020). Getting Involved: The Extent and Impact of Patient and Public Involvement in the Swedish Health System. *Health Economics, Policy and Law*, 15 (3): 325–340. doi:10.1017/S174413311900015X

Freire, P. (1970). *Pedagogy of the Oppressed*. New York: Continuum.

Kent, H. and Read, J. (1998). Measuring Consumer Participation in Mental Health Services: Are Attitudes Related to Professional Orientation? *Int J Social Psychiatry*, 44 (4): 295–310. https://doi.org/10.1177/002076409804400406.

Kiili, J., Itäpuisto, M., Moilanen, J., Svenlin, A. R. and Malinen, K. E. (2021). 'Professionals' Views on Children's Service User Involvement. *Journal of Children's Services*, 16 (2): 145–158. https://doi.org/10.1108/JCS-10-2020-0069

Kirby, P., Lanyon, C., Cronin, K. and Sinclair, R. (2003). *Building a Culture of Participation: Involving Children and Young People in Policy, Service Planning, Delivery and Evaluation: Handbook*. London: Department for Education and Skills.

Lee, S. K., Thompson, S. C. and Amorin-Wood, D. (2009). One Service, Many Voices: Enhancing Consumer Participation in a Primary Health Service for Multicultural Women. *Quality in Primary Care*, 17 (1): 63–69.

Lukes, S. (2005). *Power: A Radical View*, 2nd edn. London: Macmillan.

McLaughlin, H., Beresford, P., Cameron, C., Casey, H. and Duffy, J. (2020). *The Routledge Handbook of Service User Involvement in Human Services Research and Education*. Abingdon: Routledge.

Montenegro, C. R. (2018). Beyond Participation: Politics, Incommensurability and the Emergence of Mental Health Service Users' Activism in Chile. *Cult Med Psychiatry*, 42 (3): 605–626. https://doi.org/10.1007/s11013-018-9576-9

Morgan, J. (2016). Participation, Empowerment, and Capacity Building: Exploring Young People's Perspectives on the Services Provided to Them by a Grassroots NGO in Sub-Saharan Africa. *Children and Youth Services Review*, 65, 175–182. https://doi.org/10.1016/j.childyouth.2016.04.012.

Morgan, J. (2023). Exploring Women's Experiences of Diagnosis of ADHD in Adulthood: A Qualitative Study, *Advances in Mental Health*, online ahead of print. https://doi.org/10.1080/18387357.2023.2268756

Morgan, J. and Choak, C. (2023). Global Public Health and Violence. In V. La Placa and J. Morgan (eds), *Social Science Perspectives on Global Public Health*. London: Routledge, 109–118.

Morgan, J. and Sengedorj, T. (2015). 'If You Were the Researcher What Would You Research?': Understanding Children's Perspectives on Educational Research in Mongolia and Zambia, *International Journal of Research and Method in Education*, 38 (2): 200–218. https://doi.org/10.1080/1743727X.2014.946498

National Voices. (2014). Prioritising Person Centred Care: Supporting Self-Management: Summarising Evidence from Systematic Reviews. Available at: https://s42139.pcdn.co/wp-content/uploads/Supporting-self-management.pdf (Accessed: 3 January 2024).

NEF. (2013). *Co-Production in Mental Health: A Literature Review*. London: NEF.

Nesta. (2013). *The Business Case for People Powered Health*. London: Nesta.

Newman, J. (2001). *Modernising Governance: New Labour, Policy and Society*. London: Sage.

NHS. (2021). *Building Strong Integrated Care Systems Everywhere: ICS Implementation Guidance on Working with People and Communities*. London: NHS England and NHS Improvement.

NHS England and Department of Health and Social Care. (2022). Working in Partnership with People and Communities: Statutory Guidance. Available at: www.england.nhs.uk/wp-content/uploads/2023/05/B1762-guidance-on-working-in-partnership-with-people-and-communities-2.pdf (Accessed: 2 January 2023).

Ocloo, J. (2018). Involving a Greater Diversity of People in Healthcare Processes. Available at: www.thekristaocloocampaign.com/files/Involving%20a%20greater%20diversity%20of%20people%20in%20healthcare%20processes%20%20Comment%20%20Health%20Service%20Journal%20(4).pdf (Accessed: 2 January 2024).

Ocloo, J., Garfield, S., Franklin, B. D. and Dawson, S. (2021). Exploring the Theory, Barriers and Enablers for Patient and Public Involvement Across Health, Social Care and Patient Safety: A Systematic Review of Reviews. *Health Res Policy Sys*, 19 (8). https://doi.org/10.1186/s12961-020-00644-3

Ocloo, J. and Matthews, R. (2016). From Tokenism to Empowerment: Progressing Patient and Public Involvement in Healthcare Improvement. *BMJ Quality and Safety*, 25 (8): 626–632. https://doi.org/10.1136/bmjqs-2015-004839

OECD. (2021). *Health for the People, by the People: Building People-Centred Health Systems*. OECD Health Policy Studies, OECD Publishing, Paris.

Parfitt, T. (2004). The Ambiguity of Participation: A Qualified Defence of Participatory Development. *Third World Quarterly*, 25 (3): 537–556. https://doi.org/10.1080/0143659042000191429

Rowlands, J. (1995). Empowerment Examined. *Development in Practice*, 5 (2): 101–107. https://doi.org/10.1080/0961452951000157074

SCIE. (2022). Developing Our Understanding of the Difference Co-production Makes in Social Care. Available at: https://www.scie.org.uk/co-production/understanding-the-difference/ (Accessed: 15 January 2024).

Storm, M., Hausken, K. and Knudsen, K. (2011). Inpatient Service Providers' Perspectives on Service User Involvement in Norwegian Community Mental Health Centres. *Int J Social Psychiatry*, 57 (6): 551–563. https://doi.org/10.1177/0020764010371270

Tambuyzer, E., Pieters, G. and Van Audenhove, C. (2014). Patient Involvement in Mental Health Care: One Size Does Not Fit All. *Health Expect*, 17 (1): 138–150. https://doi.org/10.1111/j.1369-7625.2011.00743.x

Tritter, J. Q. (2009). Revolution or Evolution: The Challenges of Conceptualizing Patient and Public Involvement in a Consumerist World. *Health Expectations*, 12 (3): 275–287. https://doi.org/10.1111/j.1369-7625.2009.00564.x

Tritter, J. Q. and McCallum, A. (2006). The Snakes and Ladders of User Involvement: Moving Beyond Arnstein. *Health Policy*, 76 (2): 156–68. 10.1016/j.healthpol.2005.05.008

Waltz, M. (2020). The Production of the 'Normal' Child: Neurodiversity and the Commodification of Parenting. In H. Bertilsdotter Rosqvist, N. Chown and A. Stenning (eds), *Neurodiversity Studies: A New Critical Paradigm*. London: Routledge, 15–26.

Waterson, J. and Morris, K. (2005). Training in 'Social' Work: Exploring Issues of Involving Users in Teaching on Social Work Degree Programmes, *Social Work Education*, 24 (6): 653–675. https://doi.org/10.1080/02615470500185093

World Health Organization. (2013). Health 2020: A European Policy Framework and Strategy for the 21st century. World Health Organization Regional Office for Europe. Available at: https://iris.who.int/handle/10665/326386 (Accessed: 2 January 2024).

PART II

CHAPTER 8

Health, Social Care, and Homelessness

....

Nicholas Pleace

INTRODUCTION

This chapter explores the interrelationships between homelessness, social care, and health systems at European level and across the OECD. The chapter starts by examining distorting tendencies in how health and social care systems have tended to respond to homelessness and the newer, more evidence-based responses that have sought to improve strategy, planning, and practice. The chapter also looks at the logistical challenges in delivering health and social care to people experiencing homelessness and the importance of system integration. The emergent evidence on the gender dynamics of homelessness, and what this means for health and social care systems, is discussed as a way of exploring how widening definitions of homelessness are influencing the design for medical and social care services.

IMAGES AND REALITIES OF HOMELESSNESS

In the nineteenth century, the politest language being used by the British referred to the 'houseless poor'; references to 'beggars', 'tramps', and 'vagabonds' were far more common in describing something that was perceived as a public order issue. The 'houseless poor' were generally contained in workhouses and casual wards from the 1840s onwards. These policies showed a grudging acceptance that there was a social problem which had to be dealt with. However, workhouses retained a heavy emphasis on blaming the people who were experiencing houseless poverty, focusing on their (presumed) alcohol addiction, criminality, mental health problems, limiting illness and disability (London, 1903/1977; Higginbotham, 2012; O'Sullivan, 2023).

This image, as O'Sullivan has argued, was a powerful and persistent one. While both understanding, and the nature of policy responses towards homelessness shifted, as the Twentieth Century advanced, the idea that homelessness – particularly people living rough – was caused by the nature of the people experiencing it, continued unabated, in

DOI: 10.4324/9781003343608-10

mainstream political, health, and welfare system practice (O'Sullivan, 2020). A shift, away from blame and towards treatment began to occur, accelerating in countries like the UK in the 1960s and 1970s, but the narratives around how homelessness was being caused by the 'nature' of the people experiencing it remained, even as some academics began to highlight deep inequalities in access to housing (Wood, 1976).

A group of American academics began questioning mainstream assumptions about the nature of homelessness in the 1990s (Snow et al., 1994; Shinn, 1997; Kuhn and Culhane, 1998). The problem, as Gowan (2010) was later to characterise it, was that all the narratives around American homelessness seemed fixated on 'sin' (for which read drug addiction and associated survival crime) and 'sickness' (for which read mental illness, often severe mental illness). One part of the equation, which Gowan later called 'systems', i.e., the way in which society, economy, and social protection systems worked, seemed to be missing. These American academics were becoming increasingly critical of the idea that homelessness was primarily caused by, and persisted because of, individual needs, characteristics, experiences, and behaviour (Culhane and Kuhn, 1998). Rather, they assumed a shift to a more structural and systemic orientated approach which transcended the individual only.

The questions these American academics had were threefold. The first was centred on assumptive approaches to homelessness, i.e., a preloaded expectation that people experiencing homelessness had multiple and complex support and treatment needs that, alongside behavioural characteristics, caused and perpetuated their homelessness. In essence, this meant research was approaching homelessness within this framework, i.e., 'expecting' to find patterns of chaotic behaviour intersecting around addiction, severe mental illness, poor physical health, and criminality. The second was methodological, in that studies were often not looking at homelessness over time. However, they were instead collecting cross-sectional or 'snapshot' data over short periods, which meant shifts in trajectories through homelessness, i.e., changes in how homelessness was experienced and exits from homelessness, were generally not studied (Snow and Anderson, 1994). The third set of questions were systemic, i.e., if someone were living on the street with a mixture of addiction and severe mental illness, was that really 'wholly' explicable in terms of their needs, characteristics, experiences and choices, or was there something wrong with mental health and other structural systems and indeed with how health, social protection and housing policy was working more generally (Shinn, 1997)?

Perhaps the defining moment in understanding a shift in much, if not all, American understanding of homelessness centres on the work of Culhane and colleagues in the 1990s (Culhane and Kuhn, 1998; Kuhn and Culhane, 1998). By shifting the focus of analysis from who was using the US homelessness shelter systems at any one point to looking at patterns of use over time, Culhane and colleagues systematically illustrated why the idea that homelessness was primarily associated with high cost, high risk populations with multiple support and treatment needs, was based on a misconception (O'Sullivan, 2020; Lee et al., 2021).

Culhane and colleagues found a small population with the expected characteristics of people experiencing homelessness was ever-present, two groups who were long-term homeless (chronically homeless) and repeatedly homeless (episodically homeless). These two groups had the expected, very high, prevalence of addiction, severe mental illness, criminality, limiting illness and disability. However, there was a much bigger group who used the homeless shelters for shorter periods of time, people who were transitionally homeless, who did not have these characteristics, but who were very poor and often destitute. Only about 20% of the population using homeless shelters fell within the long-term and repeatedly homeless groups. The other 80% were transitionally homeless. As a result of only collecting data over short periods of time, people experiencing homelessness, who had multiple and complex treatment and support needs and those who were long-term and repeatedly homeless, had been significantly oversampled by mistake.

For example, a US city shelter system provided the equivalent of 340,151 stays (i.e., how many nights were available over the course of a year). Ten per cent of people experiencing homelessness in those shelters were long term (chronic) homeless and they consumed 50% of those stays, while another 10% who were repeatedly (episodic) homeless consumed another 33% of stays. Twenty per cent of the shelter using population were consuming more than 80% of shelter resources because they were not exiting homelessness, while some 80% of people experiencing homelessness using the shelter system, were only using 17% of stays (Kuhn and Culhane, 1998). When other researchers began to look, this same broad pattern emerged in the UK, Ireland, and other European countries, as well as in Australia (Jones and Pleace, 2010; Scutella et al., 2012; O'Sullivan, 2020).

The implications of these findings were twofold. First, there was evidence of a highly vulnerable population experiencing homelessness on a sustained and recurrent basis, which raised profound questions about the effectiveness of existing policy and practice and shifted the focus to social determinants. Second, there was a lot of homelessness experience that health, social care, and broader social protection systems were missing, as they focused on what (distorted) evidence informed them about a supposedly entirely high cost, elevated risk homeless population. This meant some elements of the need for health and social care among people experiencing homelessness were being neglected. This point is revisited below.

During the 2000s and 2010s, two further developments occurred. The first was evidence that the nature and extent of homelessness looked like it mirrored the nature and extent of national social protection and public health systems. In Scandinavian countries, with the partial exception of an increasingly neoliberal Sweden, very extensive welfare systems appeared to be generating homelessness in a specific form, i.e., a very small social problem strongly associated with recurrent and sustained homelessness among people with high and complex treatment and support needs (Benjaminsen and Andrade, 2015). Elsewhere in Europe and across the wider OECD, where health and welfare systems were comparatively weaker, homelessness looked increasingly like the patterns that Culhane and others had found in the USA, i.e., a small group with multiple and complex needs, alongside a much bigger, very poor, indeed destitute, population also experiencing homelessness (Bramley and Fitzpatrick, 2018). Alongside this, migrant homelessness, particularly among undocumented migrants, looked different again, as what characterised this population did not seem to be linked to individual characteristics, support, or treatment needs, nor experiences, but an inability to access any publicly funded services beyond very basic and limited help (Mostowska, 2014).

A major paradigm shift occurred in responses to homelessness in the USA, which centred on the Housing First model during the 2010s (Padgett et al., 2016). Existing homelessness systems used a linear model, whereby someone with homelessness associated with multiple and complex needs was slowly moved from what could be ward-like settings to an increasingly home-like environment, being trained, treated, and supported to a point where they should be able live independently by the end of linear residential treatment processes. These approaches had been copied from those initially developed to close long-stay mental hospitals. However, mental health services had subsequently abandoned linear residential treatment as expensive, and often ineffective, and replaced it with a housing-led approach which used mobile support from a multi-disciplinary team. Rather than training someone to be 'housing ready', these systems housed ex-psychiatric patients more or less straight away and then provided tailored, intensive, interdisciplinary case management support, over which the ex-psychiatric patient exercised very considerable control. It was this shift in practice that Housing First now followed in redesigning US homelessness services (Tsemberis, 2010).

Advocates of Housing First argued for the replacement of linear model homelessness services with a housing-based model, using a multi-disciplinary team offering intensive case management, within a consumer choice (co-productive) framework (Padgett et al., 2016). Success rates, in the US, seemed spectacular, with Housing First, keeping people with multiple and complex needs out of homelessness for at least a year (and often more) in 80% plus of cases, compared to rates of 40-60% for most of the linear services (Pleace, 2008). Randomised controlled trials in Canada (Goering et al, 2014) and France (DIHAL, 2016), alongside a significant amount of observational research, confirmed the relative effectiveness of Housing First across much of the EU and OECD in reducing homelessness among people with multiple and complex needs (Pleace et al., 2019).

Finland, pursuing its own model of housing led, and integrated homelessness strategy, was the first country in the Global North to show sustained reductions in long-term and recurrent homelessness associated with high and complex treatment needs (Y Foundation, 2017). Finnish terminology, which also used the phrase Housing First, referred to a much broader strategic integration of health, social care, social housing, and homelessness services within the same sort of housing-led framework that was the core idea of Housing First. Again, there was an emphasis on choice and control for people experiencing homelessness. One key aspect of this was the use of harm reduction rather than abstinence-based approaches to addiction in Finland, which was also a feature of the US Housing First model. In a context in which relatively extensive social protection systems seemed to prevent wider homelessness associated with poverty and destitution, a pattern also witnessed in Norway and Denmark (O'Sullivan et al., 2023), talk of Finland ending homelessness has been sounding increasingly realistic (Kaakinen, 2023).

In much of the EU and wider OECD, a systemic shift towards Housing First models, that use choice-based (co-productive) multi-disciplinary teams within a housing-led framework is underway. This progress is not uniform. The paradigm shift, a new way of thinking about homelessness, both as a problem associated with multiple and complex needs, to which Housing First is perceived as the effective response, and as a wider, largely socio-economic problem, stemming from deep social inequalities and destitution, is reflected in strategic developments, like the European Platform to Combat Homelessness, which all 27 EU Member States have agreed (European Commission, 2021). However, some medical research still follows the longstanding assumption that homelessness is invariably about multiple and complex needs, as does some homelessness research. The same inconsistencies exist across policy and practice, which can mean health and social care services are sometimes out of kilter with what the evidence base reports around the realities of homelessness (O'Sullivan et al., 2020).

POLICY AND PRACTICE AROUND HEALTH AND SOCIAL CARE FOR PEOPLE EXPERIENCING HOMELESSNESS

Generalising about policy and practice around social care and health policy and practice for people experiencing homelessness is challenging. Alongside shifting understanding of what homelessness is, systems are often highly devolved, i.e., there is more likely to be a lot of variable municipal/regional policy and practice in any given EU or OECD country than a single, national policy. The larger the country is, the greater the likelihood is that there will not be a single strategy around homelessness and mental health, homelessness, and addiction, Housing First, or indeed around homelessness, health, and social care in general (Pleace, 2023a). This said, it is possible to talk about the various kinds of system integration and practice that are in place to address health and social care needs among people experiencing homelessness. These are broadly categorised in Box 8.1.

BOX 8.1 SYSTEM INTEGRATION AND PRACTICE TO ADDRESS HEALTH AND SOCIAL CARE NEEDS FOR PEOPLE EXPERIENCING HOMELESSNESS

- Specialist healthcare, psychiatric and addiction services that were built to engage with people living rough (on the street) and in emergency shelters, which can include older services that are generally not integrated into a wider homelessness strategy.
- Health navigator services, which are health-led interventions that are designed to reduce repeated use of accident and emergency (A&E)/emergency room (ER) services and other emergency services, e.g., mental health and addiction crisis services and improve detection and treatment for serious conditions. These approaches emphasise joint working with other systems and services, including social care, the homelessness sector, and where present, social landlords.
- Housing First and housing-led services that are designed to work with health and social care services, including addiction and mental health teams, alongside other social protection systems (and where present, social/public housing) through intensive case management and multidisciplinary teams.
- High intensity supported housing services, which in the European, North American, and Australian contexts, refers to temporary and permanent congregate and communal housing which offers onsite treatment, support, and case management. This can include adoption of medical and social work practice into homelessness services, including trauma informed care (TIC) and psychologically informed environments (PIE).

It is important to note that while variation in national health and social care systems can be considerable, the difference in homelessness strategies, services, and systems, including access to, and integration of health and social care, can be profound. There are countries in the EU/OECD where, if there is any organised policy and service response to homelessness at all, it will be confined to major cities. Therefore, what is often required is an integrated national legislative framework that works and joins up with other housing and health services to support those who experience homelessness, beyond major cities and localities (Pleace et al., 2020).

Much of the specialist medical provision that has been developed tends to reflect images of homelessness that centre on associations with multiple and complex needs, again centred on the idea of strong associations between addiction and severe mental illness and homelessness. Some of this is simply administrative lag, explicable by individual services and models which predated shifting understanding of what homelessness is, but there is also a cultural lag, the image of homelessness as always being equated with people characterised by 'sin' (addiction) combined with 'sickness' (poor mental health) has sometimes proven hard to shift (Gowan, 2010; O'Sullivan et al., 2020).

The results from specialist healthcare services for people experiencing homelessness, again posited on the expectation of mental illness and addiction, were often poor when these services operated in isolation. The core challenge for 'street medicine' services is threefold: first, among those who are long-term or repeatedly homeless, needs can be acute, multiple, and complex; second, conditions in emergency shelters and living rough are not conducive to wellbeing and certainly not to recovery from mental or physical illness and third, continuity of care can be hard to maintain, i.e., people may not maintain contact for long enough for treatment to work (Kertesz et al., 2021; Kopanitsa et al., 2023). The old shorthand for this, when attempts were being made to treat people sleeping rough (street homeless) in the UK in the 1980s and 1990s summarised the problem neatly: 'You cannot treat someone living in a cardboard box' (Pleace and Quilgars, 1996). Equally, offering short term accommodation to detoxify someone or to treat a disease like tuberculosis tends to result in low success rates, if they can only return to living rough or emergency shelters (Pleace, 2008).

For these reasons, street-based or fixed site medical services can choose to operate in close strategic coordination with other services, so that mental health, addiction, other treatment, and social care needs, are simultaneously addressed within a holistic package of case management support, a model which has been used in Amsterdam (Kasper, 2018). There is also Canadian guidance on how these forms of specialist outreach teams and medical clinics should work in terms of the treatment they offer and their coordination with other services (Pottie et al., 2020).

Health navigator services also work through collaboration with other types of services and one example of good practice is Pathway in the UK (see www.pathway. org.uk). The Pathway model is designed to ensure that the National Health Service (NHS) does not discharge someone who has been in hospital into a situation of homelessness. The approach uses specialist general practitioners (GPs/doctors) who have experience with treating people experiencing homelessness, supported by experienced nursing staff and housing specialists, who connect patients with housing and homelessness services in the community.

An integral part of the approach is a team of Care Navigators who have 'lived experience' of homelessness, and who provide peer support, and there may be, depending on how the team is structured, dedicated social work, occupational therapy, and mental health practitioners. Pathway is designed to coordinate with other health, social care, and homelessness and housing services. Support begins at the point someone enters hospital from a situation of homelessness, helping them understand and navigate their treatment, and providing help as needed. The goal is that a holistic package of treatment, social care, housing related support and (at least) a stable and suitable form of accommodation is in place before someone leaves hospital (Cornes et al, 2021). Drawing on some of the lessons of Pathway, the UK's National Institute for Clinical Excellence has issued guidance on integration of health and social care for people experiencing homelessness (NICE, 2022).

A similar example, which has been explored through the European CANCERLESS project led by academics in Vienna (Carmichael et al., 2022), uses a 'navigator' model to enable access and continuity of care to people experiencing homelessness who have cancer. This model, like Pathway, is not a separate form of service like a 'street medicine' model, rather it is an adaptation and enhancement of existing, mainstream, health services to enable access to successful treatment for people experiencing homelessness. In the field of European social work, there have been similar developments. Practice has been adapted to better understand and respond to the needs of people experiencing homelessness (Gerull, 2023). Like Pathway and similar models in health systems, this represents an adaptation of mainstream services, adding to, and changing practice and responses, to enable a better response to homelessness, rather than building separate 'homelessness social work' services that would be akin to (equally separated) older models of street medicine.

European responses towards the health and social care needs of people experiencing homelessness, who have high and complex needs, in north-western Europe are increasingly focused on using intensive case management services within a Housing First model. This means there is increasing integration with health and social care services in two senses. The first is that the line between homelessness, health, and social care/social work service has become deliberately blurred by approaches which use multidisciplinary teams within a coordinated case management model and the second is that these services also seek to 'mainstream' access to health and social care, as part of a process of wider resettlement and reintegration. Housing First has much in common with a health led model like Pathway and, in turn, Pathway closely reflects the core aspects of Housing First. Services are increasingly integrated, coordinated, and housing-led or focused. In a context like France or Denmark, Housing First and related services are simultaneously the homelessness strategy and the health and social care strategy as it relates to homelessness (Pleace et al., 2019).

The idea of discrete homelessness services, in the sense of specialist provision, remains in place for people experiencing homelessness with extremely high needs.

Housing First can, where resources permit, be scaled up from an intensive case management model to assertive community treatment (ACT, an integrated interdisciplinary team that is part of the Housing First model) (Tsemberis, 2010). However, even in countries like Finland and Denmark, where housing-led services are widespread, some use of specialist accommodation remains. The Danish Skaeve Huse model, of small scale, intensively supported congregate housing is one example of services which are used when risks around independent living in ordinary housing, as in a Housing First service, are assessed as too great (Benjaminsen, 2018).

WIDER DIMENSIONS OF HOMELESSNESS

Understanding of the gender dynamics of homelessness as an agentic and structural phenomenon is still evolving, but distinct patterns have become apparent that were long missed by researchers expecting a population of lone men with high rates of addiction and mental illness. Women are much more likely to experience homelessness with their children, much more likely to experience homelessness triggered by domestic abuse and to have experienced trauma as a result. Women also experience homelessness differently. They are more likely to experience 'hidden' homelessness, i.e., relying on precarious arrangements like 'sofa surfing' between the homes of relatives, friends, and acquaintances, and only becoming formally recognised as homeless, including with their children, when the precarious arrangements of hidden homelessness are exhausted and they have to approach homelessness services (Bretherton, 2017; Bretherton, 2020; Bretherton and Mayock, 2021).

A key point here is that women lone parents and their children, form the bulk of what is referred to as 'family' homelessness in EU Member States and the wider OECD (Baptista et al, 2017), including the UK (Fitzpatrick and Pleace, 2012; Quilgars and Pleace, 2023) and USA (Batko and Culhane, 2023). The women heading these homeless families are not presenting with high rates of severe mental illness or addiction. Their main characteristic is poverty, and in many cases, the effects of traumatic experiences, associated with domestic abuse, i.e., they need different kinds of health services.

As understanding of homelessness and gender shifts, questions about the effectiveness of health and social care service responses arise. A key question centres on the treatment and care needs of women experiencing homelessness. An effective strategic response to women's homelessness and homelessness among women lone parents with dependent children has, for example, to consider integration of domestic abuse and criminal justice systems and the potential modification of systems and services, for example, building specific 'Housing First for Women' services (Quilgars et al., 2021). The other major factor here is children experiencing homelessness. In much of the EU and the wider OECD, the risks are not those of rough sleeping (street homelessness) but of prolonged stays in emergency and temporary accommodation, which may be inadequate and risky to health. Both women on their own, and women with children, are also in a state of disconnection and precarity while homeless, i.e., health and social care systems are structured around people being at fixed points, which means a stable, recognised address. This is not just a matter of having a fixed point of contact (less of an issue than it was as smartphones are near ubiquitous in the EU/OECD), it also extends to the fundamentals in how health and social care are organised.

Much of the so-called Global North uses local connection rules to orchestrate access to non-emergency health services and social care/social work (still called social services in most countries). This means a precariously accommodated homeless woman and her children, who is having to move herself, or who is being moved by services between different emergency accommodation, is at risk of being disconnected from health and social care services. She will also be having to make new arrangements every time she happens to encounter an administrative boundary. Equally, there may be wider impacts on her children as disruption to education occurs, as schools are often organised on a similar 'catchment-area' basis. The poverty that is at the core of all homelessness becomes important again, both in the sense that a woman-headed homeless family cannot exercise choice over where they live and, even if contact with health, social care and other services like schools can be maintained if they move away, transport costs can be prohibitive (Baptista et al., 2015).

There is a broader point here, which extends to the associations between poverty and recognising homelessness as often being a bigger social problem than a relatively small number of people with high and complex treatment needs who are living rough and in emergency shelters. The social gradient of health, i.e., the increased risk of serious illness and mortality at an earlier age is also present for the very poor and destitute populations who are at heightened risk of homelessness. Again, there are additional risks inherent in homelessness itself, including disruption to health and social care contact, and poor continuity of care, all of which stems from a lack of a settled, adequate, and affordable home.

CONCLUSION

Homelessness has become a 'moving target' (Lee et al., 2021) in much of the EU and wider OECD. Understanding has shifted towards greater recognition of homelessness existing primarily in association with destitution; with only smaller subpopulations, mainly experiencing recurrent and sustained homelessness, being characterised by the high rates of addiction and severe mental illness that were once thought synonymous with homelessness (O'Sullivan, 2020). Alongside this, the ways in which health and social care services have been designed for people experiencing homelessness are undergoing change. This change is happening at two levels. The first is that 'housing ready' or linear models, which were designed to use special congregate and communal accommodation to train and support someone with multiple and complex needs to be able to live independently, have been largely eclipsed by more effective Housing First models. Housing First is not perfect, but outcomes in terms of ending homelessness among people with high and complex needs are generally better than for other models of homelessness service (Aubry et al., 2021). The second change is that 'street medicine' and dedicated homelessness clinic models have been similarly left behind, both in the sense that failures were linked to these services operating in isolation from social care, housing, and homelessness services and other systems of support. This led to their changing into more coordinated and integrated responses, and in the arrival of approaches like Pathway, which while clinician-led, has a great deal in common with Housing First.

In essence, the idea of separate responses to the health and social care needs of people experiencing homelessness is fading away and being replaced by enhanced strategic integration. This development will in turn be reinforced by wider definitions and wider recognition of the dimensions of homelessness, the need for health and social care systems that can locate, recognise, and respond to the needs of homeless families – needs which are very different from longstanding ideas of who people experiencing homelessness are – and to recognise the specific needs of women experiencing homelessness, will be the first of many examples.

The importance of the absence of a stable, adequate, affordable home cannot be exaggerated. One issue here is the ways in which that lack of stability undermines continuity and access to social care and medical treatment. However, inadequate, and insecure housing undermines health (Marmot et al., 2020) and without a decent, affordable, and secure home, the effectiveness of social and healthcare services is always going to be compromised.

RESEARCH POINTS AND REFLECTIVE EXERCISES

- Read the European summary report (Pleace, 2023a). Which basic principles should underpin a coherent and effective social and healthcare strategy for people experiencing homelessness across the most developed economies?
- Read the evidence review on the women's homelessness (Bretherton and Mayock, 2021). What specific needs do women have in relation to health and social care services and how should strategic and programme approaches take this into account?
- Read the following about homelessness and COVID 19 and reflect upon policy responses (Pleace et al., 2021; Parsell et al., 2022; Pleace, 2023b).

REFERENCES

Aubry, T., Roebuck, M., Loubiere, S., Tinland, A., Nelson, G., et al. (2021). A Tale of Two Countries: A Comparison of Multi-Site Randomised Controlled Trials of Pathways Housing First Conducted in Canada and France. *European Journal of Homelessness*, 15 (3): 25–44.

Baptista, I., Benjaminsen, L., O'Sullivan, E. and Pleace, N. (2015). *Local Connection Rules and Homelessness in Europe*. Brussels: FEANTSA.

Baptista, I., Benjaminsen, L., Busch-Geertsema, V. and Pleace, N. (2017). *Family Homelessness in Europe*. Brussels: FEANTSA.

Batko, S. and Culhane, D. P. (2023). Homelessness in the United States. In J. Bretherton and N. Pleace (eds), *The Routledge Handbook of Homelessness*. London: Routledge, 413–422.

Benjaminsen, L. and Andrade, S. B. (2015). Testing a Typology of Homelessness Across Welfare Regimes: Shelter Use in Denmark and the USA. *Housing Studies*, 30 (6): 858–876. https://doi.org/10.1080/02673037.2014.982517

Benjaminsen, L. (2018). Housing First in Denmark: An Analysis of the Coverage Rate Among Homeless People and Types of Shelter Users. *Social Inclusion*, 6 (3): 327–336. https://doi.org/10.17645/si.v6i3.1539

Bramley, G. and Fitzpatrick, S. (2018). Homelessness in the UK: Who is Most at Risk? *Housing Studies*, 33 (1): 96–116. https://doi.org/10.1080/02673037.2017.1344957

Bretherton, J. (2017). Reconsidering Gender in Homelessness. *European Journal of Homelessness*, 11 (1): 1–21.

Bretherton, J. (2020). Women's Experiences of Homelessness: A Longitudinal Study. *Social Policy and Society*, 19 (2): 255–270. https://doi.org/10.1017/S1474746419000423

Bretherton, J. and Mayock, P. (2021). *Women's Homelessness: European Evidence Review* Brussels: FEANTSA.

Cornes, M., Aldridge, R. W., Biswell, E., Byng, R., Clark, M., et al. (2021). Improving Care Transfers for Homeless Patients After Hospital Discharge: A Realist Evaluation. *Health Services and Delivery Research*, 9 (17). https://doi.org/10.3310/hsdr09170

Culhane, D. P. and Kuhn, R. (1998). Patterns and Determinants of Public Shelter Utilization Among Homeless Adults in New York City and Philadelphia. *Journal of Policy Analysis and Management: The Journal of the Association for Public Policy Analysis and Management*, 17 (1): 23–43. https://doi.org/10.1002/(SICI)1520-6688(199824)17:1<23::AID-PAM2>3.0.CO;2-J

DIHAL. (2016). *The Experimental Programme Un Chez- Soi D'abord Housing First Main Results - 2011/2015*. Paris: DIHAL.

European Commission. (2021). European Platform on Combatting Homelessness – Preview. Available at: https://ec.europa.eu/social/main.jsp?catId=1550&langId=en&preview=cHJldkVt cGxQb3J0YWwhMjAxMjAyMTVwcmV2aWV3V3 (Accessed: 22 September 2024).

Fitzpatrick, S. and Pleace, N. (2012). The Statutory Homelessness System in England: A Fair and Effective Rights-Based Model? *Housing Studies*, 27 (2): 232–225. https://doi.org/10.1080/02673037.2012.632622

Goering, P., Veldhuizen, S., Watson, A., Adair, C., Kopp, B., et al. (2014). *National at Home/Chez Soi Final Report*. Calgary, AB: Mental Health Commission of Canada.

Higginbotham, P. (2012). *Life in a Victorian Workhouse*. London: Pitkin.

Jones, A. and Pleace, N. (2010). *A Review of Single Homelessness in the UK 2000–2010*. London: Crisis.

Kaakinen, J. (2023). *HOME: Report on the Measures Needed to End Homelessness by 2027 (English Translation)*. Helsinki: Y Foundation.

Kertesz, S. G., DeRussy, A. J., Kim, Y. I., Hoge, A. E., Austin, E. L., et al. (2021). Comparison of Patient Experience Between Primary Care Settings Tailored for Homeless Clientele and Mainstream Care Settings. *Medical Care*, 59 (6): 495–503. https://doi.org/10.1097/MLR.0000000000001548

Kopanitsa, V., McWilliams, S., Leung, R., Schischa, B., Sarela, S., et al. (2023). A Systematic Scoping Review of Primary Health Care Service Outreach for Homeless Populations. *Family Practice*, 40 (1): 138–151. https://doi.org/10.1093/fampra/cmac075

Kuhn, R. and Culhane, D. P. (1998). Applying Cluster Analysis to Test a Typology of Homelessness by Pattern of Shelter Utilization: Results from the Analysis of Administrative Data. *American Journal of Community Psychology*, 26 (2): 207–232. https://doi.org/10.1023/A:1022176402357

Lee, B. A., Shinn, M. and Culhane, D. P. (2021). Homelessness as a Moving Target. *The Annals of the American Academy of Political and Social Science*, 693 (1): 8–26. https://doi.org/10.1177/0002716221997038

London, J. (1903/1977). *The People of the Abyss*. London: The Journeyman Press.

Marmot, M., Allen, J., Boyce, T., Goldblatt, P. and Morrison J. (2020). *Health Equity in England: The Marmot Review 10 Years On*. London: Institute of Health Equity. Available at: health.org. uk/publications/reports/the-marmot-review-10-years-on (Accessed: 13 February 2024).

Mostowska, M. (2014). 'We Shouldn't but We Do...': Framing the Strategies for Helping Homeless EU Migrants in Copenhagen and Dublin. *The British Journal of Social Work*, 44 (1): i18–i34. https://doi.org/10.1093/bjsw/bcu043

NICE. (2022). Integrated health and social care for people experiencing homelessness. Available at: www.nice.org.uk/guidance/ng214 (Accessed: 22 September 2024).

O'Sullivan, E. (2020). *Reimagining Homelessness*. Bristol: Policy Press.

O'Sullivan, E., Pleace, N., Busch-Geertsema, V. and Hrast, M. F. (2020). Distorting Tendencies in Understanding Homelessness in Europe. *European Journal of Homelessness*, 14 (3): 109–135. Available at: www.feantsaresearch.org/public/user/Observatory/2020/EJH/EJH_14-3_A6_v03.pdf

O'Sullivan, E. (2023). Historical Perspectives on Homelessness. In J. Bretherton and N. Pleace (eds), *The Routledge Handbook of Homelessness*. London: Routledge, 13–23.

O'Sullivan, E., Benjaminsen, L., Busch-Geertsema, V., Filipovič Hrast, M., Pleace, N., et al. (2023). *Homelessness in the European Union*. Policy Department for Citizens' Rights and Constitutional Affairs, Directorate-General for Internal Policies, PE 755.915, Brussels: European Parliament.

Padgett, D. K., Henwood, B. F. and Tsemberis, S. (2016). *Housing First: Ending Homelessness, Transforming Systems and Changing Lives*. Oxford: Oxford University Press.

Parsell, C., Clarke, A. and Kuskoff, E. (2022). Understanding Responses to Homelessness During COVID-19: An Examination of Australia. *Housing Studies*, 38 (1): 8–21. doi:10.1080/02673037.2020.1829564

Pleace, N. (2008). *Effective Services for Substance Misuse and Homelessness in Scotland: Evidence from an International Review*. Edinburgh: Scottish Government.

Pleace, N. (2018). *Using Housing First in Integrated Homelessness Strategies*. London: St Mungo's.

Pleace, N. (2023a). *Social and Healthcare Services for Homeless People: A Discussion Paper*. Brussels: European Commission.

Pleace, N. (2023b). COVID-19. In J. Bretherton and N. Pleace (eds), *The Routledge Handbook of Homelessness*. London: Routledge, 71–82.

Pleace, N., Baptista, I., Benjaminsen, L. and Busch-Geertsema, V. (2020). *Staffing Homelessness Services in Europe*. Brussels: FEANTSA.

Pleace, N., Baptista, I., Benjaminsen, L., Busch-Geertsema, V., O'Sullivan, E., et al. (2021). *European Homelessness and COVID 19*. Brussels: FEANTSA.

Pleace, N., Baptista, I. and Knutagård, M. (2019). *Housing First in Europe: An Overview of Implementation, Strategy and Fidelity*. Brussels: Housing First Hub Europe.

Pleace, N. and Quilgars, D. (1996). *Health and Homelessness in London*. London: The King's Fund.

Pottie, K., Kendall, C. E., Aubry, T., Magwood, O., Andermann, A., et al. (2020). Clinical Guideline for Homeless and Vulnerably Housed People, and People with Lived Homelessness Experience. *CMAJ: Canadian Medical Association Journal*, 192 (10): E240. https://doi.org/10.1503/cmaj.190777

Quilgars, D., Bretherton, J. and Pleace, N. (2021). *Housing First for Women: A Five-Year Evaluation of the Manchester Jigsaw Support Project*. York: University of York.

Quilgars, D. and Pleace, N. (2023). Children and Families. In J Bretherton and N. Pleace (eds), *The Routledge Handbook of Homelessness*. London: Routledge, 180–190.

Scutella, R., Johnson, G., Moschion, J., Tseng, Y. P. and Wooden, M. (2013). Understanding Lifetime Homeless Duration: Investigating Wave 1 Findings from the Journeys Home Project. *Australian Journal of Social Issues*, 48 (1): 83–110. https://doi.org/10.1002/j.1839-4655.2013.tb00272.x

Shinn, M. (1997). Family Homelessness: State or Trait? *American Journal of Community Psychology*, 25 (6): 755–769. https://doi.org/10.1023/A:1022209028188

Snow, D. A., Anderson, L. and Koegel, P. (1994). Distorting Tendencies in Research on the Homeless. *American Behavioural Scientist*, 37 (4): 461–475. https://doi.org/10.1177/0002764294037004004

Wood, S. M. (1976). Camberwell Reception Centre: A Consideration of the Need for Health and Social Services of Homeless, Single Men. *Journal of Social Policy*, 5 (4): 389–399. https://doi.org/10.1017/S0047279400005018

Y Foundation. (2017). *A Home of Your Own: Housing First and Ending Homelessness in Finland*. Helsinki: Y Foundation.

CHAPTER 9

Domestic Violence and Abuse

....

Dana Sammut and Caroline Bradbury-Jones

INTRODUCTION

In the UK, domestic violence and abuse (DVA) is defined as any incident or pattern of violent, controlling, or threatening behaviour inflicted by a current or former intimate partner (Domestic Abuse [Scotland] Act, 2018) and/or family member (Violence Against Women, Domestic Abuse and Sexual Violence [Wales] Act, 2015; Domestic Abuse Act, 2021; Domestic Abuse and Civil Proceedings Act [Northern Ireland], 2021). The perpetration of DVA can encompass physical, psychological, sexual, economic, or digital forms of abuse, and its effects are often felt by other family members, including children, even when they are not the primary targets. While many definitions of DVA include specific forms of abuse, perpetrated by extended family members – including 'honour'-based violence, forced marriage, and female genital mutilation (FGM) – these often carry separate legal definitions and policy expectations, and so will not be captured within this chapter. Health and social care professionals play an integral role in recognising and responding to DVA, and frequently serve as the first point of contact for individuals experiencing abuse. This chapter presents an overview of DVA policy and practice across OECD countries, with reference to relevant global frameworks and conventions.

THE GLOBAL CONTEXT

While DVA is not exclusive to any gender, women worldwide are disproportionately the victims of male-perpetrated violence (WHO, 2021a). It is for this reason that DVA is often regarded as a gendered crime, reflecting a broader gender imbalance, rooted in societal norms and power dynamics. Globally, cultural values can influence what is deemed acceptable within relationships and families, sometimes perpetuating harmful practices, or discouraging survivors from seeking help. For example, data from the OECD (2023a) indicate that 30% of women aged 15 to 49 consider it acceptable for husbands to use physical violence against their wives,

DOI: 10.4324/9781003343608-11

ranging from an average of 9% in Europe to 38% in Africa. Socio-economic factors, legal systems, and historical legacies, underlie the social acceptability of DVA, which is often a byproduct of long-established structural hierarchies that reinforce restrictive gender norms.

Globally, women living in regions with high social acceptance of DVA assume a heavier burden of unpaid domestic work, face greater barriers to employment, and have fewer legal freedoms to divorce, inherit, and access justice systems (OECD, 2023a). These structural disadvantages perpetuate a cycle where gender biases become ingrained in societal consciousness, including within health and social care systems. The resulting disparity in health outcomes for women and gender minorities has been well-researched, with evidence highlighting inferior care, symptom dismissal, and mistreatment or harassment as causal factors (Heise et al., 2019). In the context of DVA, discriminatory laws and societal norms can mean that some forms of violence, such as marital rape, go unrecognised by survivors and service providers alike (Deosthali et al., 2022).

Structural gender biases are often implicit, and their effects are not limited to non-OECD economies. Evidence from Europe (Feresin, 2020), North America (Epstein and Goodman, 2019) and Australasia (Elizabeth, 2020) shows that women are regularly dismissed and disempowered by the legal, health and social systems they encounter following abuse, with many studies attributing this to professionals' endorsement of harmful gender stereotypes and DVA myths (consciously or otherwise). These include the beliefs that women are complicit in their own abuse (Taylor et al., 2013), and that mothers fabricate stories to alienate children from their fathers (Birchall and Choudhry, 2022), neither of which is accepted by the scientific community (see O'Donohue et al., 2016 on 'parental alienation syndrome'). A recent report from the England and Wales charity SafeLives (2021) indicates that survivors who encounter these prejudices can experience retraumatisation and feel discouraged from seeking help again.

STRATEGIES AND POLICY FRAMEWORKS ACROSS THE OECD

Understanding the prevalence of DVA across OECD member countries is a complex undertaking, in part, due to issues of data completeness and reliability. The stigma associated with DVA, together with a pervasive mistrust towards institutional systems, means that many survivors do not formally report their experiences. Legal definitions of DVA also vary from country to country: for example, Austria, Portugal, and Spain do not include economic violence (Council of Europe, 2022a). In addition, while several international standards and monitoring instruments exist, their adoption across OECD countries is not always consistent.

Most notably, there is the Council of Europe's 2011 Convention on Preventing and Combating Violence Against Women and Domestic Violence, or the Istanbul Convention, which provides specific guidance on policy integration for state actors and non-governmental partners. It includes a particular focus on DVA and obliges ratified states to implement measures in accordance with four key action areas, known as the four 'P's:

- **Prevention:** Describes measures such as awareness-raising campaigns, involving the media in efforts to combat harmful gender stereotypes, and training professionals whose work involves contact with survivors.
- **Protection:** Includes efforts to make DVA services such as shelters and helplines accessible and free to service users, and strategies to empower survivors to know their rights and available sources of support.
- **Prosecution:** Urges states to criminalise various forms of violence against women, including stalking, sexual violence, and harassment, and stipulates that investigations and legal proceedings must respect survivors' privacy and avoid victim-blaming.
- **Policy integration:** Calls for integrated policies that require a cooperative approach from multiple government and non-government entities.

(Council of Europe, 2011)

As of October 2023, the Istanbul Convention has been signed and/or ratified by 26 OECD countries (see Table 9.1); however, a recent report from independent monitoring body GREVIO (Group of Experts on Action Against Violence Against Women and Domestic Violence) found that many countries are failing to uphold best practice standards (Council of Europe, 2022b). The OECD (2023b) has argued that more needs to be done to integrate service delivery for DVA survivors across health and social care sectors.

INTEGRATED SERVICE DELIVERY

The OECD (2023b) describes integrated service delivery (ISD) as a means of ensuring that individuals who experience abuse receive coordinated care across various sectors, including health, housing, social services, and the justice system. The pervasive nature of DVA means that survivors often have complex needs that extend beyond their immediate physical safety. Some may turn to the police and seek legal help, particularly when children are involved. Many also share financial and housing links to their perpetrators, and a lack of access to money and suitable accommodation can represent a significant barrier to leaving abusive relationships (Women's Aid, 2020). Evidence from England and Wales suggests that more than half (52%) of DVA survivors need support to attain safe and stable living environments, with many facing additional barriers due to their complex needs, for example, physical disability, mental ill-health, and immigration-related concerns (SafeLives, 2018). Since the passage of the Domestic Abuse Act 2021, local authorities in England have a legal duty to provide accommodation-based support to DVA survivors and their children. However, recent data show that many women continue to be excluded from services because of gatekeeping practices, most commonly from housing officers, which introduce unnecessary hurdles for those seeking support (Solace Women's

TABLE 9.1 Policies and Strategies to Address Violence against Women and/or Domestic Violence and Abuse across the OECD

	Context			Policy, practice, and awareness							
				Violence against women strategies included in national policy				Specific DVA practices included in clinical guidelines			
								Recommended by WHO*		Not recommended by WHO*	
	Istanbul Convention[1]	Lifetime prevalence of DVA[2†]	Attitudes towards DVA[3†]	Media campaigns/ awareness raising initiatives[46]	Multi-sectoral action plan[5‡]	Training programme for health providers[6‡]	Risk assessment/ management processes and main actors[7§]	First-line support for survivors[8‖]	Selective screening/ clinical enquiry[9¶]	Mandatory reporting[10#]	Universal screening[11††]
Australia	N/A	23.0	6.8	Yes	Yes	Yes	Unknown	Unknown	Unknown	Unknown	Unknown
Austria	Ratified	15.0	4.0	Yes	Yes	Unknown	Yes – P	Unknown	Unknown	Unknown	Unknown
Belgium	Ratified	22.0	2.5	Unknown	Yes	Yes	No	Unknown	Unknown	Unknown	Unknown
Canada	N/A	44.1	13.6	Unknown	Yes	Yes	Unknown	Unknown	Unknown	Unknown	Unknown
Chile	N/A	21.0	31.3	Yes	Yes	Yes	Unknown	Yes	Yes	Yes	Yes
Colombia	N/A	30.0	12.3	No	Yes	Yes	Unknown	Yes	No	No	No
Costa Rica	N/A	27.0	3.0	Yes	Yes	Yes	Unknown	Yes	Yes	Yes	No
Czechia	Signed	22.0	2.6	Yes	Yes	Yes	Yes – P, VSS	Unknown	Unknown	Unknown	Unknown
Denmark	Ratified	23.0	0.0	Unknown	Yes	Yes	Y – P	Yes	Unknown	Unknown	Unknown
Estonia	Ratified	21.0	17.8	Yes	Yes	Yes	Yes – P, PPS, SS, SW, VSS	Yes	No	Yes	No
Finland	Ratified	23.0	13.2	Yes	Yes	Unknown	Yes – HP, P, SS, VSS	No	No	Yes	Yes
France	Ratified	22.0	5.5	Yes	Yes	Yes	No	Yes	Yes	No	Yes
Germany	Ratified	21.0	2.5	Unknown	Yes	Yes	No	Unknown	Unknown	Unknown	Unknown
Greece	Ratified	18.0	5.0	Unknown	Yes	Unknown	No	Unknown	Unknown	Unknown	Unknown
Hungary	Signed	19.0	11.5	Unknown	Yes	Yes	Yes – Varies by institution type	Unknown	Unknown	Unknown	Unknown
Iceland	Ratified	21.0	Unknown	Unknown	Yes	Unknown	Unknown	Unknown	Unknown	Unknown	Unknown
Ireland	Ratified	16.0	1.4	Unknown	Yes	Yes	Yes – HP, P, PPS, SS	Unknown	Unknown	Unknown	Unknown
Israel	Neither signed nor ratified	Unknown	14.9	Yes	Unknown	Unknown	Unknown	Yes	Yes	Yes	Yes
Italy	Ratified	16.0	6.1	Yes	Yes	Unknown	No	Yes	Yes	Yes	No
Japan	N/A	20.0	7.8	Unknown	Yes	Unknown	Unknown	Unknown	Unknown	Unknown	Unknown
Korea	N/A	16.5	41.1	Unknown	Unknown	Unknown	Unknown	Unknown	Unknown	Unknown	Unknown

(Continued)

TABLE 9.1 Policies and Strategies to Address Violence against Women and/or Domestic Violence and Abuse across the OECD (Continued)

	Context			Policy, practice, and awareness								
					Violence against women strategies included in national policy			Specific DVA practices included in clinical guidelines				
								Recommended by WHO*		Not recommended by WHO*		
	Istanbul Convention[1]	Lifetime prevalence of DVA[2†]	Attitudes towards DVA[3†]	Media campaigns/awareness raising initiatives[4§]	Multi-sectoral action plan[5‡]	Training programme for health providers[6‡]	Risk assessment/management processes and main actors[7§]	First-line support for survivors[8¶]	Selective screening/clinical enquiry[9¶]	Mandatory reporting[10¶]	Universal screening[11¶]
Latvia	Signed	25.0	1.9	Yes	Unknown	Yes	No	Unknown	Unknown	Unknown	Unknown
Lithuania	Signed	22.0	1.4	Yes	Yes	Unknown	Yes – P	Yes	Yes	Yes	Yes
Luxembourg	Ratified	20.0	4.0	Yes	Yes	Partially	No	Yes	Yes	No	Yes
Mexico	N/A	24.0	31.8	Yes	Yes	Yes	Unknown	Yes	Yes	Yes	No
Netherlands	Ratified	21.0	7.1	Unknown	Yes	Unknown	Yes – HP, SW, VSS	Unknown	Unknown	Unknown	Unknown
New Zealand	N/A	23.0	2.9	Unknown	Yes	Yes	Unknown	Unknown	Unknown	Unknown	Unknown
Norway	Ratified	20.0	11.1	Yes	Yes	Unknown	Unknown	Yes	Yes	No	Yes
Poland	Ratified	13.0	9.7	No	Yes	Unknown	Yes – HP, P, SS, VSS	Yes	Yes	Yes	Yes
Portugal	Ratified	18.0	2.5	Yes	Yes	Unknown	Unknown	Yes	Yes	Yes	Yes
Slovak Republic	Signed	18.0	5.5	Yes	Yes	Yes	Yes – P, VSS	Unknown	Unknown	Unknown	Unknown
Slovenia	Ratified	18.0	17.1	No	Yes	Yes	Yes – P, SW, VSS	No	Yes	Yes	Yes
Spain	Ratified	15.0	9.6	Yes	Yes	Yes	Yes – P, PPS, VSS	Yes	Yes	Yes	Yes
Sweden	Ratified	21.0	13.1	Yes	Yes	Unknown	Yes – P, PPS, SS, VSS	Unknown	Unknown	Unknown	Unknown
Switzerland	Ratified	12.0	14.1	Unknown	Yes	Unknown	Unknown	Unknown	Unknown	Unknown	Unknown
Türkiye	Denounced	32.0	6.0	Yes	Yes	Yes	Yes – P, SS	Yes	Yes	Yes	Unknown
United Kingdom	Ratified	24.0	12.3	Unknown	Yes	Yes	Yes – P, VSS	Unknown	Unknown	Unknown	Unknown
United States	N/A	26.0	13.9	Unknown	Unknown	Yes	Unknown	Unknown	Unknown	Unknown	Unknown

Abbreviations: DVA = domestic violence and abuse; N/A = not applicable; WHO = World Health Organization. For main actor abbreviations, see footnote 7.

'Unknown' indicates that data were unavailable, unclear, and/or unusable (e.g., due to issues of translation) from the cited sources.

1   Council of Europe (2023a). 'N/A' indicates Council of Europe non-member states. Israel, an observer state, was invited to accede the Istanbul Convention in 2022, but as of October 2023, it had neither signed nor ratified the treaty (Council of Europe, 2023b).

2   The percentage of women who have experienced physical and/or sexual violence from an intimate partner at some time in their life.

3   The percentage of women who agree that a husband/partner is justified in beating his wife/partner under certain circumstances.

4   Violence against women mass media campaigns or awareness raising initiatives are available in national policy.

5   Existence of a multisectoral action plan for violence against women. This refers to policies or strategies that span multiple sectors, including government and non-government institutions, and that encompass gender equality measures inclusive of violence (see WHO, 2021b).

6   Violence against women training programme for health sector workers is available in policy. 'Yes' indicates the availability of a comprehensive training programme; 'Partially' indicates the availability of a policy that omits certain information (see WHO, 2021b).

7   Risk assessment/management processes are standardised and/or regulated at national level. Main actors: HP = health providers; P = police; PPS = prison and/or probation services; SS = social services; SW = social workers; VSS = victim support services. Social services and social workers captured separately as per the original dataset(s). Only main actors subject to standardised and/or regulated processes, as indicated in cited sources, are included. Not an exhaustive list; see cited sources for complete data. Risk assessment/management processes differ across the four UK nations (see European Institute for Gender Equality, 2019).

8   Where available, national-level clinical guidelines/protocols include the provision of first-line support to survivors by health providers. This includes respecting survivors' autonomy, listening without pressure, offering comfort, and making connections to other services (see WHO, 2021b).

9   Where available, national-level clinical guidelines/protocols include selective or clinical enquiry for DVA by health providers. This involves asking questions when a patient presents with signs or symptoms of DVA (see WHO, 2021b).

10 Where available, national-level clinical guidelines/protocols include mandatory reporting of DVA by health providers. This can apply to actual or suspected DVA, regardless of survivor consent (see WHO, 2021b).

11 Where available, national-level clinical guidelines/protocols include universal screening for DVA by health providers. This involves asking women about DVA in *all* healthcare encounters, regardless of signs/symptoms or concerns (see WHO, 2021b).

*   WHO clinical and policy guidelines (2013).

†   Data obtained from OECD (2023c) except for Korea (lifetime prevalence), which was obtained from OECD (2020). Note that OECD violence against women indicator data stem from other primary sources and may have been collected at an earlier date. The values presented here reflect those described by the cited OECD sources, accessed in October and November 2023. UK data on DVA lifetime prevalence pertain to the four nations of England, Scotland, Wales and Northern Ireland, while DVA attitudes data pertain to Great Britain only (England, Scotland and Wales).

‡   Data obtained from WHO Sexual, Reproductive, Maternal, Newborn, Child and Adolescent Health Survey (2018–2019), publicly available (see WHO, 2023). UK data pertain to the four nations of England, Scotland, Wales and Northern Ireland.

§   Data obtained from the European Institute for Gender Equality (2019) and OECD (2023b). In cases of discrepancy, OECD (2023b) data prioritised for recency.

¶   Data obtained from WHO Sexual, Reproductive, Maternal, Newborn, Child and Adolescent Health Survey (2018–2019), available on request from WHO.

Aid, 2022). These practices range from requiring police corroboration of applicants' experiences of abuse – despite government guidance advising against this – to inappropriately enforcing 'local connection' rules, where survivors are made to reside in the same area as their abuser(s) (Women's Aid, 2020). Some local authorities have even been known to approach perpetrators directly to obtain evidence. In a survey administered by London-based charity Solace Women's Aid (2022), 11% of frontline DVA workers and housing providers reported seeing this type of gatekeeping. Beyond the emotional traumas inflicted by having their testimonies dismissed or doubted, this practice exposes survivors to the considerable risk of retaliatory violence.

Many organisations have called for consistency in the training provided to housing officers and other statutory agency workers, to improve duty awareness, and reduce the harms caused by trauma-insensitive practices. However, these obligations must also extend to other professional groups who encounter DVA in their work. Health and social care workers are often the first professional point of contact for survivors, and with the move towards ISD, having an awareness of the 'bigger picture' of DVA and its related services, will mean that professionals are better placed to support, guide, and advocate. At a minimum, these efforts can help to mitigate the barriers survivors face as they attempt to navigate multiple, disjointed services, at a time when many, are at their most vulnerable. In some cases, effective professional support can mean the difference between life and death. Unfortunately, UK evidence shows that survivors rarely receive the support they need when they first reach out to professionals. A 2015 review of DVA data from England and Wales found that it took most survivors (85% of 5,358) five attempts within a 12-month period to finally receive effective help (SafeLives, 2015). This statistic only captures those who approached the police, emergency department staff, and/or general practitioners, and the figure would likely be higher, if it included other help-seeking avenues, such as housing and children's social services.

Clearly, strategies are needed to improve service integration and increase professionals' ability to respond effectively, in the context of local and national policy frameworks, to elevate standards of care in the UK. Exploring how other nations handle service integration and professional responses can offer valuable insights for the UK, revealing opportunities to innovate and tailor solutions specific to UK challenges.

BOX 9.1 CASE STUDY

Elena, 32, and her 10-year-old daughter, Rosa, were brought to the attention of social services after Rosa's school reported consistent absences and concerns about her development. Rosa has cerebral palsy and uses a walker to help with mobility issues, and over the years, her condition has often resulted in time off school for hospital appointments and other planned treatments. However, Elena – who was usually proactive about keeping the school informed – has been notably less communicative recently. One teacher observed that the absences had increased since Elena and Rosa moved in with Elena's new partner, Mark, three months earlier.

When a social worker, Natalie, makes a home visit, she finds that living conditions in the second-floor flat are poorly suited to Rosa's needs. Elena discloses that Mark has become overbearing, often undermining her decisions for Rosa's care and dictating how finances, including adaptations for the flat, should be handled. She also confides to Natalie that Mark has created a narrative, suggesting Elena is 'exaggerating' Rosa's needs for sympathy, causing her to question her own judgment.

After reading the case study, imagine that you are the professional responding to Elena and consider the following:

- What words or phrases might you use to describe the abuse Elena is experiencing?
- Can you identify any risk factors that could increase Elena's susceptibility to abuse? How might these issues intersect and consequently shape the options available to her and Rosa?
- How is Rosa likely to be impacted by Mark's behaviour towards Elena?
- What actions would you take in this scenario?

For more information, you can access guidance from SafeLives (2015) for UK professionals who do not work in DVA specialist services.

LEARNING FOR THE UK

Table 9.1 provides an overview of selected DVA and other violence against women policies and strategies across all 38 OECD member states. The policy indicators captured in this table are by no means a comprehensive summary of each country's efforts to address DVA, nor do the missing data necessarily represent gaps in the countries' policy frameworks. However, these data do provide an opportunity to review the characteristics of certain strategies in place across the OECD and consider the implications of these approaches – both positive and negative – for health and social care professionals in the UK.

BOX 9.2 EXAMINING PATTERNS

Take a moment to examine the patterns in Table 9.1. Do any aspects stand out to you as particularly significant? Write down your observations and consider how these patterns might inform your understanding of the issues presented. Once you have noted your thoughts, continue reading the text below.

AWARENESS RAISING, MULTI-SECTORAL COLLABORATION, AND PROFESSIONAL TRAINING

Of the 23 countries where data were available on the existence of public awareness campaigns to transform gender attitudes, only three did not have at least one such intervention included in national policy. However, while awareness raising is highlighted in the Istanbul Convention as a key component of prevention, evidence demonstrates that media campaigns are often ineffective in isolation (WHO, 2019). Instead, strategies which actively engage communities and deliver targeted education have shown promising outcomes for challenging harmful attitudes, with international evidence linking these strategies to reduced DVA incidence (Leight et al., 2023). Such interventions include education initiatives for 'at risk' groups, including pregnant women (Miller et al., 2011) and adolescents (Wolfe et al., 2009), and social marketing or edutainment developed for specific audiences (De Filippo et al., 2023).

In some cases, awareness campaigns have been developed to target professional groups – including law enforcement, legal, education, healthcare, and social workers – independent of the formal in-service training these groups receive. A 2017 report by GREVIO highlighted the role of such campaigns in improving police and social workers' responses to stalking and rape in Denmark, noting that Danish law enforcement agents do not typically receive training on these issues, before entering the workforce (Council of Europe, 2017). However, it is also important to note that measures like this should complement, and not replace, standardised protocols, and formal education for professionals.

Despite all 22 OECD countries with available data indicating that health provider training is included in their national policies, the quality and implementation of training can vary considerably. In-service training on DVA, and the wider forms of violence against women, has yet to be made compulsory for health and social care professionals in many countries throughout Europe, although some have passed laws to address this (Council of Europe, 2022a). Other countries, including Sweden, have focused their efforts on educating student cohorts before they enter the workforce (Council of Europe, 2019). A 2018 UK study found that, while most medical schools delivered some teaching on DVA, most teaching leads considered it insufficient (Potter and Feder, 2018), a conclusion echoed in research on other pre-graduate professional groups (Sammut et al., 2022). Yet, regardless of when and where education is delivered, there is little doubt about the need for robust training in this area, particularly in the context of enhancing service integration.

Multi-agency cooperation has reportedly been hampered in some countries due to differences in professionals' understanding of violence against women. In Belgium, for example, this has been attributed to the failure of some services to emphasise gender dynamics in their training, resulting in a misalignment in the objectives and priorities of professionals working in different sectors (Council of Europe, 2020). Similar training gaps in Finland, Italy, and Spain's health and social care sectors have been linked to less effective support for survivors, with GREVIO citing Finnish professionals' limited awareness as contributing to discrimination against survivors from cultural minorities and those with disabilities (Council of Europe, 2022a).

In a report on DVA service integration, the OECD (2023b) highlighted guidelines from Australia's National Research Organisation for Women's Safety (ANROWS, 2016) which, among other priorities, emphasises the need for shared principles among partnering agencies. To achieve this goal, innovative approaches have been introduced across OECD member states, including formalised networking strategies in Canada, hospital-based multidisciplinary centres in Korea, and co-located services (where multiple sector providers operate from one location) across much of Europe and North America (Council of Europe, 2022a). Another approach can be seen in Denmark, where professionals who provide specialist support to survivors (for example, in women's refuges) deliver training to other sectors, including law enforcement and social services (Council of Europe, 2017). Beyond the benefits of establishing multisectoral connections, the expertise of these professionals means they are uniquely positioned to educate and guide other disciplines, situating key information about DVA in the context of its 'big picture'.

SPECIFIC PRACTICES INCLUDED IN CLINICAL GUIDELINES

Though several OECD countries have national policies for addressing violence against women within the health sector, many include practices, which do not align with WHO (2013) guidelines. As shown in Table 9.1, countries with available data indicated, often, that mandatory reporting and universal screening were included in their national clinical guidelines. In Türkiye, for example, all public institutions that provide support to survivors are legally mandated to report violence to law enforcement and the courts, regardless of risk level or consent (Council of Europe, 2022a). Practices such as these are known to affect women's help-seeking behaviours, and they are discouraged by numerous specialised agencies including GREVIO and WHO. Similar mandatory reporting obligations, including among health professionals, have been identified in Italy and the Netherlands (Council of Europe, 2022a). In contrast, several health sector policies include the provision of first-line support, which outlines minimum care standards, and centres on the principles of survivor-centred care, including respect for privacy and autonomy.

BOX 9.3 DELIVERING FIRST-LINE SUPPORT

In its 2013 clinical guidelines, WHO introduced the mnemonic 'LIVES' – Listen, Inquire about needs, Validate survivor's experience, Enhance her safety, and facilitate Support – to guide professionals in delivering first-line support. Consider how you would follow these steps upon receiving an abuse disclosure, including any barriers you might encounter and how these could be addressed.

Universal screening for DVA also diverges from WHO (2013) recommendations. This approach involves healthcare providers routinely asking all women about violence, regardless of whether any signs or symptoms suggest abuse. While studies have shown that screening does increase DVA identification, many argue that there is insufficient evidence to justify universal screening across all healthcare settings (O'Doherty et al., 2015). Among other issues, this approach demands a level of expertise that would be difficult for professionals to achieve considering widespread training challenges. Expecting an undertrained workforce to ask all women about DVA also risks turning screening into a tick-box exercise, causing staff to become overstretched, and potentially reducing the effectiveness of their responses to survivors who do disclose abuse (WHO, 2013). England's National Institute for Health and Care Excellence (NICE) has issued guidance (PH50) and quality standards (QS116) recommending that clinicians adopt a targeted approach (or 'selective enquiry') in most clinical settings, based on concerns or clinical presentation. However, universal screening is recommended in high-risk areas such as emergency, maternity, sexual health, substance abuse, mental health, and child and vulnerable adult services. Several tools exist to facilitate DVA screening, and many countries have standardised risk assessment strategies at the national level, within and outside of the health sector, as shown in Table 9.1.

BOX 9.4 DVA RISK FACTORS

The risk factors associated with DVA can be classified in a number of ways. One approach considers risk in terms of individual, relational, community, and societal circumstances, while other classifications focus on the distinction between dynamic (changeable) and static (unchangeable) risk. For this activity, begin by writing a list of DVA risk factors that you might encounter in practice, using the first classification framework to capture risks at multiple levels. Next, identify which factors are dynamic and which are static, and consider how they might influence one another across different levels, from individual to societal. For more information, see the European Institute for Gender Equality (2019) report.

BOX 9.5 IDENTIFYING RECOMMENDATIONS

- *All* professionals who encounter DVA need access to consistent and regular training opportunities. This education can (and ideally should) begin before they enter workforce, and where possible, involve groups with specialist knowledge.
- Strategies for fostering effective multiagency cooperation, including formalised networking and co-located services, can provide an important step towards streamlining support for survivors.
- Effective DVA prevention requires integrated strategies that combine public awareness campaigns with community mobilisation and targeted group education. In all cases, strategies should include a focus on intersectional discrimination and emphasise the importance of accommodating diverse needs.
- Above all, a survivor-centred approach is essential. While interpretations of 'best practice' may vary, this guiding principle remains constant. An awareness of how to provide first-line support can serve as a useful starting point for students and professionals.

CONCLUSION

This chapter has provided an overview of DVA policy and practice across the OECD, focusing on selected issues that relate to the practice of health and social care workers. As the first point of contact for many survivors, these professionals serve not only as responders, but also as advocates, educators, and intermediaries among a network of wider support services. By critically examining global policies and evidence, professionals will be better placed to innovate survivor-centred practices that reflect the best of international approaches. The ultimate goal of these efforts is to foster an environment in which all survivors are met with the support, respect, and resources they need to navigate their journey towards safety and healing.

RESEARCH POINTS AND REFLECTIVE EXERCISES

- Consider the possible sources of support available to individuals who are experiencing DVA and write down a list of organisations (national and local to you) that could be potential referral points for service users. If unsure, you can refer to statutory guidance issued by the Home Office (2022).
- Please read McKinlay et al.'s (2023) paper, then reflect upon the impact of COVID-19 on DVA in the UK.
- Please read chapter 5 of Home Office (2022), and then discuss the importance of an understanding of intersectionality in understanding survivors' experiences of DVA, and barriers to accessing services.

REFERENCES

ANROWS. (2016). Meta-evaluation of Existing Interagency Partnerships, Collaboration, Coordination and/or Integrated Interventions and Service Responses to Violence against Women. Available at: www.anrows.org.au/publication/meta-evaluation-of-existing-interagency-partnerships-collaboration-coordination-and-or-integrated-interventions-and-service-responses-to-violence-against-women-final-report/ (Accessed: 30 October 2023).

Birchall, J. and Choudhry, S. (2022). 'I was Punished for Telling the Truth': How Allegations of Parental Alienation are used to Silence, Sideline and Disempower Survivors of Domestic Abuse in Family Law Proceedings. *Journal of Gender-Based Violence*, 6 (1): 115–131. https://doi.org/10.1332/239868021X16287966471815

Council of Europe. (2011). Explanatory Report to the Council of Europe Convention on Preventing and Combating Violence Against Women and Domestic Violence. Available at: https://rm.coe.int/1680a48903 (Accessed: 29 October 2023).

Council of Europe. (2017). GREVIO Baseline Evaluation Report: Denmark. Available at: https://rm.coe.int/grevio-first-baseline-report-on-denmark/16807688ae (Accessed: 30 October 2023).

Council of Europe. (2019). GREVIO Baseline Evaluation Report: Sweden. Available at: https://rm.coe.int/grevio-inf-2018-15-eng-final/168091e686 (Accessed: 30 October 2023).

Council of Europe. (2020). GREVIO Baseline Evaluation Report: Belgium. Available at: https://rm.coe.int/grevio-report-on-belgium/16809f9a2c (Accessed: 30 October 2023).

Council of Europe. (2022a). Midterm Horizontal Review of GREVIO Baseline Evaluation Reports. Available at: https://rm.coe.int/prems-010522-gbr-grevio-mid-term-horizontal-review-rev-february-2022/1680a58499 (Accessed: 20 September 2023).

Council of Europe. (2022b). 3rd General Report on GREVIO's Activities - January to December 2021. Available at: https://rm.coe.int/prems-055022-gbr-2574-rapportmultiannuelgrevio-texte-web-16x24/1680a6e183 (Accessed: 17 September 2023).

Council of Europe. (2023a). Chart of Signatures and Ratifications of Treaty 210. Available at: www.coe.int/en/web/conventions/full-list (Accessed: 17 September 2023).

Council of Europe. (2023b). Treaty List for a Specific State: Israel. Available at: www.coe.int/en/web/conventions/full-list (Accessed: 29 October 2023).

De Filippo A., Bellatin, P., Tietz, N., Grant, E., Whitefield, A., et al. (2023). Effects of Digital Chatbot on Gender Attitudes and Exposure to Intimate Partner Violence Among Young Women in South Africa. *PLOS Digital Health*, 16 (2): 10; e0000358. https://doi.org/10.1371/journal.pdig.0000358

Deosthali, P. B., Rege, S. and Arora, S. (2022). Women's Experiences of Marital Rape and Sexual Violence Within Marriage in India: Evidence from Service Records. *Sexual and Reproductive Health Matters*, 29 (2). https://doi.org/10.1080/26410397.2022.2048455

Domestic Abuse (Scotland) Act. (2018). Available at: www.legislation.gov.uk/asp/2018/5/contents/enacted (Accessed: 7 November 2023).

Domestic Abuse Act. (2021). Available at: www.legislation.gov.uk/ukpga/2021/17/part/1/enacted (Accessed: 9 September 2023).

Domestic Abuse and Civil Proceedings Act (Northern Ireland). (2021). Available at: www.legislation.gov.uk/nia/2021/2/contents (Accessed: 7 November 2023).

Elizabeth, V. (2020). The Affective Burden of Separated Mothers in PA(S) Inflected Custody Law Systems: A New Zealand Case Study. *Journal of Social Welfare and Family Law*, 42 (1): 118–129. https://doi.org/10.1080/09649069.2020.1701943

Epstein, D. and Goodman, L. (2019). Discounting Women: Doubting Domestic Violence Survivors' Credibility and Dismissing Their Experiences. Georgetown Law Faculty Publications and Other Works. Available at: https://scholarship.law.georgetown.edu/facpub/2037 (Accessed: 2 November 2023).

European Institute for Gender Equality. (2019). *Risk Assessment and Management of Intimate Partner Violence in the EU*. Available at: https://data.europa.eu/doi/10.2839/39960 (Accessed: 2 November 2023).

Feresin, M. (2020). Parental Alienation (Syndrome) in Child Custody Cases: Survivors' Experiences and the Logic of Psychosocial and Legal Services in Italy. *Journal of Social Welfare and Family Law*, 42 (1): 56–67. https://doi.org/10.1080/09649069.2019.1701924

Heise, L., Greene M. E., Opper, N., Stavropoulou, M., Harper, C., et al. (2019). Gender Inequality and Restrictive Gender Norms: Framing the Challenges to Health. *The Lancet*, 393 (10189): 2440–2454. https://doi.org/10.1016/S0140-6736(19)30652-X

Home Office. (2022). Domestic Abuse Statutory Guidance. Available at: www.gov.uk/government/consultations/domestic-abuse-act-statutory-guidance (Accessed: 16 October 2023).

Leight, J., Cullen, C., Ranganathan M. and Yakubovich A. (2023). Effectiveness of Community Mobilisation and Group-Based Interventions for Preventing Intimate Partner Violence Against Women in Low- and Middle-Income Countries: A Systematic Review and Meta-Analysis. *Journal of Global Health,* 20 (3): 04115. https://doi.org/10.7189/jogh.13.04115.

McKinlay, A. R., Simon, Y. R., May, T., Fancourt, D. and Burton, A. (2023). How Did UK Social Distancing Restrictions Affect the Lives of Women Experiencing Intimate Partner Violence During the COVID-19 Pandemic?: A Qualitative Exploration of Survivor Views. *BMC Public Health*, 23 (1): 123. https://doi.org/10.1186/s12889-023-14987-3

Miller, E., Decker, M. R., McCauley, H. L., Tancredi, D. J., Levenson, R. R., et al. (2011). A Family Planning Clinic Partner Violence Intervention to Reduce Risk Associated with Reproductive Coercion. *Contraception*, 83 (3): 274–280. https://doi.org/10.1016/j.contraception.2010.07.013

National Institute for Health and Care Excellence. (2014). Domestic Violence and Abuse: Multi-Agency Working. PH50. Available at: www.nice.org.uk/guidance/ph50 (Accessed: 2 November 2023).

National Institute for Health and Care Excellence. (2016). Domestic Violence and Abuse. QS116. Available at: www.nice.org.uk/guidance/qs116 (Accessed: 2 November 2023).

O'Doherty L., Hegarty, K., Ramsay, J., Davidson, L. L., Feder, G., et al. (2015). Screening Women for Intimate Partner Violence in Healthcare Settings. *Cochrane Database of Systematic Reviews* 2015, 7: CD007007. https://doi.org/10.1002/14651858.CD007007.pub3

O'Donohue, W., Benuto, L. T. and Bennett, N. (2016). Examining the Validity of Parental Alienation Syndrome. *Journal of Child Custody*, 13: (2–3): 113–125. https://doi.org/10.1080/15379418.2016.1217758

OECD. (2020). Gender, Institutions and Development (Edition 2019): OECD International Development Statistics (database). Available at: https://doi.org/10.1787/ba5dbd30-en (Accessed: 26 October 2023).

OECD. (2023a). Gender, Institutions and Development (Edition 2023): OECD International Development Statistics (database). Available at: https://doi.org/10.1787/7b0af638-en (Accessed: 14 September 2023).

OECD. (2023b). Supporting Lives Free from Intimate Partner Violence: Towards Better Integration of Services for Victims/Survivors. Available at: https://doi.org/10.1787/d61633e7-en (Accessed: 26 October 2023).

OECD. (2023c). Violence Against Women (Indicator). Available at: https://doi.org/10.1787/7f420b4b-en (Accessed: 26 October 2023).

Potter, L. C. and Feder, G. (2018) Domestic violence teaching in UK medical Schools: A Cross-Sectional Study. *The Clinical Teacher*, 15 (5): 382–386. https://doi.org/10.1111/tct.12706

SafeLives. (2015). Getting it Right First Time. Available at: https://safelives.org.uk/policy-evidence/getting-it-right-first-time (Accessed: 16 October 2023).

SafeLives. (2018). Safe at Home: Homelessness and Domestic Abuse. Available at: https://safelives.org.uk/spotlight-5-homelessness-and-domestic-abuse (Accessed: 15 October 2023).

SafeLives. (2021). Understanding Court Support for Victims of Domestic Abuse. Available at: https://domesticabusecommissioner.uk/wp-content/uploads/2021/06/Court-Support-Mapping-Report-DAC-Office-and-SafeLives.pdf (Accessed: 17 September 2023).

Sammut, D., Ferrer, L., Gorham, E., Hegarty, K., Kuruppu, J., et al. (2022). Healthcare Students' and Educators' Views on the Integration of Gender-Based Violence Education into the Curriculum: A Qualitative Inquiry in Three Countries. *Journal of Family Violence*, 38: 1469–1481. https://doi.org/10.1007/s10896-022-00441-2

Solace Women's Aid. (2022). Priority Need for Housing for Survivors of Domestic Abuse: One Year On. Available at: www.solacewomensaid.org/policy-campaigns/safe-housing-survivors (Accessed: 16 October 2023).

Taylor, J., Bradbury-Jones, C., Kroll, T. and Duncan, F. (2013) Health Professionals' Beliefs about Domestic Abuse and the Issue of Disclosure: A Critical Incident Technique Study, *Health and Social Care in the Community*, 21(5): 489–499. https://doi.org/10.1111/hsc.12037

Violence against Women, Domestic Abuse and Sexual Violence (Wales) Act. (2015). Available at: www.legislation.gov.uk/anaw/2015/3/contents/enacted (Accessed: 7 November 2023).

Wolfe, D. A., Crooks, C., Jaffe, P., Chiodo, D., Hughes R., et al. (2009). A School-Based Program to Prevent Adolescent Dating Violence: A Cluster Randomized Trial. *Archives of Pediatrics and Adolescent Medicine*, 163 (8): 692–699. https://doi.org/10.1001/archpediatrics.2009.69

Women's Aid. (2020). The Domestic Abuse Report 2020: The Hidden Housing Crisis. Available at: www.womensaid.org.uk/wp-content/uploads/2020/06/The-Domestic-Abuse-Report-2020-The-Hidden-Housing-Crisis.pdf (Accessed: 15 October 2023).

WHO. (2013) Responding to Intimate Partner Violence and Sexual Violence against Women: WHO Clinical and Policy Guidelines. Available at: https://iris.who.int/handle/10665/85240 (Accessed: 28 October 2023).

WHO. (2019). RESPECT Women: Preventing Violence Against Women. Available at: https://iris.who.int/bitstream/handle/10665/312261/WHO-RHR-18.19-eng.pdf (Accessed: 30 October 2023).

WHO. (2021a). Violence Against Women Prevalence Estimates, 2018. Available at: https://apps.who.int/iris/handle/10665/341337 (Accessed: 9 September 2023).

WHO. (2021b). Addressing Violence against Women in Health and Multisectoral Policies: A Global Status Report. Available at: https://iris.who.int/bitstream/handle/10665/350245/9789240040458-eng.pdf?sequence=1 (Accessed: 28 October 2023).

WHO. (2023). Sexual and Reproductive Health and Rights: National Policies. Available at: https://platform.who.int/data/sexual-and-reproductive-health-and-rights/national-policies (Accessed: 28 October 2023).

CHAPTER 10

Substance Use and Policy across the OECD

....

John Foster and Betsy Thom

INTRODUCTION

UK substance use policy is often dependent upon what is politically acceptable and expedient. Arguably, this is encapsulated in the attitudes of wider society to drugs and drug users. The first section of the chapter will contrast recent English and Scottish alcohol policy focusing upon minimum unit pricing. The second section will focus upon differences between the UK and Portuguese illicit drug policy. The latter is far more permissive. The chapter focuses on the recent UK decision to criminalise nitrous oxide use and introduce some contemporary UK data concerning drug-related mortality trends. It will conclude by drawing lessons for UK substance use policy and provide some further reading suggestions and areas to be developed for a more nuanced understanding of minimum unit pricing and the impact of criminalising different types of drugs and drug users.

MINIMUM UNIT PRICING: SCOTTISH AND ENGLISH POLICY

In 2007, concern about heavy alcohol consumption and a high prevalence of alcohol-related harms in Scotland prompted a newly established advocacy group, Scottish Health Action on Alcohol Problems (SHAAP) to suggest a 'novel'[1] pricing policy – minimum unit pricing (MUP) – to control the availability of cheap alcohol (Butler et al., 2017). The idea was that a MUP of 50p per unit of alcohol would address problems, associated with the consumption of cheap alcohol, and would specifically target heavy drinkers, rather than the population as a whole (Holmes et al., 2014). The policy was supported by the Scottish National Party (SNP) and public health advocates, and an Alcohol Minimum Pricing (Scotland) Bill was passed in 2012. There was fierce opposition from influential sectors of the alcohol industry, in particular from the Scottish Whiskey Association, and a debate around whether the

DOI: 10.4324/9781003343608-12

intervention was a 'whole population' measure, intended to lower consumption and related harms in the population as a whole, or an intervention targeted at heavier drinkers with negligible impact on moderate drinkers. A lengthy legal battle ensued involving the Scottish courts, the European Court of Justice, and the UK Supreme Court. Finally, in 2017, the UK Supreme Court ruled in favour of MUP, and it was implemented in May 2018 (Butler et al., 2017).

The situation in England was quite different. Although MUP was announced as UK Government policy in the 2012 Alcohol Strategy, by July 2013, the UK Government announced it was abandoning the policy. The reason given was because it did not have 'enough concrete evidence that [it] would be effective in reducing harms associated with problem drinking ... without penalising people who drink responsibly ... we are not rejecting MUP – merely delaying it until we have conclusive evidence that it will be effective' (Home Office, 2013; Nicholls and Greenaway, 2015). Analyses of the failure to implement MUP in England highlight some key differences between the policy contexts and the dynamics of policy stakeholders in the two countries (Hawkins and McCambridge, 2020).

As a devolved nation, Scotland has the power to make laws on certain issues, while other issues are reserved matters, which can only be decided by the UK government. Regarding alcohol policy, fiscal measures, such as taxation on alcohol and restrictions on broadcast advertising, are reserved so the Scottish Government is unable to use those methods to address alcohol consumption. However, they do assert control over public health policy and, based on the argument that MUP addressed a public health problem and was legal under European Union (EU) trade regulations, it became formal government policy in Scotland. We briefly note three specific ways in which differences between the two countries influenced the fate of MUP, the political context, the acceptance of evidence for MUP, and stakeholder influence.

Political Context

The political context differed markedly between the two countries and influenced how alcohol- related issues were perceived. It has been argued that the Scottish government had already recognised the problems related to alcohol consumption and had concerns over the rates of alcohol-related liver cirrhosis deaths, which exceeded the rates in most other western European countries (Leon and McCambridge, 2006). However, there was little action until SNP came to power in May 2007 as a minority government. The SNP allied itself to the public health perspective on alcohol. It framed the alcohol issue as a public health problem which would be responsive to price, availability, and marketing restrictions[2] and soon after becoming a majority government in 2011, passed the Alcohol (Minimum Pricing) (Scotland) Bill in 2012.

In England, by comparison, alcohol was framed largely as crime related. Placed under the Home Office by the 2010 coalition government, the focus was on alcohol fuelled public disorder and the potential for licensing reform to address the problems (Butler et al., 2017). However, issues of price were not entirely ignored. In 2007, the Department of Health commissioned a research group at Sheffield University to examine the evidence on the relationship between alcohol-related harm, price, and promotions (Booth et al., 2008). The work of the group had an important influence on Scottish policy but failed to provide sufficient evidence to change government thinking in England.

Acceptance of the Evidence for MUP

Evidence for MUP emerged from work commissioned in 2007 by the UK Department of Health. A research team at Sheffield University was asked to model the effects of implementing different pricing and promotion options, including setting a minimum unit price. They concluded that, irrespective of income, moderate drinkers were little affected by a minimum unit price of £0·45, with the greatest effects noted for harmful drinkers. Large reductions in consumption in this group would coincide with substantial health gains in morbidity and mortality, related to reduced alcohol consumption. (Holmes et al., 2014). The research proved to be controversial as the prospective econometric modelling approach was perceived as divorced from 'real-world' circumstances. However, further support for MUP came from Canada, which had already implemented a form of minimum alcohol pricing, although different approaches were adopted across the various Canadian provinces (Stockwell et al., 2013; Zao et al., 2013). Based on the Canadian experience, Stockwell et al. (2013) concluded that, 'comprehensive and simultaneous increases in minimum prices across all beverage types and adjusted for alcohol content have a strong impact on total alcohol consumption. Further, this type of policy is close to the ideal of a fixed minimum price for a unit of alcohol as is being proposed in the UK' (p. 13).

The evidence was not without dispute. A review of 26 peer reviewed studies and seven studies from grey literature cast doubt on the strength of the evidence for MUP. It found that the overall quality of the evidence was variable. A considerable proportion of the evidence base had been produced by a small number of research teams, and the quantitative uncertainty in many estimates or forecasts, was often poorly communicated outside the academic literature (Boniface et al., 2017). Nonetheless, it was generally agreed that price-based alcohol policy interventions, such as MUP, are likely to reduce alcohol consumption, alcohol-related morbidity, and mortality.

The evidence from the modelling studies appeared at first to sway UK government policy in that the coalition government announced support for MUP in 2012. However, as mentioned above, intention did not translate to action; the policy was abandoned and attention shifted to issues of alcohol-related disorder rather than health (Butler et al., 2017). In Scotland, by contrast, there had been a consolidation of evidence from various sources since the start of the millennium. The World Health Organization (WHO) principles and a publication by Babor et al. (2003) fed into the growing support for a public health vision of alcohol policy and influenced the recommendations of an influential report from an expert group convened in 2007. Their report recommended setting a minimum price based on the strength of the alcohol (Gillan and McNaughton, 2007). Although the subsequent path towards inclusion of MUP on to the policy agenda was not entirely smooth, the scene was set, and the available evidence became the basis for further action (Katikireddi et al., 2014a).

Stakeholder Influence

Several researchers have considered the multiple influences on MUP policy and why it became government policy in Scotland but not in England – research evidence is only one factor. How different stakeholder groups interpret the evidence, use it to gain public and policy attention, and build on it to construct a convincing argument for their preferred policy option is extremely important.[3] Fergie et al. (2018) divide the stakeholder groups into two camps – opponents and proponents of MUP. Keeping in mind that governments are, themselves, stakeholders, two large stakeholder coalitions assumed a key part in this process, the alcohol industry and public health advocates.

These coalitions both included a range of different organisations, charities, and interest groups. In the case of the industry, the majority opposed MUP but some, for instance, the Scottish Licensed Trade Association, supported MUP. Public health advocates, for example, the Alcohol Health Alliance (England) and Scottish Health Action on Alcohol (Scotland) were positioned on the proponent side. Both opponents and proponents used similar techniques to gain support for their views, providing a consistent view of the evidence, aiming to influence public opinion and lobbying governments. These stakeholder groups operated across England and Scotland, but in the former, industry pressure had higher influence, while in the latter, public health advocates proved stronger (Katikireddi et al., 2014b; McCambridge et al., 2014).

PORTUGUESE DRUG POLICY VERSUS THE UK DECISION TO CRIMINALISE NITROUS OXIDE USE

Before drawing comparisons between Portuguese and UK drug policy approaches, the chapter will briefly discuss the tension between abstinence-based treatments and harm reduction. Ideally, drug treatment services should aim to encourage service users to become drug free, but for many, this is an extremely difficult and an unrealistic goal to achieve. Hence, many drugs treatment services work on a principle of harm reduction. Harm Reduction International (2022) state that 'harm reduction refers to policies, programmes, and practices that aim to minimise the negative health, social and legal impacts associated with drug use, policies and laws. It focuses on positive change and on working with people without judgement, coercion, discrimination, or requiring that people stop using drugs as a precondition of support'. Tackling drugs is perceived as a public health issue rather than a criminal justice one. It was this shift that underpinned the UK's response to HIV/AIDS (Stimson, 1990). Harm reduction for drug users typically assumes the form of substitute prescribing, the provision of condoms, or clean injection works. However, there is another aspect to harm reduction which is often forgotten and encapsulated in Marlatt's (1996) paper

'Come as You Are', based on a Nirvana song; his point being that one of the key aims of harm reduction was to keep drug users in contact with drug services. Public Health England (2018) found that every one pound invested in drug services saved four pounds in social, economic, health and criminal justice costs. Over 10 years, this figure increases to £21.

The Portuguese Situation

In 2001, Portugal decriminalised drug use and moved towards treating drug use as a health-related challenge rather than a criminal justice one. This meant that the personal use of drugs would no longer carry a prison sentence or a criminal record. 'Personal use' was defined as less than 1 gram for heroin, 2 grams for cocaine and 25 grams of 'herbal cannabis' (EMCDDA, 2015). These drugs can be confiscated and there can be some administrative sanctions or community service. As part of these changes, district-level panels were established consisting of legal, health, and social support professionals, who could suspend some of these sanctions. The aim was to educate drug users as to the risks and encourage referral to drug treatment services (Stevens and Hughes, 2016). Portugal was not the first country to decriminalise drugs, but it is perceived as the template for others to follow (Talking Drugs, Release, and IDPC 2020). Over thirty countries have now introduced some form of decriminalisation (City Wide, 2024).

Why Was Harm Reduction Introduced?

Portugal was an authoritarian dictatorship, ruled by Antonio de Oliveira Salazar, until 1968, and the first penal drug-related offences were introduced in 1970 under what was termed the New State (Estado Novo). This regime ended in 1974, and in 1976, a new Portuguese Constitution was enacted. At least in part, these greater freedoms resulted in more visible drug use. The reaction of the Portuguese government was to set up several organisations to understand the rise in drug use and respond to it. In 1981, the first reports of the HIV/AIDS virus were reported in the USA. Portugal was particularly negatively hit by the HIV/AIDS epidemic because of a rise in heroin use during the 1990s. By 1999, Portugal had the highest rate of HIV in intravenous (IV) drug users in the European Union. At this point, there were 2,000 new cases per year; the population of Portugal was circa 10 million.

It was estimated that in Europe, there were 50,000–100,000 heroin users at the turn of the century (EMCDDA, 2020a). This led to the first National Strategy for the Fight Against Drugs based on harm reduction principles which eventually led to the decriminalisation of drug use. It is also important to note that the drugs market across Europe is now characterised by the relatively widespread availability of a broader range of drugs than previous, which are often available at high potency and purity. Also, increased drug availability has been accompanied by a wider diversity in the substances on the illicit drug market, which has exposed consumers to a broader spectrum of psychoactive substances, for example, new synthetic drugs, where knowledge of the health impact cannot yet be determined. The person who was responsible for driving the decriminalisation policy was Dr Joel Castel-Branco-Goulao, and he has stated that one of the main reasons that harm reduction initiatives were acceptable, was that heroin use in particular was spread throughout society. Ferreira (2017) provides a 'Guardian Long Read', which describes the situation at the turn of the century in the Algarvein Portuguese health services.

What was the Impact of the Policy Change?

This section is indebted to Transform (2021) which provides the graphs, tables, and statistics which are referred to here in their peer-reviewed report.

- **Drug related deaths:** From 2000 to 2005, these rates decreased from 0.5% per 100,000 population to 1.5%. Over the following years, drug deaths have risen, but there have also been falls, and they remain below the 2001 levels (EMCDDA, 2020b). The 2001 Portuguese drug death rates were comparable to the EU average but from 2001–2011 EU rates increased while Portuguese rates decreased. Since 2011, both Portuguese and EU rates have risen, but in 2019, the Portuguese death rates were six deaths per million compared to an EU average of 23.7 per million.
- **Crime:** In 2001, 70% of reported Portuguese crime was linked to drug use, well above the European average at the time. Over the past 20 years in the EU, the proportion of the drug-related offences rose from 14% to 18%. The 2019 Portuguese figure was 15.9%, again below the European average (Council of Europe, 2022). Most of this decline occurred in the first decade since decriminalisation, but there are some possible issues with the data that should be acknowledged. Firstly, there has been a rise in the Portuguese prison population, which means that the percentage drop in drug related offences, may not be a reduction in reality. Félix et al. (2017) suggests there has been a reduction in drug seizures; however, again these figures must be treated with some caution. The reduction in seizures may be a result of fewer drugs being in circulation or a result of reduced police activity.
- **Drug use:** Over the past two decades, levels of Portuguese drug use have consistently scored below the European average. This is particularly marked in the age range 15–34 (EMCDDA, 2020c). However, these figures have been criticised, and it is now believed that the WHO and United Nations Office on Drugs and Crime figures, which focus upon drug use within the past 12 months, and last month respectively, are more reliable indicators (Hughes and Stevens, 2012). These suggest a small rise in drug use especially in the past year, mainly in drug users aged over 25 (SICAD, 2014). However, consumption figures are not necessarily an indicator of risk and Portugal now has more 'high risk' opioid users than most European counterparts (EMCDDA, 2020d). This is lower than in 2001 when decriminalisation was enacted. Furthermore, data from Portuguese substance misuse treatment services suggest that 90%

of individual cases are not problematic (SICAD, 2020). There has also been a shift towards drug education specifically focused on school age children and drug use in Portuguese children is lower than most European countries. This is now a consistent trend (ESPAD, 2019).

- **HIV and hepatitis B and C transmission:** The main driver of the decriminalisation policy was the spread of HIV/AIDS in Portugal. In 2001, over half of the new HIV diagnoses was due to IV use in Europe were Portuguese. The primary response to this was to introduce programmes providing clean injection works with the aim of reducing infections. By 2019, the equivalent percentage of new EU HIV diagnoses in Portugal was less than 2% (European Centres for Disease Prevention and Control, 2020). Hepatitis B and C rates have decreased consistently since 2001 (EMCDDA, 2020e).

- **Treatment and harm reduction:** Linked to Portuguese drugs decriminalisation was a commitment to expanding treatment services. Between 2000 and 2009 the number of outpatient treatment units increased from 50 to 79 (Stevens and Hughes, 2016) but the numbers of individuals in drug treatment services reduced (SICAD, 2020). The most likely explanation for this is a reduction in resources, following the global financial crisis, and a reduction in overall problematic drug use. EMCDDA data indicate that admissions for opioid users have fallen while cannabis users have increased (EMCDDA, 2019). Despite this, the level of individuals on opioid substitution in Portugal (a form of harm reduction) is higher than the European average (EMCDDA, 2020d). Harm reduction is key to Portuguese drug policy, but despite this, the number of syringes being distributed, has halved since 2003. However, the latest annual figures of 1.3 million is still one of the highest in the EU (EMCDDA, 2020f).

Comparison with UK

In this section, we will briefly consider the recent UK policy concerning a specific drug, namely nitrous oxide, and thereafter introduce some recent UK drug mortality and morbidity data.

Nitrous Oxide

In contrast to Portugal, UK politicians have found it difficult to encourage any policies which condone illicit drug use. The Home Office (2023) provides the rationale for making nitrous oxide a Class C drug. This is an invisible gas also known as 'laughing' gas and it can be misused to achieve a 'high'. It can cause neurological damage and there is a risk of suffocation and death. However, the main driver for the change, is anti-social behaviour, and the litter presented from discarded balloons and cannisters (Home Office, 2023). Data from the NHS in 2021 (NHS Digital, 2022) found that nitrous oxide was the third most used drug in England and Wales in 16–59-year-olds. The Office for National Statistics (2022) confirmed that nitrous oxide is a very popular drug with young people. It will now be a criminal offence to inhale nitrous oxide with the intention of getting 'high'. In reality, this means being in possession of a nitrous oxide cannister for anything other than dental or medical purposes. There will then be a tariff of increasing penalties.

Unlawful possession can result in an 'unlimited fine', visible community service, or a caution, all resulting in a criminal record. Serious repeat offenders can face up to two years in prison or an unlimited fine or both. Supplying the drug can result in up to 14 years in prison (repeat offenders) or an unlimited fine or both (Home Office, 2023). In a narrative review of the international evidence, Van Amsterdam et al. (2022) confirmed that nitrous oxide use, particularly in young people, was becoming increasingly problematic, and they recommended limiting availability. However, the BMJ (2023) reports that several experts have raised some concerns. Most notably, the Advisory Council for the Misuse of Drugs (ACMD), have expressed strong reservations against the decision to make nitrous oxide a Class C drug on the grounds that this is not evidence based. Although no longer part of the ACMD, Professor David Nutt (head of the Centre for Neuropharmacology, Imperial College London) expands on the reasoning of the ACMD (Science Media Centre, 2023). He pointed out that in the UK, there is one death per year in the UK from around one million nitrous oxide users compared to 28,000 deaths annually in 40 million users of alcohol. Another concern he outlined was that if individuals were discouraged from using small easy to detect cannisters, they may achieve their 'high' from larger gas cylinders, which will contain larger doses of nitrous oxide, and be harder to detect. It is also possible that the individuals could transfer their drug use to other more harmful drugs, such as cannabis, amphetamines, or legal highs.

Another commentator who has expressed concerns is Dr David Caldicott, a senior lecturer at the Australia University Medical School (Science Media Centre, 2023). His concern is that criminalising nitrous oxide use is 'less' about 'medical concern' but is 'social control'. He pointed out that zero tolerance drug policies rarely work because individuals use drugs, because they like the drug effects, and enforcement is extremely difficult, especially with younger people. He also points out, that it is common for many young people to take substances to achieve a 'high', but most transition out of this, on their own volition. Legislation, therefore, is often problematic as it may create potential criminals out of people who are likely to be transient nitrous oxide users. Although, some individuals may proceed to problematic drug users, most do not. Moreover, the Home Office (2023) have reported that nitrous oxide use has fallen from 2020 to 2022 (Home Office, 2023). As previously stated, the ACMD has not recommended making nitrous oxide a Class C drug because there is insufficient evidence of its health harms. It is informative to look at the Home Office (2023) for the government response. This document makes it clear that the government are entitled to look at other factors. They are explicit that the main rationale for the change is tackling anti-social behaviour. Most worryingly, they are ignoring the concerns of Dr Caldicottt, that this is often a self-limiting developmental stage, and potentially creating criminals, whose only criminal behavour is their transient drug use.

Mortality and Social Inequalities

To conclude we will consider some concerning recent UK drug data. Figures from the Office of National Statistics (2023a) have shown a rise in drug-related deaths in England and Wales to record levels. There has been a slight fall in male deaths, but female deaths have increased, and this is particularly marked for drug-related suicides. Most of the deaths were the result of a mixture of substances, and opiates were still implicated in nearly half of the deaths, but the biggest increase was in cocaine related deaths. These have now increased for 11 successive years as cocaine has become more affordable (as it has become increasingly available) and potent.

There is also a strong link in drug-related mortality with health and social inequalities and the largest percentage of deaths were in northwest and northeast England. The age range with the most deaths was 40–49 and this is rising. The most likely explanation for this is that these were opiate users born in the 1970s and the premature death rates are related to poor mental health, respiratory, and cardiovascular function, which are exacerbated by continuing drug use. This makes them particularly vulnerable to accidental overdoses. Also, coroners are likely to record the death as being related to the physical cause, meaning that reported drug related deaths are likely to be an underestimate. It should be noted that the increase in drug-related deaths is in the context of an overall fall in drug use (Office of National Statistics, 2023b). There are also heightened links between poverty, deprivation, increasing inequalities, and problem drug use, which may be connected to fragile family bonds, psychological discomfort, fewer employment opportunities, and less community resources and social capital. Poverty often also increases the harm for a given level of drug use. Marginalisation and stigma of low-income and vulnerable groups, more susceptible to drug use, also assume a role, and can encompass closes processes of social control among family and friends, actions by health and social care services, and policy decisions made by governments (Room, 2005).

The Black Report (GovUK, 2021) was commissioned to advise the government how to effectively respond to the increasing drug-related deaths and the main recommendation is to increase the availability of drug treatment. This is in the context of long-term austerity and reductions to local authority drug and alcohol services of 29% since 2010 (Rehab UK, 2022) and only 50% of those, who might benefit, are in in contact with treatment services (Office for Health Improvement and Disparities, 2024). The chapter concludes with a quote from the policy officer of Transform who are a charity campaigning for greater drug decriminalisation in response to the latest drug mortality statistics.

> Both this government and Labour need to rethink their 'tough on drugs' position as we mark another devastating record in drug-related deaths. Their current policies are causing harm to people in our communities. Instead, they must treat drug policy as a health issue, stop criminalising people who use drugs and start exploring legal regulations.
>
> *(Kincova, 2023)*

CONCLUSION

Despite the claim that policy is, and must be, 'evidence-based', MUP illustrates clearly, the importance of the wider political context, and how policy decisions are the outcome of a complex process, influenced by a range of factors, other than the findings from research studies. Portuguese drug policy, based upon treating drug use as a health, rather than a 'criminal concern' has witnessed drug use and drug mortality/morbidity rates in Portugal which are consistently lower than most EU countries. In contrast, the UK has recently decided to make nitrous oxide use a criminal offence primarily because it presents a public nuisance. UK drug policy occurs within the context of two main political parties finding it difficult to be 'soft' on drugs and with drug treatment being focused on those who are dependent. The recent drug-related mortality statistics suggests this may be misguided.

RESEARCH POINTS AND REFLECTIVE EXERCISES

* Explore how Wales and Northern Ireland have approached the idea of using minimum unit pricing. What has influenced their policy decisions and what are the implications for health and social care service provision?
* Many people feel the reason some types of drugs are criminalised, and others are not, relates to risk and are evidence based. Over time certain drugs have emerged as legal and good (alcohol) and bad (heroin) for varied reasons, often rooted in racism, class and fear of the other (nitrous oxide). Please read Gossop (2013) to gain insight into some of these issues and how they have informed much of UK and US drug policies.
* National drug statistics are collected through the Office of National Statistics. Please look at these two-web links (Office of National Statistics, 2021; 2023c) to gain an appreciation into how national public health data is collected.

NOTES

1   You can find out more about how taxation and pricing has been used as a way of regulating alcohol production, distribution and consumption – and how and why different forms of regulation have been used across the centuries (see Yeomans, 2019).
2   Recommendations proposed by the World Health Organization (see WHO, 2012). The latest evidence for the recommended actions is discussed in WHO (2021).
3   Based on an analysis of newspaper coverage, Fergie et al. (2018) provide a good overview of the different stakeholder groups involved in the MUP debates.

REFERENCES

Babor, T. F., Casswell, S., Graham, K., Huckle, T. and Livingston, M., et al. (2003). *Alcohol: No Ordinary Commodity. Research and Public Policy*, 3rd edn. Oxford: Oxford University Press.
BMJ. (2023). Experts Condemn Government's Decision to Criminalise Nitrous Oxide as 'Not Evidence Based'. *BMJ*, 380: 723. doi: https://doi.org/10.1136/bmj.p723
Boniface, S., Scannell, J. W. and Marlow, S. (2017). Evidence for the Effectiveness of Minimum Unit Pricing of Alcohol: A Systematic Review and Assessment Using the Bradford Hill Criteria for Causality. *BMJ Open* 7: e013497. doi:10.1136/bmjopen-2016-013497 1

Booth, A., Meier, P., Stockwell, T., Sutton, A., Wilkinson, A., et al. (2008). *Independent Review of the Effects of Alcohol Pricing and Promotion: Systematic Reviews.* Sheffield: School of Health and Related Research, University of Sheffield.

Butler, S., Elmeland, K., Nicholls, J. and Thom, B. (2017). *Alcohol, Power and Public Health.* London: Routledge.

City Wide. (2024). Which Countries have Decriminalised and How? Available at: www.citywide.ie/decriminalisation/countries.html (Accessed: 16 January 2024).

Council of Europe. (2022). Council of Europe Annual Penal Statistics. Available at: https://wp.unil.ch/space/space-i/annual-reports/ (Accessed: 12 January 2024).

EMCDDA. (2000). National Report 2000: Portugal. Available at: www.emcdda.europa.eu/html.cfm/index34675EN.html_en (Accessed: 16 January 2024).

EMCDDA. (2015). Threshold Quantities for Drug Offences. Available at: www.emcdda.europa.eu/publications/topic-overviews/threshold-quantities-for-drug-offences/html_en (Accessed: 1 December 2023).

EMCDDA. (2019). Portugal Country Drug Report 2019. Available at: www.emcdda.europa.eu/publications/country-drug-reports/2019/portugal_en (Accessed: 2 December 2023).

EMCDDA. (2020a). Statistical Bulletin 2020 – Overdose Deaths. Available at: www.emcdda.europa.eu/data/stats2020 (Accessed: 20 December 2023).

EMCDDA. (2020b). Statistical Bulletin 2020 – Prevalence of Drug Use. Available at: www.emcdda.europa.eu/data/stats2020/gps_en (Accessed: 20 December 2023).

EMCDDA. (2020c). Statistical Bulletin 2020 – Problem Drug Use. Available at: www.emcdda.europa.eu/data/stats2020/pdu_en (Accessed: 16 January 2024).

EMCDDA. (2020d). Statistical Bulletin 2020 – Drug-Related Infectious Diseases. Available at: www.emcdda.europa.eu/data/stats2020/drid_en (Accessed: 20 December 2023).

EMCDDA. (2020e). Statistical Bulletin 2020 – Health and Social Responses. Available at: www.emcdda.europa.eu/data/stats2020/hsr_en (Accessed: 21 December 2023).

EMCDDA. (2020f). *European Drug Report 2020: Key Issues.* Luxembourg: Publications Office of the European Union.

ESPAD. (2019). Results from the European School Survey Project on Alcohol and Other Drugs. Available at: www.emcdda.europa.eu/publications/joint-publications/espad-report-2019_en (Accessed: 1 December 2023).

European Centres for Disease Prevention and Control. (2020). HIV/AIDS Surveillance in Europe Available at: www.ecdc.europa.eu/sites/default/files/documents/hiv-surveillance-report-2020.pdf (Accessed: 12 January 2024).

Félix, S., Tavares, A. and Portugal, P. (2017). Going After the Addiction, Not the Addicted: The Impact of Drug Decriminalization in Portugal. Available at: https://docs.iza.org/dp10895.pdf (Accessed: 22 November 2023).

Fergie, G., Leifeld, P., Hawkins, B. and Hilton, S. (2018). Mapping Discourse Coalitions in the Minimum Unit Pricing for Alcohol Debate: A Discourse Network Analysis of UK Newspaper Coverage. *Addiction*, 114 (4): 741–753 https://doi.org/10.1111/add.14514.

Ferreira S. (2017). Portugal's Radical Drugs Policy is Working: Why hasn't the World Copied It? The Guardian, 5 December. Available at: www.theguardian.com/news/2017/dec/05/portugals-radical-drugs-policy-is-working-why-hasnt-the-world-copied-it (Accessed: 22 November 2023).

Gillan, E. and McNaughton, P. (2007). Alcohol: Price, Policy, and Public Health, SHAAP. Available at: www.shaap.org.uk/images/UserFiles/File/Price%20Report%20-%20Summary.pdf (Accessed: 22 November 2023).

Gossop, M. (2013). *Living With Drugs*, 7th edn. London: Routledge/Taylor and Francis Group.

GovUK. (2021). Independent Report: Review of Drugs – Phase Two. Available at: www.gov.uk/government/publications/review-of-drugs-phase-two-report (Accessed: 22 November 2023).

Harm Reduction International. (2022). What is Harm-Reduction? Available at: https://hri.global/what-is-harm-reduction/(Accessed: 22 October 2023).

Hawkins, B. and McCambridge, J. (2020). Policy Windows and Multiple Streams: An Analysis of Alcohol Pricing Policy in England. *Policy and Politics*, 48 (2): 315–333. https://doi.org/10.1332/030557319X15724461566370

Holmes, J., Meng, Y., Meier, P., Brennan, A., Angus, C., et al. (2014). Effects of Minimum Unit Pricing for Alcohol on Different Income and Socioeconomic Groups: A Modelling Study. *Lancet*, 383: 1655–1664. https://doi.org/10.1016/S0140-6736(13)62417-4

Home Office. (2013). Next Steps Following the Consultation on Delivering the Government's Alcohol Strategy. Available at: https://data.parliament.uk/DepositedPapers/Files/DEP2013-1301/Alcohol_consultation_response_report_v3.pdf (Accessed: 12 October 2023).

Home Office. (2023). Media Fact Sheet: Nitrous Oxide Ban. Available at: https://homeofficemedia.blog.gov.uk/2023/10/18/media-fact-sheet-nitrous-oxide-ban/ (Accessed: 22 October 2023).

Hughes, C. E. and Stevens, A. (2012). A Resounding Success or a Disastrous Failure: Re-Examining the Interpretation of Evidence on the Portuguese Decriminalisation of Illicit Drugs. *Drug and Alcohol Review*, 31(1): 101–113. https://doi.org/10.1111/j.1465-3362.2011.00383.x.

Katikireddi, S. V., Bond, L. and Hilton. S. (2014a). Changing Policy Framing as a Deliberate Strategy for Public Health Advocacy: A Qualitative Policy Case Study of Minimum Unit Pricing of Alcohol. *Milbank Quarterly*, 92 (2): 250–283. https://doi.org/10.1111/1468-0009.12057.

Katikireddi, S. V. Hilton, S., Bonell, C. and Bond, L. (2014b). Understanding the Development of Minimum Unit Pricing of Alcohol in Scotland: A Qualitative Study of the Policy Process. *PLoS ONE*, 269 (3): e91185. https://doi.org/10.1371/journal.pone.0091185.

Kincova, E. (2023) Rising Drug Deaths Show Why UK Government (and Opposition) Must Rethink Their 'Tough on Drugs' Position. Press Release, 19 December. Available at: https://twitter.com/TransformDrugs/status/1737157404968579100 (Accessed: 2 September 2023).

Leon, D. A. and McCambridge, J. (2006). Liver Cirrhosis Mortality Rates in Britain from 1950 to 2002: An Analysis of Routine Data. *The Lancet*, 7: 367 (9504): 52–56. https://doi.org/10.1016/S0140-6736(06)67924-5.

Marlatt, G. A. (1996). Harm Reduction: Come as You Are. *Addictive Behaviors*, 21 (6): 779–788. https://doi.org/10.1016/0306-4603(96)00042-1.

McCambridge, J., Hawkins, B. and Holden, C. (2014). The Challenge Corporate Lobbying Poses to Reducing Society's Alcohol Problems: Insights from UK Evidence on Minimum Unit Pricing. *Addiction*, 109 (2): 199–205. https://doi.org/10.1111/add.12380.

NHS Digital. (2022). Smoking Drinking and Drug Use among Young People in England, 2021. Available at: https://digital.nhs.uk/data-and-information/publications/statistical/smoking-drinking-and-drug-use-among-young-people-in-england/2021/part-8-drug-use-prevalence-and-consumption#:~:text=In%202021%2C%2018%25%20(confidence,down%20from%2024%25%20in%202018.&text=17%25%20of%20boys%20and%2019,fell%20from%2025%25%20in%202018 (Accessed: 12 October 2023).

Nicholls, J. and Greenaway, J. (2015). What is the Problem? Evidence, Politics and Alcohol Policy in England and Wales, 2010–2014. *Drugs: Education Prevention and Policy*, 22 (2): 135–142. https://doi.org/10.3109/09687637.2014.993923

Office for Health Improvement and Disparities. (2024). Fingertips: Public Health Data. Available at: https://fingertips.phe.org.uk/search/drug (Accessed: 12 October 2023).

Office of National Statistics. (2021). Looking After and Using Data for Public Benefit. Available at: www.ons.gov.uk/aboutus/transparencyandgovernance/datastrategy/lookingafterandusingdataforpublicbenefit#:~:text=The%20statistics%20are%20for%20the,and%20Wales%20every%2010%20years (Accessed: 1 October 2023).

Office of National Statistics. (2022). Drug Misuse in England and Wales: Ending June 2022. Available at: www.ons.gov.uk/peoplepopulationandcommunity/crimeandjustice/

articles/drugmisuseinenglandandwales/yearendingjune2022#:~:text=the%20last%20 year-,In%20the%20year%20ending%20June%202022%2C%202.6%25%20of%20 adults%20aged,ending%20March%202020%20(2.1%25) (Accessed: 1 October 2023).

Office of National Statistics. (2023a). Deaths Related to Drug Poisoning in England and Wales: 2022. Available at: www.ons.gov.uk/peoplepopulationandcommunity/birthsdeath sandmarriages/deaths/bulletins/deathsrelatedtodrugpoisoninginenglandandwales/2022 registrations#drug-poisonings-in-england-and-wales (Accessed: 9 October 2023).

Office of National Statistics. (2023b). Census 2021: Data and Analysis from Census 2021: Drug Misuse in England and Wales: Year Ending March 2023. Available at: www.ons.gov.uk/ peoplepopulationandcommunity/crimeandjustice/articles/drugmisuseinenglandandwales/ yearendingmarch2023#:%7E:text=1.-,Main%20points,(around%201.1%20million%20 people) (Accessed: 9 October 2023).

Office of National Statistics. (2023c). How We Collect and Use Data at the ONS. Available at: www.ons.gov.uk/aboutus/usingpublicdatatoproducestatistics/howwecollectandusedata attheons (Accessed: 1 October 2023).

Public Health England. (2018). Alcohol and Drug Prevention, Treatment and Recovery: Why Invest? Available at: www.gov.uk/government/publications/alcohol-and-drug-prevention-treatment-and-recovery-why-invest/alcohol-and-drug-prevention-treatment-and-recovery-why-invest#:~:text=Investing%20in%20drug%20and%20alcohol%20 treatment%20saves%20money&text=Alcohol%20treatment%20reflects%20a%20 return,%C2%A321%20over%2010%20years (Accessed: 1 October 2023).

Rehab UK. (2022). The Impact of 10 Years of Cuts to Addiction Services. Available at: https:// rehabsuk.com/blog/the-impact-of-10-years-of-cuts-to-addiction-services/ (Accessed: 1 August 2023).

Room, R. (2005). Stigma, Social Inequality and Alcohol and Drug Use. *Drug Alcohol Rev*, 24 (2): 143–155. https://doi.org/10.1080/09595230500102434.

Science Media Centre. (2023). Expert Reaction to the News that the Government are to Ban Nitrous Oxide/Laughing Gas as Part of Their Antisocial Behaviour Action Plan. Available at: www.sciencemediacentre.org/expert-reaction-to-the-news-that-the-government-are-to-ban-nitrous-oxide-laughing-gas-as-part-of-their-antisocial-behaviour-action-plan/ (Accessed: 1 August 2023).

SICAD. (2014). Statistical Synopsis: Portugal 2014. Available at: www.sicad.pt/PT/ EstatisticaInvestigacao/Documents/Sinopse%20Estatistica_2014_EN.pdf (Accessed: 1 August 2023).

SICAD. (2020). Statistical Bulletin 2018: Illicit Substances. P7. Available at: www. sicad.pt/BK/EstatisticaInvestigacao/Documents/2020/sinopses/SinopseEstatistica18_ substanciasIlicitas_EN.pdf (Accessed: 1 August 2023).

Stevens, A. and Hughes, C. (2016). Decriminalization and Public Health: Drug and Drug Addiction Policies in Portugal. Available at: www.cairn.info/revue-mouvements-2016-2-page-22.htm (Accessed: 2 August 2023).

Stimson, G. (1990). AIDS and HIV: The Challenge for British Drug Services. *Addiction*, 85 (3): 329–339. https://doi.org/10.1111/j.1360-0443.1990.tb00645.x

Stockwell, T., Zhao, J., Martin, G., Macdonald, S., Valance, K., et al. (2013). Minimum Alcohol Prices and Outlet Densities in British Columbia, Canada: Estimated Impacts on Alcohol Attributable Hospital Admissions. *American Journal of Public Health*, 103 (11): 2014–2020. https://doi.org/10.2105/AJPH.2013.301289

Talking Drugs, Release, and IDPC. (2020). 29 Countries. 49 Models of Drug Decriminalisation. One Handy Web-Tool. Available at: www.talkingdrugs.org/decriminalisation/ (Accessed: 1 August 2023).

Transform. (2021). Drug Decriminalisation in Portugal: Setting the Record Straight. Available at: https://transformdrugs.org/publications/drug-decriminalisation-in-portugal-setting-the-record-straight (Accessed: 25 August 2023).

van Amsterdam, J. G., Nabben, T. and van den Brink, W. (2022). Increasing Recreational Nitrous Oxide Use: Should We Worry? A Narrative Review. *Journal of Psychopharmacology*, 36 (8): 943–950. https://doi.org/10.1177/02698811221082442.

WHO. (2012). European Action Plan to Reduce the Harmful Use of Alcohol 2012–2020 WHO. Available at: www.who.int/europe/publications/i/item/9789289002868 (Accessed: 25 August 2023).

WHO. (2021). Making the WHO European Region SAFER: Developments in Alcohol Control Policies, 2010–2019. Available at: www.who.int/europe/publications/i/item/9789289055048 (Accessed: 25 August 2023).

Yeomans, H. (2019). Regulating Drinking through Alcohol Taxation and Minimum Unit Pricing: A Historical Perspective on Alcohol Pricing Interventions. Regulation and Governance. *Regulation and Governance*, 13 (1): 3–17. https://doi.org/10.1111/rego.12149

Zhao, J., Stockwell, T., Martin, G., Macdonald, S., Valance, K., et al. (2013). The Relationship between Changes to Minimum Alcohol Price, Outlet Densities and Alcohol-Related Death in British Columbia 2002-09. *Addiction*, 108 (6): 1059–1069. https://doi.org/10.1111/add.12139

CHAPTER 11

Health Inequalities and People with Intellectual Disabilities

....

Genevieve Breau

INTRODUCTION

Health and social care for people with intellectual disabilities (often called learning disabilities in the UK) has been shaped by professionals' understanding of disability and how society perceives disabled people. These understandings are often influenced by the medical model of disability. The process of deinstitutionalisation over the past decades, across many countries in the OECD, led to the closing of large institutions and an increase in community-based care for people with intellectual disabilities. Deinstitutionalisation has had a profound impact on how health and social care is delivered to people with intellectual disabilities and may have contributed to the health inequalities they experience. This chapter explores the biomedical model and social models of disability before continuing to discuss deinstitutionalisation and health inequalities for people with intellectual disabilities across the OECD. The concluding section explores reasonable adjustments and initiatives which have been implemented in Australia, Canada, and England to support people with intellectual disabilities in accessing healthcare.

MODELS OF DISABILITY

The biomedical model has been highly influential in how disability has been perceived in western societies and tends to place emphasis on disability as a pathogen which is outside of the 'norm', impacting on a person's 'functioning' and thus requiring medical interventions from 'expert' medical professionals. This medicalisation of disability has led to the equating of disability with dependency, reduced well-being, suffering and ill-health (Krahn et al., 2006) with its focus on 'compulsory able-bodiedness and able-mindedness' (McRuer and Berube, 2006). Moreover, the biomedical model of disability is often perceived as a deficit model, which stresses

DOI: 10.4324/9781003343608-13

individual medically diagnosed impairment as the cause of disability, overlooking how social factors can disable people. Barnes (2016), for example, highlights how in the case of wellbeing, disability per se does not necessarily result in reduced wellbeing. Rather wellbeing for disabled people can be impacted by societal stigma around disability and responses to disability, including dehumanising representations and social inequalities. The biomedical model, therefore, while useful, can often negate how social determinants, social hierarchies, hegemonic social norms, and attitudes, discrimination, stigma, and health inequalities, influence approaches to disability, and the inequities which emerge.

The social model of disability is an alternative to the biomedical model. However, conceptualisations of the model vary across countries, and thus, there are several models which appear under the definition of social models of disability. For example, Nordic countries, often influenced by normalisation theory (see below for a discussion), focus more on a social relative model of disability (although again, there will be differences across Nordic countries) which views disability as existing on a continuum in which the individual and their environment interact. This means that the same individual may have differing experiences because some environments or contexts may create barriers for them, and others may not. Thus, disability in the Nordic models tends to be relative, depending upon context, and occurs when there is a lack of synergy between the person and their environment (Goodley, 2017). This model can be perceived to have impacted definitions of disability such as the 'International Classification of Functioning Disability and Health' (ICF) (WHO, 2002) which defines disability as resulting from the interaction between a person and their environment.

The minority rights model, originating in the USA, is linked to the disability rights movement and focuses on activism and developing positive group identity. The model posits that it is the minority status of disabled people, which leads to their devaluation in society, loss of rights, oppression, discrimination, and segregation. Emphasis is placed on supporting the rights of disabled people to have their voices heard and to initiate systematic change. Disability in the minority rights model 'is not a personal defect or deficiency [but is] primarily the product of a disabling environment' (Hahn, 1991:17); with societal negative attitudes to disability influencing social policies. which in turn, influence the environments, which disabled people live in and how disabled people are responded to.

The social model of disability in the UK (Oliver, 1990) differentiates between impairment (defined as 'significant bodily differences culturally marked as "abnormal"'(Thomas, 2004: 25) and disability (defined as 'the loss or limitation of opportunities to take part in the normal life of the community on an equal level with others due to physical and social barriers') (Barnes, 1991: 2). The model highlights that having an impairment is not inherently disabling with Oliver and Barnes (2012: 22) stating that the model 'breaks the causal link between impairment and disability (with impairment) not the cause of disabled people's economic and social disadvantage'. Rather, disability is perceived as a social construct with people being disabled because of societal failures to remove structural and materialist barriers which oppress and disempower disabled people by limiting social inclusion, opportunities, and participation in society. Disability is, thus, a socially produced injustice and not located within the individual. For the UK social model of disability, structural change is needed to remove these barriers to participation through adaptations, positive action, and attitudinal changes. The focus on the differentiation between impairment and disability in the UK social model of disability, however, has been critiqued with some arguing that impairment itself can seriously limit activity and be disabling, regardless of adjustments made (Shakespeare and Watson, 2001). While there are differences between the social models of disability, they all highlight societal factors, external to the individual, and the impact of disabling environments including attitudes as key to understanding limitations placed on the participation and inclusion of disabled people in society which in turn impact on their wellbeing and quality of life.

BOX 11.1 DEFINITIONS OF DISABILITY

The UK Equality Act (2010) defines disability 'as a physical or mental impairment that has a "substantial" and "long-term" negative effect on [an individual's] ability to do normal daily activities'. This definition has been critiqued as being overly medical and prioritising 'normality' by not considering the social construction of normality (Bunbury, 2019).

The can be contrasted with the human rights and social model influenced definition of the UN Convention on the Rights of Disabled People (United Nations Department of Economic and Social Affairs, 2006) which states that 'disability is an evolving concept and … results from the interaction between persons with impairments and attitudinal and environmental barriers that hinders their full and effective participation in society on an equal basis with others'.

INTELLECTUAL DISABILITIES: DEINSTITUTIONALISATION AND HEALTH INEQUALITIES

Intellectual disabilities are defined, by the World Health Organization (WHO, 2023), as significantly reduced ability to learn new or complex information, and learn or apply new skills, arising before adulthood. It is estimated that 1% of the global population has intellectual disabilities with 85% of this number receiving a diagnosis of mild intellectual disabilities. The remainder of people are diagnosed with moderate or severe/profound intellectual disabilities (APA, 2021). Some individuals with more moderate or severe intellectual disabilities may also have co-occurring health conditions, such as cerebral palsy, autism, and/or visual or hearing impairment. There are multiple causes for intellectual disabilities, which may not be identifiable in each person diagnosed (APA, 2021).

Traditionally, people with intellectual disabilities lived at home in their communities, with families caring for them. However, this changed in many countries across Europe and North America in the eighteenth and nineteenth centuries, with the advent of industrialisation and the rise of capitalism, the era of enlightenment, and the increasing dominance of the biomedical model. For example, Foucault (1975) argues that the rise of the scientific model led to medical professionals exercising considerable power to define reality and what was perceived as 'normal' or 'deviant'. These processes of normalisation, classification, and categorisation led to the exclusion of people deemed 'deviant' in institutions such as asylums (Foucault, 2009). However, over time, concerns were raised regarding whether institutions were best equipped to provide care. For example, both Goffman (1961) and Barton (1959) detailed the negative impacts of institutionalisation on both those who lived in and those who worked in institutions, with Goffman (1961) demonstrating how residents of 'total institutions' were dehumanised and stripped of their identity and choices to comply with the efficient operation of the institution.

The deinstitutionalisation process in many high-income countries (i.e., UK, Canada, Australia, United States) began in the 1950s with dramatic increases in deinstitutionalisation during the 1970s and 1980s. Deinstitutionalisation refers to the process by which people with intellectual disabilities or other conditions (such as mental health or physical disabilities) were moved by government agencies from large institutions to the community, living either with family members, or in smaller facilities staffed by social care providers. This shift from institutional care to community care was underpinned by multiple factors, including a focus on reducing costs as institutional care was perceived as being overly expensive, and theories of human rights, social inclusion, normalisation, and participation. Normalisation theory posits, for example, that the inclusion of people with intellectual disabilities in society, as opposed to in institutions, will bring about increased community participation, quality of life, and self-esteem through 'making available [the] patterns and conditions of everyday life which are as close as possible to the norms and patterns of the mainstream of society' (Wolfensberger, 1972: 28). While social inclusion and human rights arguments focused on the morality of the segregation of citizens from the rest of society, emphasising the often-poor conditions that they lived in and an individual's right to self-determination, human dignity, and choice as well as participation in their communities as full citizens (Committee on the Rights of Persons with Disabilities, 2023).

Although deinstitutionalisation has been on the policy radar for many years, a 2020 report (Šiška and Beadle-Brown, 2020) illustrated that across the European Union approximately 1.5 million people were still living in institutions; with people with intellectual disabilities and complex needs being the most likely to be residents. Worryingly, they highlight little change in these figures over the past 10 years, with small-scale residential units being a minority in terms of care provision. Increases in institutional care were also evident for disabled adults, for example, in France, Lithuania, Luxembourg and Portugal, with no change reported in Poland, Romania, Hungary, Greece, Austria, Bulgaria, Cyprus, and Denmark. Policy on deinstitutionalisation was also found to differ across countries regardless of the type of welfare state, with policy in Ireland and Norway, influenced by the medical model of disability, with poor implementation of policy being evident in Ireland, Italy, Czechia, and

Sweden, and a lack of spending on housing and support evident among most countries. Poor integration of services and partnership working between health, social care, and other agencies, was also reported in Sweden, Ireland, and Germany (Šiška et al., 2018).

Research has highlighted several benefits of community-based living for people with intellectual disabilities including improved quality of life (McCarron et al., 2019) and acquisition of skills (Bredewold et al., 2020). However, deinstitutionalisation and increases in community living can also be associated with some unintended consequences including increases in isolation and victimisation (Bredewold et al., 2020), and potential increases in health inequalities due to lack of access to and responsiveness from mainstream population-based health services. In relation to health inequalities, a study in Australia found that people with intellectual disabilities had higher levels of mortality including preventable deaths, had an increased risk of attending emergency departments, as well as psychiatric readmissions (Reppermund et al., 2019). Another literature review across countries found higher levels of chronic diseases, including diabetes, obesity, cardiovascular diseases, and arthritis, with an increased risk of co-morbidity (Krahn and Fox, 2014).

The COVID-19 pandemic also had a major impact on the health of adults with intellectual disabilities (Jeste et al., 2020; Totsikas et al., 2021) which was compounded by difficulties in accessing health and social care services during this period as well as health conditions which put them at more risk of mortality. However, it should be borne in mind that many of these pre-existing health conditions may be a result of inequality in relation to the social determinants of health, with people with intellectual disabilities, more likely to live in poor housing, in poverty, and have high levels of unmet healthcare need, all contributing to potential pre-existing conditions (Sullivan et al., 2022). Moreover, the association above between increases in isolation and victimisation, rather than being a consequence of deinsitutionalistion itself, could be reflective of societal views towards people with intellectual disabilities. This then leads to increased victimisation, as well as a lack of appropriate funding, to provide support systems to overcome isolation.

The UN Convention on the Rights of Disabled People (United Nations Department of Economic and Social Affairs, 2006) states that 'community services and facilities for the general population [should be] available on an equal basis to persons with disabilities and [should be] responsive to their needs'. However, research indicates that there are issues surrounding availability and responsiveness of mainstream health services for people with intellectual disabilities, leading to unmet need, and contributing to health inequalities - with a report into health inequalities in Australia stating that 'People with intellectual disability are subject to systemic neglect in the Australian health system' (Royal Commission into Violence, Abuse, Neglect and Exploitation of People with Disability, 2020). Research in England has also shown that adults with intellectual disabilities are more likely to die from preventable deaths, which may be associated with a lack of diagnosis, and difficulties in accessing healthcare (Hosking et al., 2016).

Health and social care professionals in mainstream services, for example, may lack training on the health needs of people with intellectual disabilities and how to make reasonable adjustments. This can reduce access to services, including routine screenings for chronic conditions, such as vision and hearing problems, and non-communicable diseases, such as cancer exacerbating health inequalities (Ervin et al., 2014). Moreover, communication differences may mean that some people with intellectual disabilities may experience difficulties in expressing their health needs or having them understood by health professionals and may experience difficulties navigating complicated health and social care systems, including complex inaccessible information (Doherty et al., 2020). In addition, people with intellectual disabilities may experience poor attitudes from staff including, not being listened to, or excluded in decision making around their own care, as well as heightened feelings of fear and embarrassment, due to medical environment, and medical procedures (Doherty et al., 2020). Unmet need may be especially the case if individuals comprise other marginalised identities, such as sexual orientation, race, and ethnicity, or low socio-economic status (Havercamp and Bonardi, 2022) with research from the USA showing that Latinx and non-Latinx black adults, with intellectual disabilities, were more likely to display poorer physical and mental health than their white counterparts (Magaña et al., 2016).

REDUCING HEALTH INEQUALITIES FOR PEOPLE WITH INTELLECTUAL DISABILITIES: REASONABLE ADJUSTMENTS

The UN Convention on the Rights of Disabled People (United Nations Department of Economic and Social Affairs, 2006) and numerous country wide legislation, such as the Americans with Disabilities Act, the Commonwealth Disability Discrimination Act of 1992 in Australia and the UK Equality Act (2010) place emphasis on 'reasonable adjustments' or 'reasonable accommodations' for disabled people, including people with intellectual disabilities. For instance, the UK Equality Act places a statutory duty on public sector organisations that these adjustments should be 'anticipatory' and planned as part of policy and practice. The reasonable adjustment duty, however, has been critiqued, as it is said to not adequately acknowledge how social factors and 'ableist' social norms can contribute to discrimination and barriers in accessing services such as healthcare. For example, while reasonable adjustment focuses on individual adjustment, which is an important part of personalised care, the focus on the individual tends to play down the societal change which is required to tackle discrimination at the structural and cultural level, including social norms. As a result, the concept of reasonable adjustments can be perceived, by some, to reinforce the biomedical model and professional power dynamics as it is often non-disabled professionals who decide what is 'reasonable' or what Oliver (1996: 166) calls 'professionals doing it … to disabled people' with the 'reasonable' being defined in relation to ableist norms, which already disadvantage disabled people (Ma, 2023). Table 11.1 documents some reasonable adjustments which have introduced in relation to people with intellectual disabilities across three countries of the OECD: England, Australia, and Canada.

TABLE 11.1 Healthcare Reasonable Adjustments: Australia, Canada, and England

Country	Examples of reasonable adjustments
Australia	Annual health checks; healthcare passports; roadmap for improving health; use of nurse navigators to ensure co-ordination of care, support self-management and improve health literacy for people with intellectual disabilities; use of direct support staff who are not health professionals to ensure that information is relayed in understandable terms; national disability insurance scheme for funding to support 'reasonable and necessary' support.
Canada	Annual health checks; health passports; recommendations for general practitioners to screen for certain long-term conditions on an annual basis for all patients identified as having intellectual disabilities in some provinces (e.g., Ontario); introduction of Disability Inclusion Action Plan, 2022 (Government of Canada, 2023).
England	Healthcare passports; use of personal health budgets to support choice of care; annual health checks; accessible literature and letters; priority appointments to see health professional; longer appointments to ensure that service user has enough time to express themselves and process information; GP learning disability register; reasonable adjustment flag; adding requirements to summary care records. There are also initiatives such as the STOMP health care pledge to reduce the over-use of psychotropic medicines for people with intellectual disabilities and autism. Following the lead in the USA, Always Events have been introduced to focus on what matters to people with intellectual disabilities in relation to experiences of care. NHS RightCare has been introduced to support people with intellectual disabilities around diabetes needs, for example. Introduction of liaison nurses and disability champions in England and Wales, with the latter acting as an advocate, for the service user, to support reasonable adjustments.

What is evident from Table 11.1 is some convergence between examples of reasonable adjustments across the three countries as consensus emerges around evidence, policy, and practice. However, what is also evident, was that there is a paucity of examples about reasonable adjustments from many OECD countries, which may indicate a lack of priority to the needs of people with intellectual disabilities.

There are some challenges however, in relation to some of the reasonable adjustments discussed in Table 11.1. For example, the use of 'reasonable adjustment flags' to highlight that an individual may have specific needs, has led to debates about the use of flags, including evidence of reluctance to use flags, among some health care workers, leading to variation across settings. There is also little evidence that 'flags' lead to improved care and issues around the exclusion of people who do not have [or want] a medical diagnosis (Kenten et al., 2019). Healthcare passports, which aim to support communication and health literacy between professionals and people with intellectual disabilities, have also been found not to be consistently used, and with information missing in the United Kingdom (Northway et al., 2017). There is also evidence that implementation varies by region in Canada (Heifetz and Lunsky, 2018) and little evidence of any short-term benefit of their use found in a systematic review (Nguyen et al., 2014). Moreover, research on reasonable adjustments in Australia have shown that knowledge about the concept is low among many healthcare professionals (Wilson et al., 2021) and that hospital liaison nurses are not evident in all facilities in England and Wales (Sheehan et al., 2016). The use of extra time for appointments may also face challenges, for example, in Canada, where some health professionals are paid a fee per appointment (Selick et al., 2018).

BOX 11.2 ANNUAL HEALTH CHECKS AND ROADMAPS

One of the many inequalities experienced by adults with intellectual disabilities is the process of diagnostic overshadowing, where chronic diseases such as cancer or type II diabetes are not diagnosed, or diagnosed at a later stage, because health professionals may not be routinely screening for chronic illnesses, and carers (both paid and unpaid) may not realize the symptoms of many chronic diseases. Diagnostic overshadowing may also occur because a health issue is attributed to a person's disability as opposed to a medical issue. Consequently, one intervention that has been widely adopted in the UK, Canada, and Australia is the provision of annual health checks for this group. Annual health assessments, which can include new disease detection, age- and gender-specific preventive screening, and health promotion (Bakker-Van Gijssel et al., 2017) have been shown to lead to increased screening and health promotion activities, are generally acceptable to people with intellectual disabilities and their carers, and can increase awareness about health needs in this population among health professionals conducting the health check (Robertson et al., 2014). In the most recent year that data was available, in 2021–2022, 71.8% of adults with intellectual disabilities in England who were registered with a general practitioner had received an annual health check (NHS Digital, 2022).

The Australian national Roadmap for Improving the Health of People with Intellectual Disability (Australian Department of Health and Care, 2022) aims to better support for people with intellectual disabilities and their families by improving health literacy and supporting self-advocacy for people. The Roadmap calls for the development of new models of healthcare, by identifying, developing, and implementing best practices and more effective use of MBS-funded items (medical services covered by the public system) such as a broader implementation of annual health checks for adults with intellectual disabilities. Within the Roadmap, there is a greater focus on continuity of care, better care coordination, and integration within the health system, and more robust support for healthcare professionals to provide improved care for people with intellectual disabilities. Finally, there is an increasing focus on oral health, capturing better healthcare utilisation data from people with intellectual disabilities, and adapting emergency preparedness due to COVID-19.

CONCLUSION

The deinstitutionalisation of people with intellectual disabilities, and the move towards community care has resulted in the provision of healthcare for this group shifting to the community, thorough the mainstream health system. Difficulties in accessing mainstream healthcare may have led to elevated levels of unmet need for this group and contributed to health inequalities. The social model of health highlights structural, attitudinal, and materialist barriers, which can disempower disabled people, and in the case of healthcare, limit access to health services. This can result in neglect and injustice, exacerbating health inequalities, and impacting on wellbeing. Although reasonable adjustments have been highlighted as key to transforming health services for people with intellectual disabilities, they are often not well implemented. Poor implementation of reasonable adjustments may be a result of a lack of time on the part of health providers, or lack of resources to provide additional individualised care. Thus, innovative ways of providing such tailored care are needed to help reduce these inequalities caused by a suboptimal delivery of reasonable adjustments.

Moreover, poor implementation may be a result of 'ableist' discriminatory attitudes, which are pervasive in society, and more workforce training on this issue should be considered. Morgan and Breau (2024) have argued, in relation to Indigenous peoples, that many interventions which attempt to improve access to healthcare by removing barriers need to be situated in an 'anti-oppressive' framework, which also tackles social exclusion and marginalisation. The minority status of people with intellectual disabilities, and the discrimination, stigma, and structural dis-empowerment, which they often face can be a substantial barrier to access quality services and needs to be addressed. Lastly, the social model of health places emphasis upon hearing the voices of disabled people themselves and healthcare reforms, policy, and practice, should be underpinned by a focus on their active involvement in decision making processes so that health systems are more responsive to their needs.

RESEARCH POINTS AND REFLECTIVE EXERCISES

- Research how health inequities experienced by people with intellectual disabilities were exacerbated during COVID 19 (for example, Henderson et al., 2022; Marquis et al., 2023). Discuss possible reasons for these increases.
- Do you agree with Marquis et al. (2023) that narratives such as the biomedical model of disability, population health approaches and health policies, which focus on economic growth, cause harm to the health of people with intellectual disabilities?
- Research 'reasonable adjustments' (for example, Fisher et al., 2022) and discuss how policy and practice in healthcare can better reflect the social models of disability.

REFERENCES

APA. (2021). What Is an Intellectual Disability? Available at: www.psychiatry.org/patients-families/intellectual-disability/what-is-intellectual-disability#:~:text=Intellectual%20 disability%20affects%20about%201,85%25%20have%20mild%20intellectual%20 disability (Accessed: 18 November 2023).

Australian Government Department of Health. (2021). National Roadmap for Improving the Health of People with Intellectual Disability. Available at: www.health.gov.au/resources/ publications/national-roadmap-for-improving-the-health-of-people-with-intellectual-disability?language=en (Accessed: 23 August 2023).

Bakker-van Gijssel, E., Lucassen, P., Olde Harman, T., Van Son, L., Assendelft, W., et al. (2017). Health Assessment Instruments for People with Intellectual Disabilities – A Systematic Review. *Research in Developmental Disabilities*, 64: 12–24. https://doi.org/10.1016/j.ridd.2017.03.002.

Barnes, C. (1991). *Disabled People in Britain and Discrimination*. London: Hurst.

Barnes, E. (2016). *The Minority Body: A Theory of Disability*. New York: Oxford University Press.

Barton, R. (1959). *Institutional Neurosis*. Bristol: Wright.

Bredewold, F., Hermus, M. and Trappenburg, M. (2020). 'Living in the Community': The Pros and Cons: A Systematic Literature Review of the Impact of Deinstitutionalisation on People with Intellectual and Psychiatric Disabilities. *Journal of Social Work*, 20 (1): 83–116. https://doi.org/10.1177/1468017318793620

Bunbury, S. (2019). Unconscious Bias and the Medical Model: How the Social Model May Hold the Key to Transformative Thinking About Disability Discrimination. *International Journal of Discrimination and the Law*, 19 (1): 26–47. https://doi.org/10.1177/1358229118820742

Committee on the Rights of People with Disabilities. (2023). Statement of the Chair of the Committee at the Closing of the Panel on Deinstitutionalization held on 18 August 2023, in Room XVII, Palais de Nations, Geneva. Available at: https://view.officeapps.live.com/op/view.aspx?src=https%3A%2F%2Fwww.ohchr.org%2Fsites%2Fdefault%2Ffiles%2Fdocuments%2Fhrbodies%2Fcrpd%2Fstatements%2F20230911-stm-deinstitutionalization.docx&wdOrigin=BROWSELINK (Accessed: 25 February 2023).

Doherty, A. J., Atherton, H., Boland, P., Hastings, R., Hives, L., et al. (2020). Barriers and Facilitators to Primary Health Care for People with Intellectual Disabilities and/or Autism: An Integrative Review. *BJGP Open*, 4 (3). bjgpopen20X101030. https://doi.org/10.3399/bjgpopen20X101030

Equality Act c1. (2010). Available at: www.legislation.gov.uk/ukpga/2010/15/contents (Accessed: 23 August 2023).

Ervin, D. A., Hennen B., Merrick, J. and Morad, M. (2014). Healthcare for Persons with Intellectual and Developmental Disability in the Community. *Frontiers in Public Health*, 2 (83). doi:10.3389/fpubh.2014.00083

Fisher, K., Desroches, M. L., Marsden, D., Rees, S., Northway, R., et al. (2022). International Nursing Actions to Reduce Health Inequities Faced by People with Intellectual and Developmental Disability. *OJIN: The Online Journal of Issues in Nursing*, 27 (3): article 7. https://doi.org/10.3912/OJIN.Vol27No03Man07

Foucault, M. (1975). *The Birth of the Clinic: An Archaeology of Medical Perception*. M. Sheridan Smith, trans. New York: Vintage Books.

Foucault, M. (2009). *History of Madness. Trans. Jonathan Murphy and Jean Khalfa, With a Foreword by Ian Hacking*. New York: Routledge.

Goffman, E. (1961). *Asylums. Essays on the Social Situation of Mental Patients and Other Inmates*. Harmondsworth: Penguin.

Goodley, D. (2017). *Disability Studies: An Interdisciplinary Introduction*. London: Sage.

Government of Canada. (2023). *Canada's Disability Inclusion Action Plan*. Available at: www.canada.ca/en/employment-social-development/programs/disability-inclusion-action-plan.html (Accessed: 1 March 2024).

Hahn, H. (1991). Alternative Views on Empowerment: Social Services and Civil Rights. *Journal of Rehabilitation*, 57 (4): 17–19.

Havercamp, S. and Bonardi, A. (2022). Special Issue Introduction: Addressing Healthcare Inequities in Intellectual Disability and Developmental Disabilities. *Intellectual and Developmental Disabilities*, 60 (6): 449–452. doi.10.1352/1934-9556-60.6.449

Heifetz, M. and Lunsky, Y. (2018). Implementation and Evaluation of Health Passport Communication Tools in Emergency Departments. *Research in Developmental Disabilities*, 72: 23–32. https://doi:10.1016/j.ridd.2017.10.010

Henderson, A., Fleming, M., Cooper, S. A., Pell, J. P., Melville, C., et al. (2022). COVID-19: Infection and Outcomes in a Population-Based Cohort of 17,173 Adults with Intellectual Disabilities Compared with the General Population. *Journal of Epidemiology and Community Health*, 76 (6): 550–555. https://doi.org/10.1136/jech-2021-218192

Hosking, F. J., Carey, I. M., Shah, S. M., Harris, T., DeWilde, S., et al. (2016). Mortality Among Adults with Intellectual Disability in England: Comparisons with the General Population. *American Journal of Public Health*, 106 (8): 1483–1490. https://doi.org/10.2105/AJPH.2016.303240

Jeste, S., Hyde, C., Distefano, C., Halladay, A., Ray, S., et al. (2020). Changes in Access to Educational and Healthcare Services for Individuals with Intellectual and Developmental Disabilities During COVID-19 Restrictions. *Journal of Intellectual Disability Research*, 64 (11): 825–833. https://doi.org/10.1111/jir.12776

Kenten, C., Wray, J., Gibson, F., Russell, J., Tuffrey-Wijne, I., et al. (2019). To Flag or Not to Flag: Identification of Children and Young People with Learning Disabilities in English Hospitals. *Journal of Applied Research in Intellectual Disabilities*, 32 (5): 1176–1183. https://doi.org/10.1111/jar.12608

Krahn, G., Hammond, L. and Turner, A. (2006). A Cascade of Disparities: Health and Health Care Access for People with Intellectual Disabilities. *Mental Retardation and Developmental Disabilities*, 12: 70–82. https://doi.org/10.1002/mrdd.20098

Krahn, G. L. and Fox, M. H. (2014). Health Disparities of Adults With Intellectual Disabilities: What Do We Know? What Do We Do? *Journal of Applied Research in Intellectual Disabilities*, 27 (5): 431–446. https://doi.org/10.1111/jar.12067

Ma, G. (2023). Critiquing Reasonable Adjustment: Calling for Positive Action to Tackle Disability Discrimination. *Disability and Society*. https://doi.org/10.1080/09687599.2023.2287407

Magaña, S., Parish, S., Morales, M. A., Li, H. and Fujiura, G. (2016). Racial and Ethnic Health Disparities Among People with Intellectual and Developmental Disabilities. *Intellect Dev Disabil*, 54 (3): 161–72. https://doi.org/10.1352/1934-9556-54.3.161

Marquis, S., O'Leary, R., Bandara, N. A. and Baumbusch, J. (2023). Health Policy Narratives Contributing to Health Inequities Experienced by People with Intellectual/Developmental Disabilities: New Evidence from COVID-19. *Clinical Ethics*, online ahead of print. https://doi.org/10.1177/14777509231196704

McCarron, M., Lombard-Vance, R., Murphy, E., May, P., Webb, N., et al. (2019). Effect of Deinstitutionalisation on Quality of Life for Adults with Intellectual Disabilities: A Systematic Review. *BMJ Open*, 9 (4): e025735. https://doi.org/10.1136/bmjopen-2018-025735

McRuer, R. and Berube, M. (2006). *Crip Theory: Cultural Signs of Queerness and Disability*. New York: New York University Press.

Morgan, J. and Breau, G. (2024). Access to Maternal Health Services for Indigenous Women in Low- and Middle-Income Countries: An Updated Integrative Review of the Literature From 2018–2023. *Rural and Remote Health*. https://doi.org/10.22605/RRH8520

Nguyen, M., Lennox, N., and Ware, R. (2014). Hand-Held Health Records for Individuals with Intellectual Disability: A Systematic Review. *J Intellect Disabil Res*, 58: 1172–1178 https://doi.org/10.1111/jir.12104

NHS Digital. (2022). Health and Care of People with Learning Disabilities Experimental Statistics 2021 to 2022. Available at: https://digital.nhs.uk/data-and-information/publications/statistical/health-and-care-of-people-with-learning-disabilities/experimental-statistics-2021-to-2022 (Accessed: 26 January 2024).

Northway, R., Rees, S., Davies, M. and Williams, S. (2017). Hospital Passports, Patient Safety and Person-Centred Care: A Review of Documents Currently Used for People with Intellectual Disabilities in the UK. *J Clin Nurs*, 26 (5): 160–168. https://doi.org/10.1111/jocn.14065.

Oliver, M. (1990). *The Politics of Disablement*. London: Red Globe Press.

Oliver, M. (1999). Capitalism, Disability and Ideology: A Materialist Critique of the Normalization Principle. In R. J. Flynn and R. A. Lemay (eds), *A Quarter-Century of Normalization and Social Role Valorization: Evolution and Impact*. Ottawa: University of Ottawa Press, 163–174.

Oliver, M. and Barnes, C. (2012). *The New Politics of Disablement*. Basingstoke: Palgrave Macmillan.

Reppermund, S., Heintze, T., Srasuebkul, P., Reeve, R., Dean, K., et al. (2019). Health and Wellbeing of People with Intellectual Disability in New South Wales, Australia: A Data Linkage Cohort. *BMJ Open*, 9: e031624. doi:10.1136/bmjopen-2019-031624

Robertson, J., Hatton, C., Emerson, C. and Baines, S. (2014). The Impact of Health Checks for People with Intellectual Disabilities: An Updated Systematic Review of Evidence. *Research in Developmental Disabilities*, 35 (10): 2450–2462. https://doi.org/10.1016/j.ridd.2014.06.007

Royal Commission into Violence, Abuse, Neglect and Exploitation of People with Disability. (2023). Final Report – Volume 6, Enabling Autonomy and Access. Available at: https://disability.royalcommission.gov.au/publications/final-report-volume-6-enabling-autonomy-and-access (Accessed: 27 February 2024).

Selick, A., Durbin, J., Casson, I., Lee, J. and Lunsky, Y. (2018). Barriers and Facilitators to Improving Health Care for Adults with Intellectual and Developmental Disabilities: What Do Staff Tell Us? *Health Promotion and Chronic Disease Prevention in Canada: Research, Policy and Practice*, 38(10): 349–357.https://doi.org/10.24095/hpcdp.38.10.01

Shakespeare, T. and Watson, N. (2001). The Social Model of Disability: An Outdated Ideology?. *Research In Social Science and Disability*, 2: 9–28. https://doi.org/10.1016/S1479-3547(01)80018-X

Sheehan, R., Gandesha, A., Hassiotis A, Gallagher, P., Burnell, M., et al. (2016). An Audit of the Quality of Inpatient Care for Adults with Learning Disability in the UK. *BMJ Open*, 6: e010480. doi:10.1136/bmjopen-2015-010480

Šiška, J., Beadle-Brown, J., Káňová, Š., and Šumníková, P. (2018). Social Inclusion Through Community Living: Current Situation, Advances and Gaps in Policy, Practice and Research. *Social Inclusion*, 6 (1): 94–109. doi: https://doi.org/10.17645/si.v6i1.1211

Šiška, J. and Beadle-Brown, J. (2020). Report on the Transition from Institutional Care to Community-Based Services in 27 EU Member States. Available at: https://isocial.cat/wp-content/uploads/2022/03/di-report-final-submitted.pdf (Accessed: 26 February 2024).

Sullivan, W. F., Björne, P., Heng, J., and Northway, R. (2022). Ethics Framework and Recommendations to Support Capabilities of People with Intellectual and Developmental Disabilities During Pandemics. *Journal of Policy and Practice in Intellectual Disabilities*, 19 (1): 116–124. https://doi.org/10.1111/jppi.12413

Thomas, C. (2004). How is Disability Understood? An Examination of Sociological Approaches. *Disability and Society*, 19 (6): 569–583. https://doi.org/10.1080/0968759042000252506

Totsikas, V., Emerson, E., Hastings, R. and Hatton, C. (2021). The Impact of the COVID-19 Pandemic on the Health of Adults with Intellectual Impairment: Evidence from Two Longitudinal UK Surveys. *Journal of Intellectual Disability Research*, 65 (10): 890–897. https://doi.org/10.1111/jir.12866

United Nations Department of Economic and Social Affairs. (2006). The United Nations Convention on the Rights of Persons with Disabilities. Available at: www.un.org/development/desa/disabilities/convention-on-the-rights-of-persons-with-disabilities/convention-on-the-rights-of-persons-with-disabilities-2.html (Accessed: 23 August 2023).

Wilson, N. J., Pracilio, A., Kersten, M., Morphet, J., Buckely, T., et al. (2021). Registered Nurses' Awareness and Implementation of Reasonable Adjustments for People with Intellectual Disability and/or Autism. *Journal of Advanced Nursing*, 78 (8): 2426–2435. https://doi.org/10.1111/jan.15171

Wolfensberger, W. P. (1972). *The Principle of Normalization in Human Services*. Toronto: National Institute on Mental Retardation.

WHO. (2002). *International Classification of Functioning, Disability and Health*. Geneva: World Health Organization.

CHAPTER 12

Women in Prison

....

Julia Morgan

INTRODUCTION

Although women comprise significantly smaller percentages of the prison population in all countries, the global rates of female imprisonment have increased (global increase of 60% for women compared to 22% for men since 2000) (Fair and Walmsley, 2022). However, there is variation between countries and regions and numbers of women imprisoned have decreased, since 2000, in Europe; the only region to show such a decrease. The needs of imprisoned women are often complex with elevated levels of vulnerability and victimisation evident. This vulnerability is compounded when women enter institutions which are primarily designed for male prisoners, meaning their needs are often overlooked. This chapter will give an overview of the numbers of women in prison across selected OECD countries before continuing to discuss imprisoned women's specific wellbeing needs.

DEMOGRAPHICS OF WOMEN IN PRISON

Globally, imprisonment rates for women are increasing. There are many reasons put forward for this, such as increases in the severity of crimes committed by women, including crimes of violence, which result in a higher likelihood of a prison sentence (Jeffries and Newbold, 2015). Alternatively, it has been argued that low level non-violent crimes and offences related to substance misuse, which are typically more likely to be associated with women, are increasingly being treated more punitively with prison sentences (Jeffries and Newbold, 2015). The United States of America (USA) has the highest incarceration rate in the world for both men and women (Prison Policy Initiative, 2021) with these high rates being a result of a policy and legislative focus on the 'war on drugs', prison industrial complexes which support neoliberal and corporate interests, and on mass incarceration (Nellis, 2023; Zhang, 2024).

In relation to women, the USA accounts for over 30% of women imprisoned globally and yet contains only 4% of the world's female population (Prison Policy Initiative, 2018). As of 2018, the rate of imprisonment for women in the USA was

DOI: 10.4324/9781003343608-14

TABLE 12.1 Rate per 100,000 Incarcerated: Selected OECD Countries

Country	Women rate per 100,000
USA	133
Costa Rica	43
Chile	42
New Zealand	35
Latva	32
Columbia	31
Australia	28
Hungary	26
Türkiye	25
Mexico	17
Korea	15
UK – England and Wales	13
UK – Scotland	13
Canada	13
Germany	9
Norway	9
Italy	8
Ireland	7
Japan	7
UK – Northern Ireland	6
Iceland	5

Source: Prison Policy Initiative (2018)

133 women imprisoned per 100,000 population (Prison Policy Initiative, 2018). The USA system is tripartite and consists of state prisons, federal prisons, and local jails with more women imprisoned in local jails (60% of whom are still awaiting trial) than in state/federal prisons (Prison Policy Initiative, 2023). Table 12.1 highlights incarceration rates for women across selected OECD countries. What can be seen from the table is that women in the USA are three times more likely than women in Costa Rica to be imprisoned (Costa Rica occupied in 2018 second place in the imprisonment of women across OECD countries), 10 times more likely to be imprisoned than women in England and Wales, and Canada, and almost 27 times more likely to be imprisoned than women in Iceland. The USA, therefore, is an outlier in relation to imprisonment rates and the rest of the OECD.

Ethnic minority women and women of colour are more likely to be imprisoned than their white or non-ethnic minority counterparts. For example, in England and Wales, in June 2023, 3,342 women had their ethnicity recorded. Women of black and 'mixed' ethnicity were much more likely to be imprisoned (black women represented 7.4% of the prison population compared to 4.2% of the general female black population, while 'mixed' ethnicity women represented 5.2% of the female prison population compared to 2.9% of the general female 'mixed'' population (Ministry of Justice, 2023a; Office for National Statistics, 2023). Asian women by contrast are less likely to be imprisoned representing 3% of women who were imprisoned compared to 9.2% of the female Asian general population while white women represented 83.3% of the female prison population compared to 81.7% of the female white general population. In England and Wales Gypsy/Traveller women comprise an estimated 6% of the prison population even though Gypsies and Travellers are estimated to make up only 0.1% of the general population (Traveller Movement, 2021). This estimate does not include Roma women as data on Roma (in prison) is not currently collected in England and Wales. Gypsy/Traveller women are normally included in the white ethnicity group for reporting purposes, and this probably explains the higher rates of white ethnicity imprisonment for women above.

In Ireland, Irish Traveller women are 18 to 22 times more likely to be imprisoned than the general population (Irish Penal Reform Trust, 2014). While in Europe, it is agreed that Roma, including Roma women, are over-represented in prison populations with one study reporting that Roma women in Spain represent 1.4% of the general population but 25% of imprisoned women (Cerezo and Díez-Ripollés, 2017). The collection of data, however, is hampered by a lack of focus on ethnicity across many countries (Fair Trials, 2020; European Roma Rights Centre 2021). Foreign nationals are also disproportionately imprisoned across Europe (Prisonwatch, 2022); with data from Norway showing that 19 per cent of women in prison were foreign nationals (Sivilombudsmannen, 2017).

Exploring the 2021 ethnicity data for the USA, for state and federal prisons, shows a similar pattern with black women being 1.6 times more likely to be imprisoned than white women and Latina women, 1.3 times more likely to be imprisoned (Monazzam and Budd, 2023). While Native American and Alaska Native women are four times as likely as white women to be imprisoned (Carson, 2022). There is considerable variation, however, by state and by age; and among younger women (aged 18–19 years old), American Indian and Alaska Native, as well as black women were more than six times more likely to be imprisoned than white women of the same age. Indigenous women are also over-represented in prisons throughout many countries across the OECD. In New Zealand, Indigenous women represent 60% of the female prison population and 48% in Canada (Penal Reform International, 2022). While in Australia, the rates of imprisonment of Aboriginal and Torres Strait Islander women are significantly increasing with these women being 19 times more likely to be imprisoned than non-Indigenous women (Australian Human Rights Commission, 2021). Structural violence, including poverty and disadvantage, as well as structural racism, including ethnic profiling, stop and search, harsher sentencing, and over-policing of communities are at the heart of these disparities (Lammy, 2017; European Roma Rights Centre, 2021).

NATURE OF OFFENCES AND VULNERABILITY OF IMPRISONED WOMEN

Globally, women are, much more likely than men, to be imprisoned for non-violent offences including theft, fraud, and drug possession and as a result tend to serve shorter sentences than men who are more likely to be sentenced for violent offences (Ministry of Justice, 2020; House of Commons Justice Committee, 2022; Penal Reform International, 2022). Some imprisoned women, however, do serve long sentences and the number of women serving an indeterminate sentence, in England and Wales, has grown from 96 in 1991, to 370 in June 2022 (Prison Reform Trust, 2023a).

While in the USA, 6,600 women were sentenced to life (with and without parole) or a virtual life sentence of 50 years or more (Nellis, 2021). Across the USA, one in every 39 imprisoned black women was serving life without parole compared to one in every 59 white women imprisoned (Nellis, 2021). Moreover, in 2022, 50 women were living on death row in the USA and eight in Japan (2021 figure), the only two countries across the OECD who still have the death penalty (Death Penalty Information Center, n.d.; Crimeinfo and Eleos Justice, 2022).

As we can see from Table 12.2, women in prison across selected OECD countries are overwhelmingly vulnerable and disadvantaged, with many experiencing co-occurring mental ill-health and substance misuse issues as well as victimisation and trauma in both childhood and in adulthood. The elevated levels of vulnerability among many women in prison indicate a gendered pathway into crime which is different for men and women, with women more likely to report prominent levels of negative life events than men and to commit crimes because of these gendered vulnerabilities (Wright and Cain, 2018). For example, research indicates that there are links between the physical abuse of women and their subsequent offending behaviours (DeHart et al., 2013).

TABLE 12.2 Vulnerability of Imprisoned Women across Selected OECD Countries

Country	Background of women
England and Wales	76% of imprisoned women reported a mental health condition compared to 51% of imprisoned men; 59% of imprisoned women reported a problem with alcohol while 37% of women report a drug problem compared with 25% of men; 26% of women, compared to 16% of men, experienced homelessness; women were more likely to be jobless (53%) than to be employed in the month before their arrest; 31% of imprisoned women had spent time in local authority care as a child compared to 24% of imprisoned men; 60% of imprisoned women survived domestic violence; 64% of women had histories of brain injuries: with most of these injuries a result of domestic violence. Women were 5 times more likely than men to self-harm and 46% of women reported having attempted suicide compared to 21% of imprisoned men (Prison Reform Trust, 2021a; 2023b; 2023c; Ministry of Justice, 2022; 2018).
Norway	Female prisoners are four times more likely than the general population to have mental health conditions. Women reported high levels of sexual abuse, 57% of female inmates had been sexually abused as an adult and 42% as a child. Women were more likely than male inmates to report substance misuse issues (Sivilombudsmannen, 2017).
USA	12% of women reported homelessness as a child; 19% were in foster care; 43% had lived as children in households who received welfare; 53% of women were unemployed before incarceration; 50% had physical/cognitive disabilities and 76% mental health illnesses (Prison Policy Initiative, 2023).
Spain	37.4% of women reported emotional abuse, 21.8% physical abuse and 19.5% sexual abuse in childhood (Caravaca-Sánchez et al., 2019). High levels of social exclusion, including poverty, previous adolescent experiences of reform schools, low levels of educational qualifications and higher likelihood of having a relative in prison (Cerezo and Díez-Ripollés, 2017).

(Continued)

TABLE 12.2 Vulnerability of Imprisoned Women across Selected OECD Countries (Continued)

Country	Background of women
Australia	Two out of three imprisoned women had received a mental health diagnosis; 48% of women had been imprisoned previously; lower levels of education were evident; higher levels of unemployment; 27% were in emergency or short-term accommodation; 7% were homeless before imprisonment; 17% had a parent or carer in prison when they were a child; 40% reported their health as fair to poor with 36% being diagnosed with a chronic condition; 86% were current smokers; 27% reported high risk alcohol consumption; 74% of women, who were new entrants to prison, reported using illicit drugs (methamphetamine the most common drug used), and 31% reported a history of self-harm (Australian Institute of Health and Welfare, 2020).
New Zealand	Three quarters of women had been victims of family violence, rape and/ or sexual assault as a child or adult. High levels of mental health issues and substance addictions, low educational achievement, high levels of poverty, unemployment, and reliance on state benefits were reported. Many also face child custody issues. In addition, Māori women face further intergenerational trauma because of colonisation (Department of Corrections, 2021).
Chile	53.4% of imprisoned women were unemployed prior to imprisonment; 57.6% had primary level education; over 60% had taken or were currently taking illicit drugs (Aboaja et al., 2023).
Switzerland	68.3% of women were not working prior to imprisonment; 70% were on the lowest income level; one in three women rated their health as poor or very poor; 43.3% reported mental health conditions; 65% mentioned pain on the day of the survey; 78.3% were current smokers; 49.2% mentioned prior illicit drug use; 85% were taking medication for physical or mental health conditions (Augsburger et al., 2022).

THE SPECIFIC NEEDS OF WOMEN IN PRISON

Women's specific needs can be overlooked in prison environments which are often designed by men, for men, who are the majority in prisons across OECD countries (United Nations, 2015). For example, Norway is often heralded as a country with high quality prisons which are inclusive, and treatment focused (Borgen Project, 2020). However, women who are imprisoned in Norway are at risk of facing 'worse conditions than men' (Sivilombudsmannen, 2017: 10) with reports of poor sanitary facilities, especially for menstruating or pregnant women; a lack of appropriate areas for physical activities; a higher likelihood of women being held in poor quality buildings and at higher security levels than needed due to a lack of female prison places; a fear of harassment and abuse in mixed sex prisons where women come into contact with male prisoners during work and leisure activities; low priority given to the needs of women in relation to work activities;

and unmet needs in health services with substance misuse programmes being said to be 'inferior' to those offered to male inmates. The poorer standard of substance misuse programmes for women in Norway is indicative of a lack of planning for the needs of imprisoned women who are more likely to have substance misuse issues and need high-quality interventions.

Moreover, the effect of imprisonment on vulnerable women with complex needs, can be overlooked in criminal justice systems, with imprisonment itself leading to what has been called 'incarceration-based trauma' (Anderson et al., 2020) which may be more significant for women because of previous experiences of victimisation. The trauma of imprisonment including lack of control, fear, loss of children, potential violence including threats, and poor conditions, including over-crowding, surveillance, and lack of privacy, may exacerbate previous trauma (for example, histories of abuse) and lead to the re-traumatisation of vulnerable women. This may have significant impacts on women's mental health, behaviour and wellbeing, with an awareness of the potential impact of imprisonment on women being key to supporting them, once in prison, and to considerations of alternative methods to custody (see Wright and Cain, 2018).

Imprisoned women also have specific needs as a high percentage are mothers who have primary caregiver responsibility for children. In the USA, 58% of women who are in federal/state prisons and 80% of women who are in jails are mothers (Maruschak et al., 2021); in England and Wales, 58% are mothers (Prison Reform Trust, 2021a) with 17,000 children impacted by maternal imprisonment (Prison Reform Trust, 2021a), while in Australia, 90% are mothers (Australian Institute of Health and Welfare, 2019) with many of these women being single parents. The imprisonment of mothers has major impacts on the maintenance of mother-child relationships, which can have a detrimental effect on women's mental health (Morgan and Leeson, 2023). This is often exacerbated because there are fewer prisons for women, which results in mothers often being placed in prisons, far from their children. Distance, cost, and time can, therefore, negatively impact children visiting their mothers, and can have long-lasting impacts on mother-child bonds, with the loss of relationships potentially leading to further trauma for women. Moreover, imprisonment can have significant impacts on children, including children having to leave their family home to live with alternative carers, an increase in caring responsibilities for children and increases in the risk of children's offending behaviours, poorer educational experiences, and emotional trauma (Leeson and Morgan, 2019; Department for Education, 2022). Mothers, in turn, may face increasing stigma, guilt, shame, and rejection by family members because of the impact of their imprisonment on their children (Morgan and Leeson, 2023). As a result, mothers may require additional help to stay connected with their children because of difficulties in children physically visiting their mothers, as well as sensitive support with maternal emotions such as ambiguous loss, guilt, and shame (Morgan and Gill, 2014; Morgan and Leeson, 2023).

Some mothers across OECD countries, however, do live with their children in prison in mother and baby units (MBUs). Reasons for this include the facilitation of breastfeeding, the rights of the child to family life, and a focus on supporting mother-child bonds as separation, especially in the early years, may lead to a range of adverse outcomes (UNHRO, 2019). Positive impacts for both mothers and children in MBU's have been shown including improved mental health, wellbeing, and mother-child relationships, with some research showing reduced reoffending rates for mothers (Dolan et al., 2019; Paynter et al., 2020). However, while MBU's are welcomed by many mothers, research from across OECD countries, shows that they can be experienced as potentially stressful (Lai et al., 2022) and disempowering, especially in relation to levels of surveillance and judgement of mothering behaviours and restrictions on the choices that mothers can make in relation to their child (Nuytiens and Jehaes, 2022; Sapkota et al., 2022). This may be exacerbated for women who are ethnic minorities and foreign nationals (Ogrizek et al., 2023). The ages that children can live with their mothers in prison are shown in Table 12.3 with considerable variation being seen.

There are concerns, however, around children living with their mothers in prison including the deprivation of children's liberty, and the impact of the prison regime, and environment on children and their development (UNHRO, 2019). The Mandela

TABLE 12.3 Age Limits for Babies/Children Living in Prison across OECD Countries

Maximum age of children	Country
Children not allowed to live in prison with their parent	Norway (not allowed in live in prison but homes outside of the prison are available where mothers/babies may live until they are 9 months old)
Up to 1 year old	Hungary, Ireland, Malta, Bulgaria
Up to 18 months old	England and Wales, Scotland, Monaco; however, in Scotland mothers on licence (released from prison with part of a sentence still to serve) may live with their children, until school age, in an 'independent living unit' outside the prison gates
Up to 2 years old	Slovenia, Romania, Cyprus, New Zealand
Up to 3 years old	Poland, Spain, Switzerland, Lithuania, Greece, Finland, Denmark, Belgium, Estonia, Austria
Up to 4 years old	Latvia
Up to 5 years old	Portugal
Up to 6 years old	Mexico, Italy
Variable ages	USA: depends on State –30 days after birth up to 2 years old
	Canada: full-time up until children turn 5/part-time till they turn 7
	Germany: high security until 3 and low security until 6 years old
	Netherlands: up to 9 months in prison and then up to 4 years old in special mother-child homes
	Australia: depends upon State – Victora – up until school age and New South Wales up until 6 years old

Rules (2015) highlight that children should only live with their mother in prison when it is in the best interests of the child and that children should have access to appropriate childcare and healthcare facilities, and should never be treated as if they, themselves, were prisoners.

BOX 12.1 ENGLAND: MOTHER AND BABY UNITS

There are six mother and baby units (MBUs) attached to female prisons in England with a capacity of 64 women/70 babies (to support multiple births). Women make an application to be accepted into a MBU and those who are unsuccessful will be separated from their babies shortly after birth. The decision for a mother to be accepted into a MBU consists of consideration of:

- whether it is in the best interests of the child;
- the necessity to maintain good order within the MBU; and
- the health and safety of other children and women on the unit.

Decisions are informed by security reports, risk assessments, health/substance misuse assessments, and Children's Services reports. There are no exclusions relating to offence or sentence types. MBU's are managed by prison staff and qualified nursery professionals and include living space and nursing facilities which are registered with OFSTED. Mothers and children should have access to the same level of health services and postnatal care that they would receive in the community. Staff should wear 'plain' clothing and facilitate the MBU as the child's home. A childcare plan should be initiated. Qualified nursery staff take care of the child when the mother is out of the unit for interventions or work. All basic equipment such as cots, nappies and toys must be provided. Mothers and children should not be locked in their rooms, and mothers on the unit are responsible for their children's daily care, including the preparation of food. Stay and play as well as parenting classes should be available. Governors are expected to give babies experiences like visits to the park and other developmental opportunities. Mothers can apply for an extension to the upper-age limit (Ministry of Justice, 2023b).

The Farmer Review (2019), however, noted the low take up of places in MBUs in England and highlighted anecdotal reports of a lack of social work support for women to be accepted into the units. Being unsuccessful in MBU applications which results in the removal of the baby from the mother's care, has been shown to lead to increases in maternal self-harm, suicide, and mental ill-health (Abbott, 2023).

Out of the 38 OECD countries only three, Costa Rica, Mexico and Columbia, do not imprison pregnant women with alternatives such as house arrests being used (Epstein et al., 2021). In all other 35 countries of the OECD, women may be imprisoned while they are pregnant. The Bangkok Rules (United Nations, 2011) encourages non-custodial sentences for pregnant women, but it is difficult to ascertain the numbers of pregnant women in prison (and the number of babies living with their mothers in prison) as data is not routinely collected across OECD countries making comparison difficult. However, for England and Wales, there were 600 pregnant women in prison in one year (Prison Reform Trust, 2021a); in Australia, in 2017, 1.8% of imprisoned women were pregnant (Australian Institute of Health and Welfare, 2019) and in the USA, 3.8% of women were pregnant in 2016–2017 (Sufrin et al., 2019). Many pregnant women in prison tend to be high-risk obstetric groups because of their vulnerable backgrounds, their histories of substance misuse, and because they are often locked in a prison cell, out of view, for a substantial amount of time, which increases the possibility of experiencing complications or giving birth without support. This has led to concerns about the wellbeing of pregnant women in prison due to prison environments, including possible violence as well as a potential lack of access to antenatal, obstetric, and postnatal care which can violate reproductive justice.

This had devastating consequences in England in 2019–2020, when two babies died because of inadequate and outdated prison maternity services, which was not equivalent to what would have been received in the community, a lack of guidance on what to do in cases of unexpected births, and a lack of recognition of the signs of early labour (McAllister, 2021a; 2021b). Concerns are also apparent across OECD nations with research in the USA highlighting a lack of prison protocols for the care of pregnant women (Prison Policy Initiative, 2019) and the 'devaluation of reproductive bodies' including the use of shackling during delivery (Kuhlik and Sufrin, 2020: 423), in Australia where women reported a lack of information on pregnancy, breastfeeding, and what to expect during labour, as well as a lack of access to nutritional food antenatal classes and postnatal care (Sapkota et al., 2022) and in New Zealand with reports of poor nutrition and hunger and a lack of treatment for substance misuse in pregnant women (Office of the Inspectorate, 2023).

To support the needs of imprisoned women, the importance of gender responsive approaches has been highlighted across many OECD countries. These gender specific approaches consider the gendered pathway or context which underpins much of female offending (Wright and Cain, 2018); with these interventions being strength-based, relational, and trauma-informed, taking on board the victimisation and vulnerability of many women who are imprisoned (Wright et al., 2012). Public Health England (2018), for example, have published gender specific standards, which outline that women in prison should have access to high quality interventions around mental health and substance misuse while New Zealand's Women's Strategy highlights that 'women's pathways to offending commonly stem from experiences of trauma' which require both gender and culturally responsive holistic programming and services (Department of Corrections, 2021:6).

Community-based sentencing or out-of-court disposals (OoCDs), in England and Wales, form part of gender responsive approaches, as imprisonment can exacerbate women's marginalisation, with women being more likely, than men, to struggle to find employment and housing on release. This in turn has been shown to impact re-offending rates (Hedderman and Joliffe, 2015; Prison Reform Trust, 2020; Justice and Home Affairs Committee 2023). Moreover, community-based treatment requirements for mental health and substance misuse may be a better option for many women, rather than short-term prison sentences, where treatment may be difficult to access because of the short length of the sentence (Ministry of Justice, 2018).

Alternative approaches to imprisonment such as OoCDs, deferred sentences, community-based sentencing, and restorative justice initiatives, may also mitigate some of the issues around pregnant women in prisons and the separation of mothers from their children (Epstein et al., 2021). In 2023, the Justice Secretary, Alex Chalk, announced that sentences up to 12 months in England and Wales will be suspended and replaced with community orders to combat over-crowding in prison (Beard, 2023). This will have a direct impact on those women in England and Wales who are imprisoned for shorter sentences.

CONCLUSION

This chapter shows that imprisoned women across many countries of the OECD are more likely to have histories of co-occurring victimisation, vulnerability, and disadvantage. Women, therefore, often enter prison with complex health and wellbeing needs as well as specific requirements in relation to pregnancy and motherhood. Prison environments are not conducive to supporting women's health and wellbeing as they are often designed for men. Hence gender responsive approaches and alternatives to female imprisonment are required which take on board the specific needs of women. These gender responsive approaches need to be underpinned by a focus on intersectionality as women may have additional needs and face additional challenges, both within prison and outside of prison, because of intersectional factors, such as ethnicity, race, social class, disability, sexuality, age, and histories of colonisation.

RESEARCH POINTS AND REFLECTIVE EXERCISES

- Why is an understanding of intersectionality important in understanding the needs of imprisoned women?
- Read the report by the Prison Reform Trust (2021b). What impacts did COVID-19 have upon the health and wellbeing of women in prison?
- Read the paper by Wright et al. (2012) on gender responsive approaches. Reflect upon appropriate gender responsive initiatives for women in the criminal justice system. Research 'abolition feminism' (e.g., Davis et al., 2022; Davis, 2003; Critical Resistance. n.d.) and reflect upon how we can re-imagine alternatives to imprisonment.

REFERENCES

Abbott, L. (2023). Birth Supporters Experiences of Attending Prisoners being Compulsorily Separated from their New-Born Babies. *International Journal of Health Promotion and Education*, online ahead of print. https://doi.org/10.1080/14635240.2023.2213201

Aboaja, A., Blackwood, D., Alvarado, R. and Grant, L. (2023). The Mental Wellbeing of Female Prisoners in Chile. *BMC Res Notes*, 16 (78). https://doi.org/10.1186/s13104-023-06342-x

Anderson, J. D., Pitner, R. O. and Wooten, N. R. (2020). A Gender-Specific Model of Trauma and Victimization in Incarcerated Women. *Journal of Human Behavior in the Social Environment*, 30 (2): 191–212, https://doi.org/10.1080/10911359.2019.1673272

Augsburger, A., Neri, C., Bodenmann, P., Gravier, B., Jaquier, V., et al. (2022). Assessing Incarcerated Women's Physical and Mental Health Status and Needs in a Swiss Prison: A Cross-Sectional Study. *Health and Justice*, 10 (1): 8. https://doi.org/10.1186/s40352-022-00171-z

Australian Human Rights Commission. (2021). *Australia's Criminal Justice System*. Australia: Human Rights Commission.

Australian Institute of Health and Welfare. (2020). *The Health and Welfare of Women in Australia's Prisons*. Canberra: AIHW.

Australian Institute of Health and Welfare. (2019). *The Health of Australia's Prisoners*. Canberra: AIHWY.

Beard, J. (2023). What is the Government Doing to Reduce Pressure on Prison Capacity? Available at: https://commonslibrary.parliament.uk/what-is-the-government-doing-to-reduce-pressure-on-prison-capacity/ (Accessed: 15 February 2024).

Borgen Project. (2020). Norway's Prison System Benefits its Economy. Available at: https://borgenproject.org/norways-prison-system/ (Accessed: 28 October 2023).

Caravaca-Sánchez, F., Fearn, N. E., Vidovic, K. R. and Vaughn, M. G. (2019). Female Prisoners in Spain: Adverse Childhood Experiences, Negative Emotional States, and Social Support, *Health and Social Work*, 44 (3): 157–166, https://doi.org/10.1093/hsw/hlz013

Carson, E. A. (2022). Prisoners in 2021 – Statistical Tables, US Department of Justice. Available at: https://bjs.ojp.gov/library/publications/prisoners-2021-statistical-tables (Accessed: 15 February 2024).

Cerezo, A. and Díez-Ripollés, J. (2017). Women in Prison in Spain: Their Criminological and Social Invisibility. In P. Van Kempen and M. Krabbe (eds), *Women in Prison: The Bangkok Rules and Beyond*. Cambridge: Intersentia, 697–722.

Crimeinfo and Eleos Justice. (2022). Imposition of the Death Penalty and its Impact: Japan. Available at: www.ohchr.org/sites/default/files/2022-05/crimeinfo-eleos-justice-reply-dp.pdf (Accessed: 1 October 2023).

Critical Resistance. n.d. CR's Abolitionist Toolkit. Available at: https://criticalresistance.org/resources/the-abolitionist-toolkit (Accessed: 23 September 2024).

Davis, A. (2003). *Are Prisons Obsolete?* New York City: Seven Stories Press.

Davis, A., Dent, G., Meiners, E. and Richie, B. (2022). *Abolition. Feminism. Now.* Chicago: Haymarket Books.

Death Penalty Information Center. (n.d). Current Female Death Row Prisoners. Available at https://deathpenaltyinfo.org/death-row/women (Accessed: 1 October 2023).

DeHart, D., Lynch, S., Belknap, J., Dass-Brailsford, P. and Green, B. (2013). Life History Models of Offending: The Role of Serious Mental Illness and Trauma in Women's Pathways to Jail. *Psychology of Women Quarterly*, 38 (1): 138–151. https://doi.org/10.1177/0361684313494357

Department for Education. (2022). *Applications to Mother and Baby Units in Prison: How Decisions are Made and the Role of Social Work. A Case Review of Social Work Decision Making (2017–2021)*. London: Department of Education.

Department of Corrections. (2021). *Wāhine: E Rere Ana Ki Te Pae Hou – Women's Strategy 2021–2025*. Wellington: Department of Corrections.

Dolan, R., Shaw, J. and Hann, M. (2019). Pregnancy in Prison, Mother and Baby Unit Admission and Impacts on Perinatal Depression and 'Quality of Life'. *The Journal of Forensic Psychiatry and Psychology*, 30 (4): 551–569. https://doi.org/10.1080/14789949.2019.1627482

Epstein, R., Brown, G. and Garcia De Frutos, M. (2021). *Why are Pregnant Women in Prison?* Coventry: Coventry University.

European Roma Rights Centre. (2021). *Justice Denied: Roma in the Criminal Justice System*. Belgium: European Roma Rights Centre.

Fair, H. and Walmsley, R. (2022). *World Female Imprisonment List*, 5th edn. London: ICPR.

Fair Trials. (2020). *Uncovering Anti-Roma Discrimination in Criminal Justice Systems in Europe*. Brussels: Fair Trials.

Farmer, L. (2019). Importance of Strengthening Female Offenders' Family and Other Relationships to Prevent Reoffending and Reduce Intergenerational Crime. Available at: www.gov.uk/government/publications/farmer-review-for-women (Accessed: 28 October 2023).

Hedderman, C. and Joliffe, D. (2015). The Impact of Prison for Women on the Edge: Paying the Price for Wrong Decisions. *Victims and Offenders: An International Journal of Evidence-Based Research, Policy and Practice*, 10 (2): 152–178. https://doi.org/10.1080/15564886.2014.953235

House of Commons Justice Committee. (2022). *Women in Prison: First Report of Session 2022–23*. London: House of Commons.

Irish Penal Reform Trust. (2014). *Travellers in the Irish Prison System: A Qualitative Study*. Dublin: Irish Penal Reform Trust.

Jeffries, S. and Newbold, G. (2015). Analysing Trends in the Imprisonment of Women in Australia and New Zealand. *Psychiatry, Psychology and Law*, 23 (2): 184–206. https://doi.org/10.1080/13218719.2015.1035619

Justice and Home Affairs Committee. (2023). *Cutting Crime: Better Community Sentences*. London: House of Lords.

Kuhlik, L. and Sufrin, C. (2020). Pregnancy, Systematic Disregard and Degradation, and Carceral Institutions. *Harvard Law and Policy Review*, 14 (2): 417–466.

Lai, C., Rossi, L. E., Scicchitano, F., Ciacchella, C., Valentini, M., et al. (2022). Motherhood in Alternative Detention Conditions: A Preliminary Case-Control Study. *Int J Environ Res Public Health*, 19 (10): 6000. https://doi.org/10.3390/ijerph19106000.

Lammy, D. (2017). *The Lammy Review: An Independent Review into the Treatment of, and Outcomes for, Black, Asian and Minority Ethnic Individuals in the Criminal Justice System*. London: Lammy Review.

Leeson, C. and Morgan, J. (2019). Children with a parent in prison England and Wales: A hidden population of young carers. *Childcare in Practice* 28(2): 196–209. https://doi.org/10.1080/13575279.2019.1680531

Maruschak, L., M., Bronson, J. and Alper, M. (2021). Parents in Prison and Their Minor Children: Survey of Prison Inmates, 2016, Bureau of Justice Statistics. Available at: https://bjs.ojp.gov/library/publications/parents-prison-and-their-minor-children-survey-prison-inmates-2016 (Accessed: 23 October 2023).

McAllister, S. (2021a). *Independent Investigation into the Death of Baby A at HMP Bronzefield on 27 September 2019*. London: PPO.

McAllister, S. (2021b). *Independent Investigation into the Death of Baby B at HMP&YOI Styal on 18 June 2020*. London: PPO.

Ministry of Justice. (2018). *Female Offender Strategy*. London: Ministry of Justice.

Ministry of Justice. (2020). *Statistics on Women and the Criminal Justice System 2019*. London: Ministry of Justice.

Ministry of Justice. (2022). *Women and the Criminal Justice System 2021*. London: Ministry of Justice.

Ministry of Justice. (2023a). *Annual Prison Population. Table 1.4: Prison Population by Type of Custody, Sex, and Ethnicity*. London: Ministry of Justice.

Ministry of Justice. (2023b). *Policy Name: Pregnancy, Mother and Baby Units (MBUs), and Maternal Separation from Children up to the Age of Two in Women's Prisons*. London: Ministry of Justice.

Monazzam, N. and Budd, K. M. (2023). Incarcerated Women and Girls. Available at: www.sentencingproject.org/fact-sheet/incarcerated-women-and-girls/#footnote-ref-5 (Accessed: 30 September 2023)

Morgan, J. and Gill, O. (2013). *Children Affected by the Imprisonment of a Family Member: A Handbook for Schools Developing Good Practice*. London: Barnardo's.

Morgan, J. and Leeson, C. (2023). Stigma, Outsider Status and Mothers in Prison. *Journal of Family Issue*s. https://doi.org/10.1177/0192513X231162975

Nellis, A. (2021). *In the Extreme: Women Serving Life without Parole and Death Sentences in the United States*. Washington, DC: The Sentencing Project.

Nellis, A. (2023). Mass Incarceration's Lifetime Guarantee. In K. M. Budd, D. C. Lane, G. W. Muschert and J. A. Smith (eds), *Beyond Bars- A Path Forward From 50 Years of Mass Incarceration in the United States*. Bristol: Policy Press, 1–10.

Nuytiens, A. and Jehaes, E. (2022). When Your Child is Your Cellmate: The 'Maternal Pains of Imprisonment' in a Belgian Prison Nursery. *Criminology and Criminal Justice*, 22 (1): 132–149. https://doi.org/10.1177/1748895820958452

Office for National Statistics. (2023). *Male and Female Populations*. London: Office for National Statistics.

Office of the Inspectorate. (2023). *Mothers and Babies Thematic Report. Prison Management of Pregnant Women and Mothers of Infants*. Wellington: Department of Corrections.

Ogrizek, A., Radjack, R., Moro, M. R. and Lachal, J. (2023). The Cultural Hybridization of Mothering in French Prison Nurseries: A Qualitative Study. *Cult Med Psychiatry*, 47 (2): 422–442. https://doi.org/10.1007/s11013-022-09782-5

Paynter, M., Jefferies, K., McKibbon, S., Martin-Misener, R., Iftene, A., et al. (2020). Mother Child Programs for Incarcerated Mothers and Children and Associated Health Outcomes: A Scoping Review. *Canadian Journal of Nursing Leadership*, 33 (1): 81–99. https://doi.org/10.12927/cjnl.2020.26189

Penal Reform International. (2022). *Global Prison Trends 2022*. Penal Reform International. Available at: www.prisonpolicy.org/blog/2019/12/05/pregnancy/ (Accessed: 24 October 2023).

Prison Policy Initiative. (2018). States of Women's Incarceration: The Global Context 2018. Available at: www.prisonpolicy.org/global/women/2018.html (Accessed: 24 October 2023)

Prison Policy Initiative. (2019). Prisons Neglect Pregnant Women in Their Healthcare Policies. Available at: www.prisonpolicy.org/blog/2019/12/05/pregnancy/ (Accessed: 24 October 2023)

Prison Policy Initiative. (2021). States of Incarceration: The Global Context 2021. Available at: www.prisonpolicy.org/global/2021.html (Accessed: 24 October 2023).

Prison Policy Initiative. (2023). Women's Mass Incarceration: The Whole Pie 2023. Available at: www.prisonpolicy.org/reports/pie2023women.html (Accessed: 24 October 2023).

Prison Reform Trust. (2020). *Working It Out: Improving Employment Opportunities for Women with Criminal Conviction*s. London: Prison Reform Trust.

Prison Reform Trust. (2021a). *Why Focus on Reducing Women's Imprisonment? England and Wales*. London: Prison Reform Trust.

Prison Reform Trust. (2021b). *Women's Experiences of Prison During the Covid-19 Lockdown Regime*. London: Prison Reform Trust.

Prison Reform Trust. (2023a). *Invisible Women: Understanding Women's Experiences of Long-Term Imprisonment Briefing 2: Hope, Health, and Staff-Prisoner Relationships*. London: Prison Reform Trust.

Prison Reform Trust. (2023b). *Prison: The Facts. Bromley Briefing Summer 2023*. London: Prison Reform Trust.

Prison Reform Trust. (2023c). *Bromley Briefings Prison Factfile: January 2023*. London: Prison Reform Trust.

Prisonwatch. (2022). Foreign Prisoners. Available at: https://prisonwatch.org/foreign-prisoners/#publications. (Accessed: 24 October 2023).

Public Health England. (2018). *Women in Prison: Standards to Improve Health and Wellbeing.* London: Public Health England.

Sapkota, D., Dennison, S., Allen, J., Gamble, J., Williams, C., et al. (2022). Navigating Pregnancy and Early Motherhood in Prison: A Thematic Analysis of Mothers' Experiences. *Health Justice*, 10 (32). https://doi.org/10.1186/s40352-022-00196-4

Sivilombudsmannen. (2017). *Women in Prison: A Thematic Report about the Conditions for Female Prisoners in Norway*: Oslo: Norwegian Parliamentary Ombudsman.

Sufrin, C., Beal, L., Clarke, J., Jones, R. and Mosher, W. D. (2019). Pregnancy Outcomes in US Prisons, 2016–2017, *American Journal of Public Health*, 109 (5): 799–805. https://doi.org/10.2105/AJPH.2019.305006

Traveller Movement. (2021). *Gypsy, Roma, and Traveller Women in Prison.* London: The Traveller Movement.

United Nations. (2011). UN Rules for the Treatment of Women Prisoners and Non-Custodial Measures for Women Offenders (The Bangkok Rules). Available at: www.unodc.org/documents/justice-and-prison-reform/Bangkok_Rules_ENG_22032015.pdf (Accessed: 19 October 2023).

United Nations. (2015). United Nations Standard Minimum Rules for the Treatment of Prisoners (the Nelson Mandela Rules). Available at: www.unodc.org/documents/justice-and-prison-reform/GA-RESOLUTION/E_ebook.pdf (Accessed: 23 October 2023).

UNHRO. (2019). Global Study on Children Deprived of Liberty. Available at: www.ohchr.org/en/treaty-bodies/crc/united-nations-global-study-children-deprived-liberty (Accessed: 23 October 2023).

Wright, E. M. and Cain, C. M. (2018). Women In Prison. In J. Wooldredge and P. Smith (eds), *The Oxford Handbook of Prisons and Imprisonment.* New York: Oxford University Press, 163–188.

Wright, E. M., Van Voorhis, P., Salisbury, E. J. and Bauman, A. (2012). Gender-Responsive Lessons Learned and Policy Implications for Women in Prison: A Review. *Criminal Justice and Behavior*, 39 (12): 1612–1632. https://doi.org/10.1177/0093854812451088

Zhang, Y. (2023). Did the Prison Industrial Complex Deliver on Its Promise? Prison Proliferation and Employment in Rural America. *The British Journal of Criminology*, 64 (1): 229–247. https://doi.org/10.1093/bjc/azad011

CHAPTER 13

End of Life Care Policy across the United Kingdom, Cyprus, and Romania

....

Panagiotis Pentaris

INTRODUCTION

End-of-life care, a critical facet of health and social care provision, addresses the complex needs of individuals in the final stages of life and extends support to their families and friends. Its formal recognition and structured development within the UK's healthcare system can be traced back to 1967, when Dame Cicely Saunders, established the first Hospice organisation, offering care to those at the end of their lives. However, the precise definition and characteristics of end-of-life care, and the concept of quality within this context, remain contested. This chapter explores the intricate landscape of end-of-life care, elucidating its historical definitions, evolving definitions, and the policy contexts in the United Kingdom, Cyprus, and Romania. It is not an exhaustive account of either, but it draws conclusions of the intricate relationships between epistemological and policy contexts in end-of-life care.

DEFINITIONAL ENQUIRIES

End-of-life care, a service designed for individuals nearing the end of their lives, typically within the last year, constitutes a pivotal aspect of health and social care provisions, addressing not only the needs of the service user, but also their families and friends (Pentaris, 2018). Its formal recognition and structured development within the UK's healthcare system can be traced back to 1967, when Dame Cicely Saunders, established the first Hospice organisation, offering care to those at the end of their lives (Zechner, 2023). However, the precise definition and characteristics of end-of-life care, and the concept of quality within this context, remain subjects of ongoing debates (Dresser, 2004).

Moreover, the interchangeable use of terms such as 'end-of-life care', 'palliative care', and 'hospice care' further complicates the delineation of these concepts, making

DOI: 10.4324/9781003343608-15

it challenging to operationalise quality of life in policy and practice (Radbruch et al., 2020; Singer and Bowman, 2002). Different organisations and institutions offer varying, but mostly similar definitions. For example, the National Hospice and Palliative Care Organization (NHPCO) in the USA defines hospice care as a model focused on compassionate, patient-tailored medical care, pain management, and emotional, and spiritual support for individuals facing serious or life-limiting illnesses (NHPCO, 2023). On the other hand, palliative care is described as a patient and family-centred approach, aiming to optimise quality of life, by addressing physical, intellectual, emotional, social, and spiritual needs (NHPCO, 2023). The World Health Organization (WHO) similarly defines palliative care as an approach, targeting patients and families in the context of life-limiting illnesses, while the Global Atlas of Palliative Care, defines hospice care as end-of-life care provided by healthcare professionals and volunteers (WHPCA/WHO, 2020). In the UK, Marie Curie characterises end-of-life care as care for individuals in the last year of their lives.

These varying descriptors and interchangeable terminology complicate the development of policies and practices, hindering a focused exploration of quality of life in end-of-life care, particularly in diverse environments. The context in which these terms are used significantly influences their meaning and application.

BOX 13.1 PALLIATIVE CARE

Consider the following definition of palliative care by the World Health Organization (WHO) and reflect on how it applies in different contexts. What are the benefits and challenges?

Palliative care is a crucial part of integrated, people-centred health services. Relieving serious health-related suffering, be it physical, psychological, social, or spiritual, is a global ethical responsibility … palliative care … has to be available at all levels of care.

(WHO, n.d.)

The roots of contemporary end-of-life care descriptors can be traced back to historical interventions from religious, philosophical, and medical perspectives in ancient Greece and the Roman Empire (Kastenbaum and Moreman, 2018). Religious and ethical considerations have played a substantial role in shaping end-of-life care throughout history, with religious leaders, nuns, and volunteers, prioritising dignity for the dying in various communities (Abel, 2013). Hospices have a long history dating back to the Fifth Century, originating from Greek-speaking Christian groups. The concept of 'pain' in the context of end-of-life care has evolved from religious interpretations of suffering as a punishment from God to a more humane and medicalised perspective. This shift has influenced the ethical understanding of caring for the dying and, subsequently, the definition of end-of-life care (Phipps, 1988). St. Joseph's Hospital innovations in the early Twentieth Century and the establishment of St. Christopher's Hospice by Dame Cicely Saunders in 1967, continued the religious foundation of end-of-life care. These initiatives reinforced the integration of ethical and moral principles into end-of-life care, emphasising the importance of dignity and compassion (Pentaris, 2018).

Recent efforts to define end-of-life care have attempted to shift away from the medicalised concepts of palliative and hospice care, focusing on more inclusive practices and service delivery. In the UK, for example, since the End-of-Life Strategy 2008, various scholarly attempts have been made to pursue evidence of the benefits. In their book, Adshead and Dechamps (2016) succinctly assert that 'end of life care is everybody's business'; and for this to be an effective argument, the prioritisation of the social model in this field is key. The social model tends to focus upon the social and economic determinants of health and social care as opposed to the biomedical model's narrow emphasis upon physical and biological processes of dying. Their argument focuses on the sentiment that a social model in end-of-life care will consider resources and networks surrounding the person and their families and friendship networks when planning care. Since the 1970s, when the social model was first emphasised (Beigel and Ghertner, 1977; Oliver, 1983), health services have engaged in a conversations about how to effectively integrate the medical model, which focuses on the individual, and a social model of care (initially focused on disability) which gives rise to the need to consider broader social circumstances, which could change health outcomes. This focus has also enabled a more extensive focus on, for instance, the broader phenomenon of 'wellbeing' as a micro and macro concept, and how it can be integrated into health and social care policy and practice, with the needs of the individual at the centre of this (La Placa et al., 2013). The gravitas of this model in disabilities is evident when looking at service cuts and how those negatively affect people living with disabilities (Oliver, 2013).

Other examples of more inclusive practices in end-of-life care refer to culture- and context-specific care planning. Various studies have highlighted the lack of a shared definition and the influence of cultural and religious views on the interpretation of end-of-life care (Mularski, 2006; Izumi et al., 2012; Gysels et al., 2013). Radbruch et al. (2020) have proposed a consensus-based definition of palliative care, which underlines a comprehensive approach to individuals of all ages, with severe health-related suffering, due to illness, especially those near the end of life. This definition centres upon improving the quality of life for patients, their families, and caregivers. This definition, as others, has a focus on the context in which it is harvested and understood; it focuses on illness and suffering, using medical language to characterise non-medical experiences, when quality of life is a state beyond the physical (Kastenbaum and Moreman, 2018; Pentaris, 2018). More recent research by Pentaris and Christodoulou (2021a) has identified four key qualities of inclusive end of life care: (a) informed decision-making; (b) respect; (c) adaptability; (d) nonjudgmental practice. All four are linked with the intent of end-of-life care policies that are introduced from time to time. Examples of those include the 'Ambitions for End-of-Life Care and the End-of-Life Care Guide', in England and Wales, or the 'Quality Health Services and Palliative Care' (WHO, 2021), while all characteristics of quality in end-of-life care are relevant to both generic and specialist skills in the area (Evans et al., 2020; Borgstrom et al., 2021; NHS England, 2016).

END-OF-LIFE CARE POLICY

WHO (2020) published a fact sheet about palliative care, underscoring that approximately 57 million people annually require palliative care, of whom around 45% are in the last year of their life. Worldwide, however, as the factsheet highlights, only 14% of the 57 million people actually receive it. These numbers were further diminished with the global COVID-19 pandemic (Pentaris, 2021). This was later recognised by the UK's Parliamentary Office of Science and Technology (POST), emphasising both the exacerbation of need during the global pandemic and the repositioning of distribution of end-of-life care outside of designated organisations such as hospices (POST, 2022). Such facts are considered when exploring how to improve the circumstances, and following WHO's recommendations, adequate policies are required to ensure equity and equality in end-of-life care, particularly in relation to accessibility for those from more deprived backgrounds (Rodin et al., 2020; Selman et al., 2022). The diverse range of descriptors used to define end-of-life care may lead to variations in the approach to care. This section provides further information about the policy context in the four nations of the UK, Cyprus, as well as Romania, highlighting both similarities and differences in their approaches. It is important to note that all three countries have radically different economies and histories, and this must be borne in mind through any comparison. As was mentioned in chapter two, Esping-Andersen (1990) developed a typology of 18 OECD welfare states based upon three tenets: decommodification, social stratification and the private–public mix and divided welfare states into three ideal regime types, Liberal, Conservative, and Social Democratic.

Whereas the UK would be categorised as Liberal, with a less developed welfare state and where principles of neoliberalism dominate attitudes to and organisation of health and social services, Romania, and Cyprus, are located within the Conservative category. Conservative regimes are more characterised by status differentiation type welfare approaches in which benefits are often earnings-related and structured towards maintaining widely held social and cultural patterns, for example, the role of the family in providing health and social care, as opposed to state or individual provision. However, as is the case throughout much of the OECD, greater pressure to increase expenditure is accompanied by less state intervention and provision through market mechanisms and services outside the state sector.

United Kingdom

The UK, comprising of four devolved nations, has developed, and implemented numerous key strategies, informing service providers and commissioners of expectations of quality of end-of-life care. It has also increasingly considered the voices and lived experiences of those at the receiving end of services to help develop more inclusive and concrete responses to the needs of those at the end of their lives and their loved ones. That said, and since 2008, when the first End of Life Strategy (Department of Health, 2008) was developed, further policies have been introduced, not merely and directly affecting end of life services, but the healthcare system altogether, considering end of life services as an integral part of it. The End-of-Life Strategy (2008) had a specific focus on adults, creating policies and guidance for the care of older individuals, as commonly palliative, hospice, and end of life care, are equated with the care of older individuals, leaving other age groups unattended (also see Pentaris, 2018). An additional limitation in previous policies has been that of focusing on cancer patients primarily, an area that was later addressed, emphasising the need that professionals and organisations shall offer equal opportunities for end-of-life care to patients, other than those facing challenges by cancer.

Having said that, policy in England specifically has only recently made it explicit that end of life care, inclusive of palliative and hospice care, where there are definitional challenges, is a part of the wider system of health and social care services. An example is the Care Act (2014) which accumulated service duties toward adults in need of services, and specifically the right of people to be assessed, and afforded the opportunity to receive those services, including carers who were not explicitly supported in policy previously. Since then, other socio-political changes which England has witnessed (Chandra and Erlingsdóttir, 2020) have led to further developments.

For example, the Health and Care Act (2022) is one of the most recent amendments to the overall health and social care legislation in England. This Act argues for the establishment of an integrated care system, which enhances partnerships of commissioners and providers of health and social care services. Palliative care, particularly, is perceived as a statutory requirement under this act; integrated care boards (ICBs) are introduced, with the responsibility to provide palliative care for all. Specifically, the 'Palliative and End of Life Care Statutory Guidance for Integrated Care Boards' (NHS England, 2022) stipulates:

> The duty [of ICBs] is intended to ensure that palliative and end of life care needs of people of all ages, with progressive illness or those nearing the end of their lives, and their loved ones and carers, receive the care and support they need to live and to die well.

In the last five years, England has significantly focused on the care of the dying and the bereaved (Pentaris, 2021), enabling the implementation of further guidance and policies which at times reiterate the same message; or on other occasions, such policies highlight areas that were previously not explicitly stated. Such examples may be found in the 'NHS England Palliative and End of Life Care National Delivery Plan 2022–2025' (NHS, 2022). This plan is set out with the aim of improving access, quality, and sustainability of services, and positive outcomes for those on the receiving end. This new and current plan and strategy sets six main ambitions for the field:

- Every person to be seen as an individual and have a personalized care plan for them.
- No discrimination on any grounds; all people experience fair access to care.
- Regular reviews of care plans to maximise comfort and wellbeing.

- Coordinated care with multidisciplinary teams.
- Well-equipped staff to deliver high quality end-of-life care.
- All community resources are used for the care of those with end-of-life needs.

In other words, this new strategy establishes the responsibility of integrated care systems to ensure the concept of 'dying well' for all people regardless of their background. The plan highlights that consideration needs to be afforded to the varied needs, based on age, and inclusive of end-of-life care for children. The above-mentioned ambitions are detailed further in the 'Ambitions for Palliative and End of Life Care: A National Framework for Local Action 2021–2026' (National Palliative and End of Life Care Partnership, 2021). This framework further highlights the principles close to which all targets set by ICBs need to be.

The new strategy and ambitions documents follow the 'NHS Long Term Plan 2019' (NHS England, 2019) which set the tone for the former two. This plan sets a focus on collaborative and personalised care and its delivery, and a commitment to palliative and end of life care, which we see evidenced in the strategy and ambitions and guidance for all ICBs. As well as the directions and guidance for integrated healthcare, there is also an emphasis upon the important contributions of the social care sector, following the recognition of the value of partnerships in palliative and end of life care. Thus, the Local Government Association (LGA), in 2020, published the End-of-Life Care Guide for all Councils in the country. This guide highlights the role of Councils in delivering high quality end of life care and supporting the provision in the community and in collaboration with the healthcare sector.

Legislation and policies in Northern Ireland, Wales, and Scotland do not fall far from those of England, following a similar pattern, and highlighting similar ambitions. The promotion of health services and provision in Wales, for example, is legislated by the National Health Service Wales Act 2006, which recognises the duty of care for all Trusts and the demand for equal opportunities and fair treatment and care for all. Yet, other aspects have not been recognised in this legislation, such as collaborative and integrated care.

The 'Health and Social Care (quality and Engagement) (Wales) Act 2020' highlights that everyone should have a voice in their care (Welsh Government, 2019). With this new Act, the Welsh Government sought to respond to the need to engage everyone, as service users, in their own care and ensure that feedback results in change and improvements. A key example of this Act is the replacement of the 'Community Health Councils by the Citizen Voice Body', which invites all citizens to share their experiences with the health and social care sectors and use the evidence to make changes as required. In other words, an attempt to integrate health and social care services, and provide more holistic approaches to service delivery, (seen from the Social Services and Well-being (Wales) Act 2014 (Social Care Wales, 2023) aligns the duty of assessing need with just provision of services by Councils.

In 2017, the 'Palliative and End of Life Care (PEoLC) Delivery Plan' was published with an update in 2021. This plan included the 'Quality Statement for Palliative and End of Life Care for Wales' (Welsh Government, 2022a), which describes what good quality palliative and end of life care services look like. This statement draws on the principle of 'active offer', referring to the engagement of patients and family members in the planning of their care, and was first introduced with the Welsh Government's 'More than Just Words Plan' (Welsh Government, 2022b). The quality statement highlights the need for developing more resilience in service provision, with a focus on coproduction, and a value-based approach, when offering services to people near the end of their lives. Specifically, the document highlights key attributes in the delivery of palliative and end of life care: safety; timely services; effectiveness; person-centred care; efficiency; and equity. Such attributes are found in the regulations for England, but also Scotland.

The Scottish Government, with the 'Palliative and end of life care: Strategic framework for Action 2015' (Scottish Government, 2015) ensured that by 2021, everyone in need of palliative and end of life care had access to it. One key difference between this strategy and that of Wales and England, is that the Scottish approach placed responsibility on service providers and the Government to ensure that all professionals in health and social care, involved with palliative and end of life services, are enabled the support they need to improve their skills, knowledge, and services in their respective sectors. This is an important policy directive as such significant policy and legislation highlights the duty of care, and the need for adequacy in expertise, when delivering the services, but fails to place responsibility on the 'systems' preparing and supporting those delivering care.

Lastly, Northern Ireland presents similar ambitions, highlighting integrated care in palliative and end of life services, among other areas, with the 'Health and Social Care Act (Northern Ireland)' 2022 (Acts of Northern Ireland Assembly, 2022). The 'Living Matters Dying Matters' (Department of Health, 2010) five-year strategy in Northern Ireland has set out principles, such as equity and accessibility, as well as collaborative working with patients, and family or friends, in palliative and end of life care. Northern Ireland led the way in proposing a fully developed 'Strategy for Children's Palliative and End of Life Care (2016)' (Department of Health, 2016), a ten-year strategy. This document sets out directions for the care of children and young people who are ill and dying, following a four-year consultation with the public since 2014. The recommendations for implementation include support for families; holistic assessments; the right to care and choice; end of life and bereavement care for all.

Across the UK, there have been initiatives in end-of-life care policies that share the following principles: accessible and fair care to all, without discrimination; well-equipped professionals at the delivery front; collaborative approaches, and holistic assessments. The progression of policy in this area is very recent (within the last five years) and hence it would be difficult to produce measures of success of these policies. However, the increasing concern with engaging the public and patients in the planning of care and delivery may only be a promising approach to positive out-comes in the future. Yet not all countries or contexts are aligned with such progress, and below we consider two further examples from Cyprus and Romania.

BOX 13.2 REFLECTIVE THOUGHTS

How does integrated care influence the lived experiences of those at the receiving end of end of life and palliative care?

How do infrastructural changes, inclusive of funding cuts, affect end of life and palliative care?

Cyprus

A key difference between the policy context of the UK and Cyprus is that of provision. In Cyprus, the underdevelopment of palliative and end of life care is evident, and most services are delivered by private and voluntary organisations, albeit some government-funded ones. Unlike the UK, the social and welfare system in Cyprus is not as advanced, but increasing demographic, economic, and societal pressures mean palliative care policy is shifting towards an integrated approach into the mainstream public healthcare system. Only recently has Cyprus developed a National Health Insurance Fund which finances services provided by a combination of public and private providers. However, health and social care spending in Cyprus remains significantly below the EU average. In 2008, the Government Bioethics Office released an opinion piece about palliative care in Cyprus (Cypriot Democracy, 2008). This focused on proposing the need for the healthcare system to ensure equal and equitable care for all when faced by terminal illnesses. This also sets the tone for how palliative, rather than end of life care, is perceived and designed in the country; focusing on cancer particularly. The General Healthcare System in 2020 established information about who might deliver services (General Healthcare System, 2020); a very brief and non-informative account which was simply a statement of what professionals are responsible for, including nurses and physicians, but excluding social services, such as social work.

Pentaris and Christodoulou (2021b) produced a first national report on evidence about end-of-life care, which along with other public consultations across the healthcare system led to a more robust and formal integration of palliative care into the healthcare sector, delineating their responsibilities. This advancement, in 2021, is too new to be able to recognise its impact. Nonetheless, it justifies the long-standing contributions and services provided by two key organisations focusing primarily on cancer patients. First, there is the 'Cyprus Anti-Cancer Society Hospice', which has provided palliative and end of life care, for over 25 years, as well as bereavement services to family and friends. Second, there is the 'Cancer Association of Cancer Patients and Friends' (PASYKAF), which offers services to cancer patients, families, and friends, but has over the years, opened its delivery to patients, with conditions other than cancer. These two non-profit, charitable organisations are the key mechanisms providing hospice, and end of life related care to those in need, while hospital care remains focused on treatment, rather than comfort and 'dying well', (which are the values which underpin the work of the former). An additional service available in the country is that of the 'St. Michael's Hospice', which is a residential and home care service to those living with terminal illnesses. The Church is a key factor in the provision of services, while the focus altogether is on adult care. It is clear from the above that little comparison can be drawn between the UK and Cyprus, apart from the different pace in which the two nations have evolved their commitment to end of life care, as well as cultural histories and perspectives. Once again, various nations progress differently and based on resources, need, and commitment (Lewis, 2007).

Romania

Lastly, the chapter considers the policy context of Romania in end-of-life care, which appears to lie in the middle of those of the UK and Cyprus. The political and economic legacy of Communism, characterised by economic dislocation, poverty, and food and fuel shortages, meant that health and social services lagged far behind those of other countries, even after the December 1989 Revolution, which overthrew the dictators, Nicolae and Elena Ceausescu. In Romania, health expenditure is still among the lowest in Europe, as is health status, and one of the most significant challenges of the Romanian healthcare system is the substantial shortages of staff due to large outflows of medical personnel to Western Europe, as well as lack of financial resources, generally. Diseases such as cancer in Romania continue to have significant stigma attached to it when compared to other countries (Pacurari et al., 2021). Mosoiu et al. (2000) also highlight that historically, the dominance of the Romanian Orthodox Church, and its emphasis upon strong religious and familial values, has tended to focus upon care in the home, by family members, compared with other forms of care. This type of palliative care is largely ignored in official costings and analyses of health and social care across Romania, as are the effects on family caregivers, even beyond initial bereavement

At large, end of life care in Romania is delivered both in hospices and hospitals. 'Hospice Casa Sperantei' is the leading organisation, pioneering palliative and end of life care developments and services in Romania. Since 2015, the country had 115 palliative care services established – 78 palliative care inpatient units; 24 home-based services; five outpatient clinics; four-day centres and four hospital teams (Mosoiu et al., 2018). Accumulatively, these services are the core of care provision in end-of-life care, with a particular focus on life-limiting illnesses and particularly cancer. This is like the focus on cancer services in Cyprus, but also in the UK nations, up until 10 years prior to writing this chapter. In 2023, the National Plan of the Combat and Control of Cancer [Planul National de Combatere si Control al Cancerului] (Ministerul Sănătăril, 2023) came to replace the Romanian Palliative Care Strategy. The latter was the product of a collaboration of and input from the National Palliative Care Association in the country, along with the Ministry of Health and other experts. This Strategy was focused on the overall provision of palliative care, specifically for cancer patients, locally, regionally, and nationally. The aim was to highlight the need for basic, specialised, and developmental services. Similarly, the recently established National Plan seeks to detail knowledge about mortality rates and categorisations of cancer, and it focuses on the need for specialised care in those areas, administering responsibility to different public services. This plan emphasises the demand for palliative care specifically, but not necessarily across age groups, albeit the recognition of child mortality, and the need for support in those areas in the future.

COMPARATIVE FINAL THOUGHTS

The UK, Romania, and Cyprus represent distinct policy contexts in the domain of end-of-life care, which seeks to provide services to a proportionate part of the population of each of the countries (Table 13.1). The UK's approach is characterised by a comprehensive and evolving strategy that has progressively incorporated palliative and end-of-life care into its broader healthcare system. The UK's policies have shifted beyond exclusive focus on older individuals and cancer patients, emphasising equal access to care for all, involving multidisciplinary teams, and promoting personalised care plans. Recent legislative changes, such as the Health and Care Act 2022, have solidified the integration of palliative care into the healthcare system and further prioritise patients' and families' voices in care planning.

Conversely, Cyprus exhibits a lag in end-of-life care development, with a significant reliance on private and voluntary organisations, particularly in palliative care provision. The policy landscape is marked by a focus on cancer patients and a slower formal integration of palliative care into the healthcare sector. Two key charitable organisations have historically provided services to cancer patients and have extended their care to other illnesses. Hospital care in Cyprus remains primarily treatment-focused rather than emphasising comfort and holistic end-of-life care. Romania, situated between the UK and Cyprus, has made considerable progress in end-of-life care. It offers a mix of hospice and hospital-based care, with a strong focus on cancer patients. Hospice Casa Sperantei, in particular, has played a pioneering role in Romania's palliative care developments. The country established numerous palliative care services across different modalities, demonstrating its commitment to offering specialised care for life-limiting illnesses. These comparisons highlight the diversity in end -of-life care policies across different nations, influenced by resources, needs, and historical contexts.

TABLE 13.1 People Needing End-of-Life or Palliative Care, by Nation

Nation	N population
UK (no data of devolved nations available)	100,000 (POST, 2022)
Cyprus	2,634–3,927 (Aristodemou & Speck, 2017)
Romania	150,000 (Mosoiu, Mitrea, and Dumitrescu, 2018)

CONCLUSION

This chapter has shed some light on the intricacies of end-of-life care and the diverse policy landscapes within the UK, Cyprus, and Romania. While end-of-life care serves as a critical aspect of healthcare provision, its definition and policy context continue to evolve, reflecting unique historical, cultural, and healthcare system-specific factors in each of these nations. For example, attitudes towards and organisation of services is different for each country, with Romania, for instance, less historically exposed to Globalisation, than the UK. The comparative insights offered in this chapter underscore the remarkable diversity in end-of-life care policies, shaped by a complex interplay of resources, needs, historical contexts, and cultural influences. As end-of-life care continues to develop as a fundamental component of health and social care policy, landscapes will continue to adapt and develop, ultimately striving to provide compassionate and quality care for individuals in the last stages of their lives and their families. End-of-life care is a multifaceted, dynamic domain, and the ongoing journey of shaping its policies and practices reflects the evolving needs and values of societies across the OECD.

RESEARCH POINTS AND REFLECTIVE EXERCISES

- Discuss in groups if there is a potentiality for a global definition of end-of-life care. Consider values, principles, cultural and traditional tendencies, and resources when discussing this point.
- The care of the dying was nurtured by groups and communities with strong religious ties, linking their faith with the ethical responsibility of looking after those in need. What should be the role of religion, belief, and faith in end-of-life care nowadays?
- How have Covid-19 and associated measures impacted on end of life and palliative care across the OECD?

REFERENCES

Abel, E. K. (2013). *The Inevitable Hour: A History of Caring for Dying Patients in America*. Baltimore, MD: Johns Hopkins University Press.

Acts of Northern Ireland Assembly. (2022). Health and Social Care Act (Northern Ireland) 2022. Available at: www.legislation.gov.uk/nia/2022/3/contents/enacted (Accessed: 24 September 2023).

Adshead, L. and Dechamps, A. (2016). End of Life Care: Everybody's Business. *Journal of Social Work Practice*, 30 (2):169–185 doi:10.1080/02650533.2016.1168379

Aristodemou, P. A. and Speck, P. W. (2017). Palliative Care Service in Cyprus, A Population-Based Needs Assessment Based on Routine Mortality Data. *Progress in Palliative Care*, 25 (5): 215–223. doi:10.1080/09699260.2017.1361627

Beigel, A. and Ghertner, S. (1977). Toward a Social Model: An Assessment of Social Factors which Influence Problem Drinking and its Treatment. In B. Kissin and H. Begleiter (eds), *The Biology of Alcoholism. Treatment and Rehabilitation of the Chronic Alcoholic, Vol. 5*. Boston, MA: Springer, 197–233.

Borgstrom, E., Cohn, S., Driessen, A., Martin, J. and Yardley, S. (2021). Multidisciplinary Team Meetings in Palliative Care: An Ethnographic Study. *BMJ Supportive and Palliative Care*. https://doi.org/10.1136/bmjspcare-2021-003267

Chandra, G. and Erlingsdóttir, I. (2020). *The Routledge Handbook of the Politics of the#Metoo Movement*. London: Routledge.

Cypriot Democracy. (2008). Palliative Care: Offering a Medical-Social System of Care to People. Available at: www.bioethics.gov.cy/Moh/cnbc/cnbc.nsf/All/48FBC3FE739E59C0C2257CB30042BD07/$file/ΓΝΩΜΗ%20ΕΕΒΚ%20για%20ΑΝΑΚΟΥΦΙΣΤΙΚΗ%20ΦΡΟΝΤΙΔΑ.pdf (Accessed: 25 September 2023).

Department of Health. (2008). End of Life Strategy: Promoting High Quality End of Life Care for all Adults, NHS England. Available at: https://assets.publishing.service.gov.uk/media/5a7ae925ed915d71db8b35aa/End_of_life_strategy.pdf (Accessed: 10 September 2023).

Department of Health. (2010). Living Matters, Dying Matters Strategy (2010). Available at: www.health-ni.gov.uk/publications/living-matters-dying-matters-strategy-2010 (Accessed: 9 September 2023).

Department of Health. (2016). A Strategy for Children's Palliative and End of Life Care 2016-26. Northern Ireland. Available at: www.health-ni.gov.uk/publications/strategy-childrens-palliative-and-end-life-care-2016-26 (Accessed: 20 September 2023).

Dresser, R. (2004). Death with Dignity: Contested Boundaries. *Journal of Palliative Care*, 20 (3): 201–206. https://doi.org/10.1177/082585970402000313

Esping-Andersen, G. (1990). *The Three Worlds of Welfare Capitalism*. London: Polity.

Evans, C. J., Bone, A. E., Yi, D., Gao, W., Morgan, M. et al., (2021). Community-Based Short-Term Integrated Palliative and Supportive Care Reduces Symptom Distress for Older People with Chronic Noncancer Conditions Compared with Usual Care: A Randomised Controlled Single-Blind Mixed Method Trial. *International Journal of Nursing Studies*, 120. Aug; 120:103978. https://doi.org/10.1016/j.ijnurstu.2021.103978.

General Healthcare System. (2020). Palliative Care: What are the Services Provided? Available at: www.gesy.org.cy/sites/Sites?d=Desktop&locale=en_US&lookuphost=/en-us/&lookuppage=hiopalliative (Accessed: 9 October 2023).

Gysels, M., Evans, N., Menaca, A., Higginson, I. J., Harding, R., et al. (2013). Diversity in Defining End of Life Care: An Obstacle or the Way Forward? *PloS one*, 8 (7): e68002. https://doi.org/10.1371/journal.pone.0068002

Health and Care Act (2022). Available at: www.legislation.gov.uk/ukpga/2022/31/contents/enacted (Accessed: 2 August 2023).

Izumi, S., Nagae, H., Sakurai, C. and Imamura, E. (2012). Defining End-of-Life Care From Perspectives of Nursing Ethics. *Nursing Ethics*, 19 (5): 608–618. https://doi.org/10.1177/0969733011436205

Kastenbaum, R. and Moreman, C. (2018). *Death, Society, and Human Experience*. London: Routledge.

La Placa, V. G., McNaught, A. and Knight, A. (2013). Discourse of Wellbeing in Research and Practice. *International Journal of Wellbeing*, 3 (1): 116–125. https://doi.org/10.5502/ijw.v3i1.7

Lewis, M. J. (2007). *Medicine and Care of the Dying: A Modern History*. Oxford: Oxford University Press.

Local Government Association. (2020). End of Life Care: Guide for Councils. Available at: www.local.gov.uk/publications/end-life-care-guide-councils (Accessed: 10 October 2023).

Ministerul Sănătăril. (2023). Planul National de Combatere si Control al Cancerului. Available at: www.ms.ro/media/documents/Planul_Na%C8%9Bional_de_Combatere_%C8%99i_Control_al_Cancerului_RIQiTXG.pdf (Accessed: 10 October 2023).

Mosoiu, D., Andrews, C. and Peroll, D. (2000). Palliative Care in Romania. *Palliative Medicine*, 14 (1): 65–67. https://doi.org/10.1191/026921600671052814

Mosoiu, D., Mitrea, N. and Dumitrescu, M. (2018). Palliative Care in Romania. *Journal of Pain and Symptom Management*, 55 (2): S6–S76. https://doi.org/10.1016/j.jpainsymman.2017.03.036

Mularski, R. A. (2006). Defining and Measuring Quality Palliative and End-of-Life Care in the Intensive Care Unit. *Critical Care Medicine*, 34 (11): S309–S316. https://doi.org/10.1097/01.CCM.0000241067.84361.46

National Health Service (Wales) Act. (2006). Available at: www.legislation.gov.uk/ukpga/2006/42/contents (Accessed: 2 August 2023).

National Palliative and End of Life Care Partnership. (2021). Ambitions for Palliative and End of Life Care: A National Framework for Local Action 2021-2026. Available at: www.england.nhs.uk/wp-content/uploads/2022/02/ambitions-for-palliative-and-end-of-life-care-2nd-edition.pdf (Accessed: 21 October 2023).

NHPCO 2023. Hospice Care Overview for Professionals. Available at: www.nhpco.org/hospice-care-overview/#:~:text=Considered%20to%20be%20the%20model,the%20patient%27s%20needs%20and%20wishes (Accessed: 13 April 2023).

NHS. (2022). End of Life Care Strategy: Good End of Life Care for All. Available at: www.esneft.nhs.uk/wp-content/uploads/2023/02/FINAL-05781-22-End-of-Life-Care-Strategy-2022-2025.pdf (Accessed: 21 October 2023).

NHS England. (2019). The NHS Long Term Plan. Available at: www.longtermplan.nhs.uk/wp-content/uploads/2019/08/nhs-long-term-plan-version-1.2.pdf (Accessed: 21 October 2023)

NHS England. (2022). Palliative and End of Life Care: Statutory Guidance for Integrated Care Boards (ICB), July 2022. Available at: www.england.nhs.uk/wp-content/uploads/2022/07/Palliative-and-End-of-Life-Care-Statutory-Guidance-for-Integrated-Care-Boards-ICBs-September-2022.pdf (Accessed: 21 October 2023).

NHS England. (2016). NHS England Specialist Level Palliative Care: Information for Commissioners April 2016. Available at: www.england.nhs.uk/wp-content/uploads/2016/04/speclst-palliatv-care-comms-guid.pdf (Accessed: 22 October 2023).

Oliver, M. (1983). *Introduction: Setting the Scene*. In. M. Oliver and B. Sapey. *Social Work with Disabled People. Practical Social Work Series*. London: Palgrave, 1–5.

Oliver, M. (2013). The Social Model of Disability: Thirty Years On. *Disability and Society*, 28 (7): 1024–1026. https://doi.org/10.1080/09687599.2013.818773

Pacurari, N., De Clercq, E., Dragomir, M., Colita, A., Wangmo, T. et al., (2021). Challenges of Pediatric Palliative Care in Romania: A Focus Groups Study. *BMC Palliat Care* 20: (178). https://doi.org/10.1186/s12904-021-00871-7

Pentaris, P. (2018). *Religious Literacy in Hospice Care: Challenges and Controversies.* London: Routledge.

Pentaris, P. (ed.). (2021). *Death, Grief and Loss in the Context of COVID-19* (1st ed.). Abingdon: Routledge. https://doi.org/10.4324/9781003125990

Pentaris, P. and Christodoulou, P. (2021a). Knowledge and Attitudes of Hospice and Palliative Care Professionals Toward Diversity and Religious Literacy in Cyprus: A Cross-Sectional Study. *Journal of Palliative Medicine*, 24 (2): 233–239. https://doi.org/10.1089/jpm.2020.0011.

Pentaris, P. and Christodoulou, P. (2021b). Qualities of Culturally and Religiously Sensitive Practice: A Cross-Sectional Study. *Journal of Palliative Care*. https://doi.org/10.1177/08258597211050742

Phipps, W. E. (1988). The Origin of Hospices/Hospitals. *Death Studies*, 12 (2): 91–99. https://doi.org/10.1080/07481188808252226

POST. (2022). Palliative and End of Life Care. POSTNOTE, 675. Available at: https://researchbriefings.files.parliament.uk/documents/POST-PN-0675/POST-PN-0675.pdf (Accessed: 15 August 2023).

Radbruch, L., De Lima, L., Knaul, F., Wenk, R., Ali, Z. et al., (2020). Redefining Palliative Care—A New Consensus-Based Definition. *Journal of Pain and Symptom Management*, 60 (4): 754–764. https://doi.org/10.1016/j.jpainsymman.2020.04.027

Rodin, G., Zimmermann, C., Rodin, D., Al-Awamer, A., Sullivan, R. et al., (2020). COVID-19, Palliative Care and Public Health. *European Journal of Cancer*, 136, 95–98. https://doi.org/10.1016/j.ejca.2020.05.023

Scottish Government. (2015). Palliative and End of Life Care: Strategic Framework for Action. Available at: www.gov.scot/publications/strategic-framework-action-palliative-end-life-care/(Accessed 29 October 2023).

Selman, L. E., Farnell, D. J. J., Longo, M., Goss, S., Seddon, K. et al., (2022). Risk Factors Associated with Poorer Experiences of End-Of-Life Care and Challenges in Early Bereavement: Results of a National Online Survey of People Bereaved During the COVID-19 Pandemic. *Palliative Medicine*, 36 (4): 717–729. https://doi.org/10.1177/02692163221074876.

Singer, P. A. and Bowman, K. W. (2002). Quality End-of-Life Care: A Global Perspective. *BMC Palliative Care*, 1 (4–10. https://doi.org/10.1186/1472-684X-1-4

Social Care Wales. (2023). Social Services and Well-being (Wales) Act 2014. Available at: https://socialcare.wales/resources-guidance/information-and-learning-hub/sswbact/overview#:~:text=The%20Social%20Services%20and%20Well%2Dbeing%20(Wales)%20Act%20came,transforming%20social%20services%20in%20Wales (Accessed: 20 August 2023).

Welsh Government. (2022a). Quality Statement for Palliative and End of Life Care for Wales. Available at: www.gov.wales/quality-statement-palliative-and-end-life-care-wales-html (Accessed: 3 August 2023).

Welsh Government. (2022b). More Than Just Words: Welsh Language Plan in Health and Social Care. Available at: www.gov.wales/more-just-words-welsh-language-plan-health-and-social-care (Accessed: 3 August 2023).

Welsh Government. (2019). Health and Social Care (Quality and Engagement) (Wales) Bill. Available at: www.gov.wales/sites/default/files/publications/2019-06/easy-read_0.pdf (Accessed: 3 August 2023).

WHO. (n.d.). Palliative care. Available at: www.who.int/health-topics/palliative-care (Accessed: 23 September 2024).

WHO. (2020). Palliative Care. Available at: www.who.int/news-room/fact-sheets/detail/palliative-care#:~:text=Each%20year%20an%20estimated%2056.8,of%20them%20living%20in%20Africa (Accessed: 13 November 2023).

WHO. (2021). Quality Health Services and Palliative Care: Practical Approaches and Resources to Support Policy, Strategy and Practice. Available at: www.who.int/publications/i/item/9789240035164 (Accessed: 3 August 2023).

WHPCA/WHO. (2020). Global Atlas of Palliative Care. Available at: https://cdn.who.int/media/docs/default-source/integrated-health-services-(ihs)/csy/palliative-care/whpca_global_atlas_p5_digital_final.pdf?sfvrsn=1b54423a_3 (Accessed: 3 August 2023).

Zechner, M. (2023). Constructing A Regime of Truth to Support Palliative Care at Risk. *European Journal of Politics and Gender*, 6 (2): 167–182. https://doi.org/10.1332/251510823X16783539965894

CHAPTER 14

Dental Services across the Four Nations of the United Kingdom

....

Charlotte Jeavons and Maria Morgan

INTRODUCTION

Diseases of the oral cavity constitute a global public health problem; they are among the most prevalent in the world, having a considerable effect on quality of life. Most oral diseases are preventable. In the UK the National Health Service (NHS) provides dental care to most of the population, although an increasing number of people are seeking privately sourced and funded care as access to NHS dental care can be problematic. Dentists are the main providers of care in the UK, but pressure is increasing for the sector to adopt a 'skill mix' approach, fully utilising the whole dental workforce, and widening the public's access to dentistry. In contrast to all other NHS services which are 'free at the point of delivery', most who access NHS dental services pay a standardised fee. Political autonomy in the form of devolution has seen significant health policy differences evolve across the four nations of the UK. This makes the dental service landscape in the UK a complex one. This chapter outlines some of the major differences between the four nations of the UK and their approach to oral and dental care.

THE NHS DENTAL SERVICE IN THE UK

Dentistry, as part of the new NHS in 1948 had three key principles: (1) no one would be prohibited from dental care due to cost, (2) dental care would be free at the point of delivery, and (3) care would be based on clinical need (National Health Service Act, 1946). Such was, and still is, the demand for dentistry that it has not been possible to deliver on these three principles and patient charges were introduced in 1952 National Health Service (Charges for Dental Treatment) Regulations. (1952). The arrangements for NHS dental care remained unchanged until the early 1990s when the contract between the NHS and dentists as independent practitioners was

DOI: 10.4324/9781003343608-16

changed (Health Departments of England, Scotland, Wales, and Northern Ireland, 1990). Many dentists were unhappy with the new arrangements leading to a rise in privately funded care as many left the NHS for good. The 1990 contract change was intended to promote preventive and continuous care and to move away from the focus of treating disease. It was intended to meet the changing needs of the population (Brocklehurst et al., 2016). From here on, the four nations of the UK started to diverge in the way NHS dental care was viewed and delivered.

Political autonomy in the form of national devolution has seen significant health policy differences evolve in England, Wales, Scotland, and Northern Ireland from 1999 onwards. It left England as the only nation of the UK legislated for solely by the UK government. Scotland and Wales have emphasised universal access to services, whereas England has pursued more top-down techniques, using targets and market-orientated mechanisms. Northern Ireland has mostly adopted policies from England, but with less emphasis on public accountability and market-type mechanisms. The Nuffield Trust (Connolly et al., 2010) and the National Audit Office (2012) have attempted to examine the performance of these divergent healthcare systems, but lack of comparable data has restricted any reliable conclusions from being drawn.

In 2006, a new dental contract was introduced in England (National Health Service (General Dental Services Contracts), 2005). This prioritised a local commissioning model of care where general dental practitioners were paid according to activity that was categorised into three bands of treatment. This replaced the 400 individually listed chargeable treatments from the 1990 contract. These bands represented different levels or 'units of dental activity' (UDA). Patient charges were also simplified to only three levels of payment. A key feature of this contract was cost containment and dental activity was capped at an agreed number of UDAs per year by local NHS commissioners. Dentists were penalised if they under or over performed against UDA targets. In addition, local dentists no longer had to provide emergency care for their patients. This responsibility now fell to local NHS primary care trusts. This contract, which shapes the way much of the dentistry in England is carried out, has been heavily criticised for failing to improve access to care and not aligning incentives to the goal of improving oral health (Steel, 2009). Local commissioning of dentistry has led to a fragmentation in services across England. Moreover, there is no universal national oral health improvement programme as there is in the other UK nations. In recognition of these issues, NHS England (2024) published a 'plan to recover and reform NHS dentistry'. The full outcomes of this will not be known for some years.

Scotland's NHS remains a separate body from the other public health systems in the UK (The Scotland Act, 1998). Primary care and secondary care have been retained as traditional integrated system with minimal involvement of the private sector or external commissioning. Similarly, to the rest of the UK, dental care is provided through three main routes: the general dental service (high-street practices), the community or salaried dental service (primary care focusing on vulnerable groups, for instance, children or people with special needs), and the hospital dental service, but crucially there are differences in how these services are funded and managed when compared to the rest of the UK. Most dentistry in Scotland is carried out by the general dental service and this still operates under the 1990 contract with a renumeration of model based on 'fee per item'. Unlike England, there is no local commissioning model and so outputs i.e., the number of chargeable dental treatments that can be performed, remains unconstrained, and therefore more able to meet changing demands. In 2005, Scotland launched a universal oral health improvement programme for children, 'ChildSmile'. This integrates general and community dental services with a focus on schools and nurseries as part of a setting-based approach.

NHS Wales operates general, salaried, and hospital dental services, similarly to the other nations. The general dental service is delivered under the same 2006 dental contract as England, but with some variation. A key issue for Wales is the degree to which the Welsh government have the capacity and expertise to operate a general dental service that is different from England (Chestnutt, 2014). As in England, primary care services that are focused on prevention as opposed to treatment are seen as desirable. The Community Dental Service in Wales has retained its traditional position as the safety net for children who have struggled to find dental care via the general dental service, or who would not have sought care elsewhere, and for people with special needs. This differs somewhat to England and Scotland's salaried service, which now largely focuses only on patients with special or complex needs. Hospital dentistry in Wales is currently vastly different to that in England. The market-place operating model has been abolished; whereas in England this has increased. In 2009 the Welsh government set out a plan for a universal oral health improvement programme like Scotland's ChildSmile, called 'Designed to Smile' (NHS Wales, 2009).

In Northern Ireland, the NHS equivalent is referred to as Health and Social Care (HSC) and underwent major reform in 2009, although the purchaser-provider model of commissioning and delivery of dental care remained. Hospital dental care in Northern Ireland is similar to much of the UK where patients are referred for specialist treatment. The community or salaried dental service provides treatment to similar patient groups as in England and there is no remit to include children who cannot access care elsewhere as in Wales. In contrast to England and Wales, where the 2006 contract limited the number of general dental practitioners, services in Northern Ireland operate under no such limits. In 2016 the HSC launched a national oral health improvement project, but on a smaller scale to, those in Scotland and Wales, called 'Happy Smiles' (Health and Social Care, 2016). Dentistry operates in a mixed economy with England and Northern Ireland having the largest private sectors. Scotland and Wales lead the way in publicly funded significant national oral health improvement programmes.

PRIMARY AND SECONDARY NHS DENTAL SERVICE IN THE UK

Significant public resources remain invested in NHS dentistry, supported by co-payments from most adults, although some are exempt from patient charges if they are in receipt of specific state-funded benefits. Children under the age of 18 do not pay for professional dental care. Broadly, there are three branches of dental service delivery.

'General dental services' (GDS) remain the main provider. General dental practices are found on the UK 'high street' and can be accessed by anyone. Referrals are not required. Most general dental practices carry out dental services under the auspices of the NHS, but in recent years this is diminishing, and more general private practices are offering services. 'Community dental services' (CDS) traditionally provide services for high-needs children, patients with special needs, population dental screening, epidemiology, and health promotion. In addition, the CDS Wales and Scotland (now known as the 'public dental service') provide a safety-net services for children who can't access the GDS. Northern Ireland does not charge patients for care or provide NHS dentistry for patients unable to access care through the GDS. 'Hospital dental services' (secondary care) accepts patients on referral from medical and dental practitioners. Consultants in other areas/specialties, including emergency dental services, also make referrals. The hospital service also provides outpatient care in special cases where there are medical considerations which make it desirable for patients to be treated in a hospital setting. Specialist hospital services are provided from two settings – local acute hospitals and dental teaching hospitals. The acute hospitals usually manage patients requiring oral and maxillofacial, orthodontic, and restorative dentistry services. The dental teaching hospitals, in addition, offer opportunities for the management of patients, training and research in a wide range of dental specialties.

ORAL EPIDEMIOLOGY IN THE FOUR NATIONS OF THE UK

Before devolution, the UK had a comprehensive dental epidemiology programme. This involved decennial surveys of children and adults commissioned by the four UK health departments, commencing in 1968. Local surveys coordinated by the British Association for the Study of Community Dentistry (BASCD), focussing on children, began in 1985/86 in England and Wales, and in 1987/88 in Scotland. Northern Ireland participated in 1993/94, although this participation has been inconsistent over the years. The surveillance of population oral health via dental epidemiology provides valuable information, which has been used to affect public health policy. It has been used to plan health services via national and regional 'Oral health needs assessments' to improve national targeting of oral health promotion and monitor effectiveness. Information gleaned from the surveys has also been used to secure funding for underserved vulnerable groups, e.g., older people in care homes and added to the knowledge base by informing the study design of research studies.

These dental epidemiological surveys comprise a dental examination, with standardised criteria carried out by trained and calibrated examiners, and an accompanying questionnaire. The primary source data generated is used to monitor the oral health of the population, unique to health surveillance, as other health disciplines rely on secondary data sources for these purposes. In recent years, dental surveys have mainly focussed on children. Some countries in the UK have started to survey other priority groups, such as older people living in care homes, people with special needs linked to disability (Public Health England, 2015), adults attending general dental practices (Public Health England, 2020), homeless people (Doughty et al., 2022) and 18–25-year-olds (Morgan and Monaghan, 2020).

Devolution has resulted in different dental policies being implemented across the constituent countries of the UK, accompanied by different approaches to dental epidemiology. Scotland and Wales have withdrawn from the decennial UK surveys and differences in interpretation of the form of consent required for dental surveys means that while the Scots continue with negative (opt-out) consent for their surveys, the Departments of Health in England and Wales have introduced the use of positive (opt-in) parental consent for participation in the BASCD coordinated surveys of children's oral health. Devolution has had a negative impact on national data comparisons, which was routine, but has now almost ceased.

The UK is the fourth most densely populated country in Europe. Within the UK, England has the highest population density and Scotland the lowest (Atkins and Dalton, 2021). Sparsely populated areas mean higher costs for providing health services. Provision of multiple facilities such as numerous small dental practices distributed across spread out villages have financial and workforce implications. Those who have financial and physical capacity to access private dentistry can do so when and where they choose. Conversely, those who rely solely on NHS care are at the mercy of politicians and policy makers who decide on the organisation of services, as such much of the population are more or less dentally disadvantaged, depending on which of the UKs four nations they reside.

The UK population is increasing and ageing with implications for population health and care needs. Also, people with a disability have higher care needs on average (Atkins and Dalton, 2021). Demands placed on health and social care are influenced by demographic and socioeconomic factors as well as advances in treatments and diagnostics. The four UK countries have different populations with unique needs. For example, Scotland, Wales, and Northern Ireland have higher average needs for health care than England (Atkins and Dalton, 2021). The provision of dental services and treatment alone is not sufficient to reduce oral health inequalities at a national level and may even widen inequalities. Moreover, the oral health gradient mirrors the UK's social gradient with lifestyle factors such as diet and smoking being strongly correlated to poverty and to (oral) health inequalities. The most recent UK national Child Dental Health Survey (NHS England, 2015) highlighted that those eligible for State funded school meals have a greater chance of having obvious decay experience. Local surveys have reported that between one quarter and one third of five-year-old children have experience of decayed, missing, or filled teeth (dmft) depending on the country being considered. England has the lowest experience of decay at 23.7%, while Northern Ireland has the highest at 34.6%. The average number of teeth affected for those with experience of decay is approximately four teeth.

TABLE 14.1 Summary of Disease Experience in Primary Dentition Using Most Recent Individual Country-Level Surveys

Country	Survey Year	Experience of decay (dmft > 0)	Mean no. teeth affected of those with dmft > 0	Range % dmft > 0 by health board	
				Lowest	Highest
England	2021/22	29.3	3.5	23.3 Southwest	38.7 Northwest
Wales	2015/16	34.2	3.58	26.3 Hywel Dda	47.3 Cwm Taf
Scotland	2020	26.5	3.94	15.4 Orkney	31.4 Greater Glasgow & Clyde
Northern Ireland	2018-19	34.6	3.86	29.4 Southern HSCT	35.8 Western HSCT

Sources: England: Office for Health Improvement and Disparities (2023a); Wales: Morgan and Monaghan (2017); Scotland: Public Health Scotland (2020); Northern Ireland: Department of Health (2023)

A key indicator which highlights the inequalities in health related to tooth decay is the number of hospitalisations for tooth extraction using a general anaesthetic. Using England as an example, during 2021/2022 there were 26,741 episodes of tooth extractions with a primary diagnosis of dental caries (tooth decay) for 0- to 19-year-olds undertaken in hospital under general anaesthesia (Office for Health Improvement and Disparities, 2022; 2023a; 2023b).The caries-related tooth extraction rate for children and young people living in the most deprived communities is nearly three and a half times more than those living in the most affluent communities, meaning those more likely to need dental treatment are also more likely to need complex and costly treatment and be reliant on NHS care. The most recent Adult Dental Health Survey in 2009 (Fuller et al., 2011) demonstrated an overall improvement in oral health. This improvement occurred mainly for the younger age groups, up to 45 years of age. For those aged over 45, the legacy of higher disease levels earlier in their life course, and various approaches to dental care, remain visible with far fewer teeth present and fewer sound teeth. Similarly to the pattern of disease reported for children, differences in adult oral health were highlighted across the UK countries. Thus, the social gradient associated with experience of oral disease persists into adulthood.

THE DIFFERENCE IN ORAL HEALTH IMPROVEMENT PROGRAMMES ACROSS THE UK

Dental surveillance in the form of regular cross sectional epidemiology surveys have highlighted unacceptable levels of dental caries in children and vulnerable adults and wide inequalities of disease across social groups in all nations of the UK. As was mentioned, in 2005 ChildSmile, a national oral health improvement programme for children was introduced in Scotland and is the most comprehensive programme. It is often held up as an example of good practice. This was followed shortly after by Designed to Smile in Wales in 2009, and then by 'Happy Smiles' in Northern Ireland (Health and Social Care, 2016; 2023). In England, the decision to implement oral health improvement programmes like this has been left to local commissioners. This means there is no universal programme, only smaller local facsimiles, which has resulted in large parts of the population not able to benefit. The number and geographic coverage of programmes of this kind is not known. This contrasts with the very different political choices made in the other nations of the UK, where government policy has favoured central co-ordination and control.

In England, the intention of giving responsibility to local commissioners, is to empower local areas to contract services, which are specifically tailored to their populations (Office for Health Improvement and Disparities, 2022). This also means that oral health improvement in England is fragmented. Economies of scale cannot be leveraged and any improvements in population oral health are very difficult to monitor and evidence. However, the recent NHS England (2024) plan to 'recover and reform dentistry' has outlined the launch of 'Smile for Life' a population wide programme modelled on the successes of the other national programmes. Initiatives such as these follow a similar model based on health improvement principles using a whole system approach. They include the following:

- Supervised toothbrushing in nurseries and primary schools.
- Universal fluoride varnish application.
- Whole school approach to health, food, and nutrition.
- Designated child friendly dental practices.
- Individualised support for parent to access dental care.

THE DENTAL AND ORAL HEALTH WORKFORCE

When NHS dentistry emerged in 1948, the workforce consisted solely of dentists and no other personnel were recognised, but in 1956, the Dentists Act (1956) was enshrined into law and the regulatory body of the General Dental Council (GDC) was born. This act also enabled the training of what were known as 'dental auxiliaries', who were also required to be registered with the GDC. Today, there are six types of 'auxiliaries': nurses, hygienists, therapists, orthodontic therapists, dental technicians, and clinical dental technicians, now collectively known as 'dental care professionals' (DCPs). These individual titles can only be used by those holding relevant qualifications recognised by the GDC. The GDC also recognises 13 areas of specialism that dentists may pursue after extended training. In 2023, there are 114,000 dental professionals registered with the GDC with dental nurses comprising approximately 60,000 of these, and who work in all areas of dentistry and across both NHS and private systems (GDC, 2023). Dental hygienists, therapists, and orthodontic therapists mostly provide private dental care, although some dental therapists are employed in NHS community dental services. Common to all DCPs, until 2013, was the inability of patients to directly access the care they provided without first being referred by a dentist. However, a contested landmark decision by the GDC in 2013 enabled this without a dentist referral (GDC, 2013a). This was known as 'direct access' and it led to the expansion of training and skills for all DCPs. In reality, dentists remain a 'gatekeeper' for NHS care because DCPs are not permitted to contract directly with the NHS and 'direct access' to dental care is a privilege enjoyed by those who can afford to pay privately.

All dentists undergo five years of dental training at an approved dental school. This enables them to practice dentistry and service the public. They form the largest part of the GDS (general dental service, or 'high street' dentistry). Dentists on one of the specialty lists, held by the GDC, have undergone more advanced post graduate training, after their initial 'bachelor's of dentistry'. Specialists practice in all areas of clinical dentistry relevant to their specialism. Those on the dental public health specialty register are an exception to this and their work can involve a combination of clinical and office-based work, such a policy making, or commissioning, and some do not practice clinically at all. Most in this position hold consultant contracts with either the NHS or local authority. The level and complexity of care which each category of registrant can provide is outlined in their 'scope of practice' (GDC, 2013b).

In 1993, The Nuffield enquiry (The Nuffield Institute, 1993) into dental education and training redefined how the dental workforce should be structured to increase access to care to meet population needs. This report advocated 'skill mix', which is a model of care that uses the whole team to deliver services. Skill mix in medicine is well established, but dentistry has lagged and need to adapt to this practice. However, population needs are changing, with more people retaining their teeth into later life, while oral health inequalities remain. There are increasing calls for greater access to affordable NHS dental care (Gov.UK, 2022) and the universal adoption of skill mix has the potential to make a significant difference by freeing up costly resources (e.g., dentists' time spent on routine care which could be better spent on more complex treatment; Brocklehurst et al., 2014; Dyer et al., 2014). This is an ongoing international debate with other countries further along in their utilisation of DCPs than the UK (Nash et al., 2008; Brocklehurst et al., 2016). One of the key tenants of the recent NHS plan to 'recover and reform dentistry' (NHS England, 2024) restated the aims of the Workforce Plan, published a year earlier (NHS England, 2023) which formally recognised the need to train more dental care professionals. The stated aim is to increase training places by 40% by 2031. This will require cultural change across the dental sector and a shift in how the public view the delivery of dentistry, but if achieved, will increase capacity within the dental workforce and increase the potential for improved access to oral care for the public.

CONCLUSION

This chapter sought to outline the complexities found in the UK regarding dental services, many of which have come about since governmental devolution of the four nations within the UK. However, underlying this complexity are stark inequalities in oral health across the UK population. It is difficult to compare how well each nation is tackling these inequalities because of the very large differences in service organisation based on each government's belief in their responsibility for oral health i.e., that this is of utility to all, and should be centrally funded and organised, or that this is better served by devolving responsibility to local authority areas, who understand their population needs. The chapter highlighted the considerable burden of dental disease by comparing child oral health data across nations and how this is being addressed in each nation. As yet, we are too early in the devolution experiment to know which approach to organising dental services, including workforce operating models, has a more desirable effect on reducing inequalities. However, it is interesting that England, (the outlier in the way oral health services are organised when comparing UK nations) has now published the intention to implement a centrally co-ordinated oral health improvement programme mirroring those in Scotland, Wales, and Northern Ireland. A return to collaborative epidemiology across the four devolved governments is needed for us to make decisions about future organisation and implementation of oral care services.

RESEARCH POINTS AND REFLECTIVE EXERCISES

- Reflect upon why enhanced access to dentistry is important across the four nations of the UK and its impact upon the health and wellbeing of British citizens?
- What causes inequality in access to dentistry and how do they feed into more general social and economic inequalities across the UK?

REFERENCES

Atkins, G. and Dalton, G. (2021). *The NHS, Schools and Social Care in the Four Nations: How do they Compare?* London: Institute for Government.

British Association for the Study of Community Dentistry. (2024). Epidemiology. Available at: www.bascd.org/activities/epidemiology/survey-resources/ (Accessed: 30 October 2023).

Brocklehurst, P., Birch, S., McDonald, R., Hill, H., O'Malley. L., et al. (2016). Determining the Optimal Model for Role Substitution in NHS Dental Services in the UK: A Mixed-Methods Study. *NIHR Journals Library*; 2016. (Health Services and Delivery Research, No. 4.22.). Available at: www.ncbi.nlm.nih.gov/books/NBK378807/ (Accessed: 29 September 2023).

Brocklehurst P., Mertz B., Jerkovic-Cosic, K., Littlewood, A. and Tickle, M. (2014). Direct Access to Midlevel Dental Providers: An Evidence Synthesis. *J Pub Health Dent*, 74: 326–335. doi.org/10.1111/jphd.12062

Chestnutt, I. (2014). Devolution and Dentistry in Wales. *Faculty Dental Journal*, 5 (3): 110–113. doi10.1308/204268514X14017784505817

Childsmile. (2005). Improving the Oral Health of Children in Scotland. Available at: www.childsmile.nhs.scot/(Accessed: 29 September 2023).

Connolly, S., Bevan, G. and Mays, N. (2010). *Funding and Performance of the Healthcare Systems in the Four Nations of the United Kingdon Before and After Devolution.* London: Nuffield Trust.

Dentists Act. (1956). Available at: https://discovery.nationalarchives.gov.uk/details/r/C3635927 (Accessed: 28 September 2023).

Department of Health. (2023). *National Dental Epidemiology Oral Health Survey Northern Ireland – Five-year-old Children in Northern Ireland (2018–2019).* Available at: www.health-ni.gov.uk/publications/national-dental-epidemiology-oral-health-survey-northern-ireland-five-year-old-children-northern (Accessed: 4 April 2024).

Doughty, J., Grossman, A., Paisi, M., Tran, C., Rodriguez, A., et al. (2022). A Survey of Dental Services in England Providing Targeted Care for People Experiencing Social Exclusion: Mapping and Dimensions of Access. *British Dental Journal*, 20: 1–8. doi.10.1038/ s41415-022-4391-7

Dyer, T. A., Brocklehurst, P., Glenny, A. M., Davies, L., Tickle, M., et al. (2014). Dental Auxiliaries for Dental Care Traditionally Provided by Dentists: Cochrane Database Systematic Review. Available at: www.cochranelibrary.com/cdsr/doi/10.1002/14651858. CD010076.pub2/full (Accessed: 29 September 2023).

Fuller, E., Steele, J., Watt, R. and Nuttall, N. (2011). Oral Health and Function – A Report from the Adult Dental Health Survey 2009. Information Centre for Health and Social Care. Available at: https://doc.ukdataservice.ac.uk/doc/6884/mrdoc/pdf/6884theme1_ oral_health_and_function.pdf (Accessed: 30 October 2023).

GDC. (2013a). Direct Access. Available at: www.gdc-uk.org/standards-guidance/standards-and-guidance/direct-access (Accessed: 28 September 2023).

GDC. (2013b). Scope of Practice. Available at: www.gdc-uk.org/docs/default-source/scope-of-practice/scope-of-practicea2afa3974b184b6a8500dd0d49f0b74f.pdf?sfvrsn=8f417ca8_7 (Accessed: 28 September 2023).

GDC. (2023). Registration Report 2023. Available at: www.gdc-uk.org/docs/default-source/registration-reports/registration-report—february-2023.pdf?sfvrsn=61731780_3 (Accessed: 29 September 2023).

Gov.UK. (2022). New Measures to Improve Access to Dental Care. Available at: www. gov.uk/government/news/new-measures-to-improve-access-to-dental-care (Accessed: 29 September 2023).

Health and Social Care. (2016). National Dental Epidemiology Oral Health Survey Northern Ireland - Five-Year-Old Children in Northern Ireland (2018-2019). Available at: www. health-ni.gov.uk/sites/default/files/publications/health/doh-ndep-oral-health-survey.PDF (Accessed: 30 October 2023).

Health and Social Care. (2023). Happy Smiles Pre-School Oral Health Programme. Available at: https://online.hscni.net/our-work/dental-services/happy-smiles/ (Accessed: 29 September 2023).

Health Departments of England, Scotland, Wales, and Northern Ireland. (1990). *The New Contract – An Operating Manual for Dentists*. London: DH.

Morgan, M. and Monaghan, N. (2017). *Picture of Oral Health 2017 – Dental Caries in 5 Year Olds (2015/16)*. Cardiff: Cardiff University.

Morgan, M. and Monaghan, N. (2020). Welsh Dental Survey of 18–25-Year-Olds Years 1 and 2 Main Report. Available at: www.cardiff.ac.uk/__data/assets/pdf_file/0010/2447677/ Wales-18-25-Dental-Survey-Report-for-Years-1-and-2-August-2020.pdf (Accessed: 30 October 2023).

Nash, D. A., Friedman, J. W., Kardos, T. B., Kardos, R. L., Schwarz, E., et al. (2008). Dental Therapists: A Global Perspective. *International Dental Journal*, 58: 61–70. doi. org/10.1111/j.1875-595X.2008.tb00177.x

National Audit Office. (2012). *Health Across the UK: A Comparison of the NHS in England, Scotland, Wales and Northern Ireland*. London. The Stationery Office.

National Health Service Act. (1946). Available at: www.parliament.uk/about/living-heritage/ transformingsociety/livinglearning/coll-9-health1/health-01/#:~:text=1946%20NHS%20 Act&text=and%20Northern%20Ireland.-,The%20first%20Minister%20of%20 Health%20was%20Aneurin%20Bevan%20MP.,diagnosis%20and%20treatment%20 of%20illness (Accessed: 28 September 2023).

National Health Service (Charges for Dental Treatment) Regulations. (1952). Available at: https:// vlex.co.uk/vid/national-health-service-charges-861201780 (Accessed: 28 September 2023).

National Health Service (General Dental Services Contracts). (2005). Regulations. Available at: www.legislation.gov.uk/uksi/2005/3361/contents (Accessed: 29 September 2023).

NHS England. (2015). Child Dental Health Survey 2013, England, Wales and Northern Ireland. Available at: https://digital.nhs.uk/data-and-information/publications/statistical/children-s-dental-health-survey/child-dental-health-survey-2013-england-wales-and-northern-ireland (Accessed: 28 September 2023).

NHS England. (2023). The Long-Term Workforce Plan 2023. Available at: www.england.nhs.uk/wp-content/uploads/2023/06/nhs-long-term-workforce-plan-v1.2.pdf (Accessed: 31 March 2024).

NHS England. (2024). Faster, Simpler, and Fairer: Our Plan to Recover and Reform NHS Dentistry. Available at: www.gov.uk/government/publications/our-plan-to-recover-and-reform-nhs-dentistry/faster-simpler-and-fairer-our-plan-to-recover-and-reform-nhs-dentistry (Accessed: 31 March 2024).

NHS Wales. (2009). Designed to Smile. Available at: https://abbhealthiertogether.cymru.nhs.uk/parentscarers/keeping-your-child-safe-and-healthy/dental-hygiene (Accessed: 1 April 2024).

Nuffield Institute. (1993). Nuffield Report: *The Education and Training of Personnel Auxiliary to Dentistry*. London: The Nuffield Institute.

Office for Health Improvement and Disparities. (2022). Child Oral Health: Applying All Our Health. Available at: www.gov.uk/government/publications/child-oral-health-applying-all-our-health/child-oral-health-applying-all-our-health (Accessed: 30 October 2023).

Office for Health Improvement and Disparities. (2023a). Hospital Tooth Extractions in 0- to 19-Year-Olds 2022. Available at: www.gov.uk/government/statistics/hospital-tooth-extractions-in-0-to-19-year-olds-2022/hospital-tooth-extractions-in-0-to-19-year-olds-2022 (Accessed: 30 October 2023).

Office for Health Improvement and Disparities. (2023b). National Dental Epidemiology Programme (NDEP) for England: Oral Health Survey of 5-Year-Old Children 2022. Available at: www.gov.uk/government/statistics/oral-health-survey-of-5-year-old-children-2022/national-dental-epidemiology-programme-ndep-for-england-oral-health-survey-of-5-year-old-children-2022 (Accessed: 30 October 2023).

Public Health England. (2015). Dental Public Health Epidemiology Programme Oral Health Survey of Five-Year-Old and 12-Year-Old Children Attending Special Support Schools 2014: A Report on the Prevalence and Severity of Dental Decay. Available at: https://webarchive.nationalarchives.gov.uk/ukgwa/20180801132959mp_/www.nwph.net/dentalhealth/specsurvey/DPHEP%20for%20England%20OH%20Survey%20Special%20Support%20Schools%202014%20Report.pdf (Accessed 1 April 2024).

Public Health England. (2020). National Dental Epidemiology Programme for England: Oral Health Survey of Adults Attending General Dental Practices 2018. Available at: https://assets.publishing.service.gov.uk/media/5ee0abb0d3bf7f1eb9646438/AiP_survey_for_England_2018.pdf (Accessed: 30 October 2023).

Public Health Scotland. (2020). Report of the 2020 Detailed Inspection Programme of Primary 1 Children and the Basic Inspection of Primary 1 and Primary 7 Children. Available at: https://publichealthscotland.scot/media/4545/2020-10-20-ndip-report.pdf (Accessed: 30 October 2023).

Scotland Act. (1998). Available at: www.legislation.gov.uk/ukpga/1998/46/contents (Accessed: 29 September 2023).

Steele, J. (2009). *NHS Dental Services in England*. London: The Stationery Office.

CHAPTER 15

Emerging Long-Term Care Systems
Learning from Comparison

....

Cassandra Simmons, Johanna Fischer, and Kai Leichsenring

INTRODUCTION

Advances and success stories in medical treatments, hygiene, and pharmacology, but also in nutrition, working and housing conditions, have contributed to an unprecedented rise in longevity globally (UN DESA, 2023). This includes the ageing of persons with chronic conditions, multimorbidity, dementia, or other cognitive impairments, and needs for long-term care (LTC), whose life expectancy has significantly increased, resulting in a growing number of persons in need and rising costs for individuals, families, and public authorities. The chapter will start with a specification of terminology and a brief historical sketch of emerging LTC systems. Quantitative trends, challenges regarding services and benefits, workforce, and financing, as well as select solutions for policy and mutual learning, will then be presented in a comparative perspective to indicate latent areas of learning. It will also trace the advances of LTC systems by focusing upon the emerging own identity, structures, processes, policies, workforce, and funding mechanisms of LTC systems in OECD countries. Given the time shifts of these processes across different countries and regions, this policy area is particularly prone to offer potential learnings from success and failure across jurisdictions.

THE EMERGENCE OF LTC SYSTEMS ACROSS THE OECD

Health systems are focused on 'curing' patients and have therefore been challenged by persons with long-term conditions, who need regular medical treatment, but mainly personal and social support to compensate for physical, sensorial, or cognitive decline, and to foster a decent quality of life under these circumstances. Such care has traditionally been provided by (female) family members who are

DOI: 10.4324/9781003343608-17

still the largest unpaid care workforce. However, the increasing quantity and the more demanding quality of care needs – in concomitance with changing family structures and more equal participation of women in the labour market – call for more professionalised and person-centred approaches to community-based long-term care.

This entails the development of a wide range of services from home care and day-care centres to support for informal carers and residential settings. These services have been rooted both within the social welfare systems and the health-care systems in countries of the Organisation of Economic Co-operation and Development (OECD) with their divergent developmental pathways and legacies. Over the past decades we have, however, witnessed developments at the interface between social and healthcare systems and between formal and informal care systems that resulted in the emergence of distinct LTC systems (Leichsenring et al., 2013; OECD, 2013).

BOX 15.1 TERMINOLOGIES OF LONG-TERM CARE

In an international context, it is still challenging to agree on a generally agreed definition of long-term care due to conceptual, cultural and language issues. In Anglo-Saxon countries, the terms social care and healthcare are widespread, with distinctions made between home and community-based care and residential care, and only the latter being called 'long-term care'. However, today there is a rather widespread consensus in international and inter-governmental organisations such as the World Health Organisation (WHO) and OECD, that a range of long-term care services and facilities must be deployed for people who need 'day-to-day help with activities such as washing and dressing, or help with household activities such as cleaning and cooking' (Oliveira Hashiguchi and Llena-Nozal, 2023). This is also reflected in the definition of LTC generally used by the European Commission and the Social Protection Committee:

> Long-term care is defined as a range of services and assistance for people who, as a result of mental and/or physical frailty and/or disability over an extended period of time, depend on help with daily living activities and/or are in need of some permanent nursing care. The daily living activities for which help is needed may be the self-care activities that a person must perform every day (Activities of Daily Living, or ADLs, such as bathing, dressing, eating, getting in and out of bed or a chair, moving around, using the toilet, and controlling bladder and bowel functions) or may be related to independent living (Instrumental Activities of Daily Living, or IADLs, such as preparing meals, managing money, shopping for groceries or personal items, performing light or heavy housework, and using a telephone).
>
> (European Union, 2021: 17)

Services to address these needs may be provided by formal care organisations that are rooted in the health sector or in the social care sector, or they may be accomplished informally (and unpaid) by families, friends, or neighbours. They may be procured within the health care setting, in specialised social care settings or in an integrated continuum of long-term care (WHO Euro, 2022, see Figure 15.1).

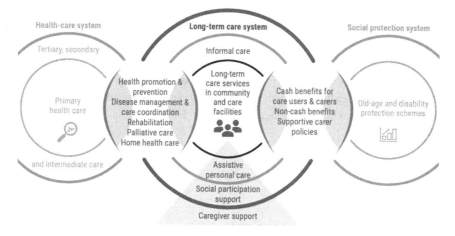

FIGURE 15.1 Emerging Long-Term Care Systems at the Interface of Health and Social Care

Source: WHO Euro (2022, p. 8)

LTC is a comparably recent field of social policy making. While public healthcare systems were already introduced since the end of the Nineteenth Century in many countries (de Carvalho and Schmid, 2023), LTC entered the policy agenda much later. Clearly, the need for assistance with daily living is not a new phenomenon but has gained salience due to social and demographic change over the past decades. Changing family structures, life courses and gender roles have, for instance, resulted in rising numbers of one-person households or growing female labour market participation. As informal care provided mostly by (female) family members is – historically and still today – an important source of care provision, the availability of (informal) care supply in the future is being jeopardised (Wittenberg, 2016).

Another crucial trend putting LTC on the agenda is global demographic ageing, that is the increasing share of older persons in countries across the world. Figure 15.2 illustrates this development for OECD countries between 2001 and 2021. In many European countries, such as Finland, Czechia, or Portugal, as well as in East Asia with Japan and Korea, the increase has been particularly substantial. Overall, in 2021, older adults comprised at least 15% of the total population in more than three quarters of OECD countries. While not every older person needs LTC, there is a strong association between old age and care needs, with a higher care prevalence of care needs among higher age groups (WHO, 2015). Statistics for the older population in England and Wales show, for instance, that 11-12% of persons aged 65 to 70 are considerably limited in their ability to carry out day-to-day activities, while in the age bracket of 80 to 84 years, this share increases to 23.7% for women and 20.5% for men (Office for National Statistics, 2023).

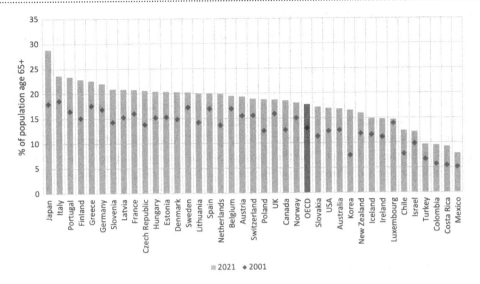

FIGURE 15.2 Share of Total Population Aged 65+ across OECD Countries over Time

Source: OECD Database (2023).

Against this backdrop, many countries have introduced policies for the provision, financing, and regulation of care services for older persons. Most OECD countries have by now established some type of public LTC scheme offering social benefits for people in need of care and/or their care givers (Fischer et al., 2023). However, these systems vary vastly, for instance, as regards their types, levels and coverage of benefits, workforce composition and financing and governance structure, as we will discuss in more detail below. Another variation refers to the extent of distinctiveness of the adopted system. Is LTC explicitly recognised as a specific social risk and a separate area of social protection or are LTC benefits 'just' incorporated as part of existing schemes in the healthcare system or social assistance legislation (Rothgang et al., 2021)? This classification can be helpful for exploring the public recognition and institutionalisation of LTC across countries and time, highlighting various stages and pathways of LTC system emergence. While most OECD countries have introduced an indistinct system in the last decades, distinct systems treating LTC as a policy field of its own are scarcer. Figure 15.3 shows a timeline of

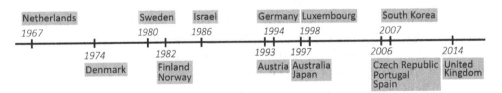

FIGURE 15.3 Timeline of Introduction Dates of Distinct Long-Term Care Systems in OECD Countries (as of 2019)

Source: Fischer et al. (2023)

Note: Year refers to date of law adoption establishing the system.

their establishment, with 16 OECD countries having introduced a distinct system by 2019. By far the first is the adoption of the Exceptional Medical Expenses Act in the Netherlands in 1967, followed by Nordic countries. These early adopters have further developed comprehensive LTC policies still today. In contrast, the UK figures as a recent example for introducing a distinct LTC system. While the country was among the first to establish initial entitlements for LTC as early as 1948 with the Social Assistance Act, 'a single, clear statute' which 'modernises over 60 years of care and support law' (Burstow, 2018, p. 313) was only adopted in England in 2014 with the Care Act.[1] Further progress in the area has been made in recent years in other parts of Europe. For instance, in 2021, a novel LTC Act introducing compulsory LTC insurance was adopted in Slovenia (Prevolnik Rupel, 2022), while in Italy, the introduction of a distinct system has been under discussion (www.pattononautosufficienza.it).

LONG-TERM CARE BENEFITS

LTC systems offer a variety of different benefit types to support persons in need of care as well as their informal care givers. One fundamental distinction can be drawn between benefits offered in-kind, that is services or assistive equipment, and direct payments made to recipients in cash, often referred to as cash-for-care schemes. Importantly, countries rely on different mixtures of benefit types in the design of their LTC policies. Some, such as Denmark or Japan, focus on service delivery, whereas others, such as Czechia or Italy provide mainly cash benefits. A third group of countries, such as Spain or Germany, offers both in-kind services and monetary payments extensively.

Taking a closer look at care services, we can broadly distinguish between institutional settings – in which care is provided for many persons in need of care jointly inside a residential care home – and home- and community-based care (HCBC) settings. The latter can include ambulatory services delivered in care recipients' own home as well as day care centres or meals-on-wheels, but also innovative, small-scale living arrangements, with integrated LTC support. Generally, policies in OECD countries tend to move away from residential services towards more HCBC, referred to as 'deinstitutionalisation'. Several reasons underly this movement away from (larger) LTC institutions: the aim to strengthen human rights by integrating persons with care needs into the community, considerations about lower costs, and persisting personal preferences for being cared for at home (Ilinca et al., 2015). Figure 15.4 illustrates this trend, showing a decreasing share of older people receiving institutional care between 2011 and 2021 for most OECD countries. Still, it also shows that the share of residential LTC users differs between countries as well, mostly ranging between one and 6% of persons aged 65 and older.

In contrast to institutional care, LTC provision at home is much more widespread in most countries. OECD data for 2021 show that the share of persons aged 65+ receiving home care services varies from more than 25% in Israel and Lithuania to

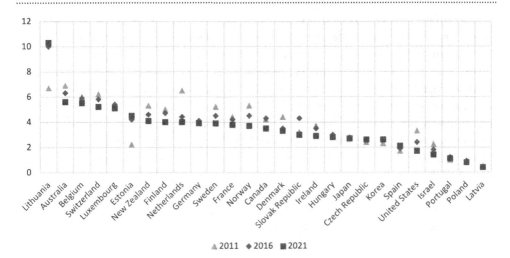

FIGURE 15.4 Share of Older People Aged 65+ Using Residential Care Services in OECD Countries over Time

Source: OECD (2023)

about 5% in France and Estonia, and even less in Portugal (see Figure 15.5). These differences reflect, for instance, the varying priorities and preferences about HCBC and formal care arrangements generally across OECD countries. As a reverse of the decreasing share of persons in residential care, home care services have increased in many countries over the past 10 years. However, the picture is not completely clear-cut. In countries such as Denmark, the Netherlands or New Zealand, home care use (as well as residential care) has decreased over time, reflecting a trend towards enhanced targeting, linked to a decreasing generosity of the LTC systems.

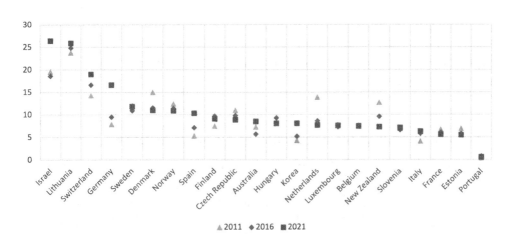

FIGURE 15.5 Share of Older People Aged 65+ Using Home Care Services across OECD Countries over Time

Source: OECD Database (2023)

In contrast to most in-kind services, cash benefits enable users the flexibility to choose and arrange their care themselves, as the money can be used in different ways. Traditionally, LTC services are more common than cash benefits, but especially from the 1990s onwards many European LTC systems have also introduced or expanded cash-for-care schemes (Da Roit and Le Bihan, 2010). On the one hand, such schemes can be aimed at supporting informal care, often provided inside the family, by offering resources to remunerate informal care givers or increasing household income. On the other hand, cash payments can strengthen users' autonomy and empower them to take own decisions about an adequate care arrangement (Da Roit and Gori, 2019). A snapshot of persons receiving LTC cash benefits within the European Union in 2019 again indicates the large discrepancy in individual entitlements, and thus in the definition of LTC needs, across countries (Figure 15.6). However, the figures must be interpreted carefully. A high number of recipients does not necessarily imply a generous system, as benefit amounts might be particularly low if large parts of the population are included (Ranci et al., 2019).

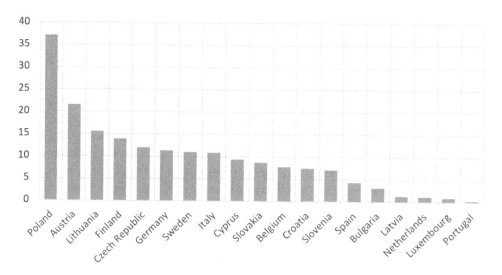

FIGURE 15.6 Share of Older People Aged 65+ Receiving a LTC Cash Benefit (2019)

Source: Pavolini (2021)

BOX 15.2 COHERENCE AND INTEGRATION OF THE BENEFIT SYSTEM

In the UK, different types of LTC benefits – including residential and HCBC services and cash payments – are available in some form as well. In 2022, 5.1% of the population aged 65+ in England received long-term social care support from local authorities, 1.9% in form of residential care and 3.2% as HCBC (NHS, 2022). Furthermore, around 1.4 million older persons in Great Britain received cash payments via the Attendance Allowance (DWP, 2023). However, public support and benefit systems are characterised by strong institutional and regional fragmentation, with different criteria for different types of benefits as well as between local authorities (Glendinning, 2013). Such fragmentation might hinder transparency regarding available support measures and therefore limit informed choice and lead to inequalities in access. Recent regulatory reforms of LTC needs assessment in Australia might provide an example of how coherence and integration of the LTC system can be strengthened. Earlier reform steps have established a national Senior's Gateway Assessment Service which developed central indicators for comparing care providers and care assessment tools as well as a central information point (website My Aged Care) for (prospective) care users, their relatives and health professionals (Theobald and Ozanne, 2016). From mid-2024 onwards, the reform goes a step further, harmonising various pre-existing care assessment processes to establishing a single assessment system for different types of LTC benefits in Australia (Department of Health and Aged Care, 2023). With the new system, people can rely on a single assessment pathway even if their needs or location changes.

THE LONG-TERM CARE WORKFORCE

The LTC workforce, comprised of care workers providing a continuum of care across a range of institutional, community, and home-based settings, are the backbone of care systems, and play a critical role in carrying out services at the point of delivery. Among the multi-professional LTC workforce are nursing staff who carry out direct medical care, personal care aides who provide help and support with activities of daily living, social workers who assist families in navigating the complex field of care, as well as care managers who oversee the provision of care and contribute to developing care plans for individuals with care needs, among others.

Matching the substantial diversity in the structure of care systems as discussed above, so too varies the characteristics of the care workforce across countries, particularly in terms of the type of education and training required of care workers, as well as their specific roles across settings. While some commonalities are present across the qualifications needed for specific care worker roles, there is no harmonisation across countries. Care workers tasked with responsibilities related to medical care (i.e., nursing, monitoring, care coordination, etc), such as nurses, are most commonly required to complete a bachelor's degree, although often without specific training on conditions of older people (OECD, 2020). By contrast, the educational requirements for personal care workers are set lower and varies significantly across countries, often mandating only a minimum education level, which may consist of vocational training, technical qualification, or simply initial training programmes. Often perceived as low-skilled work, many countries do not require personal care workers to be licensed or certified as having the necessary skills (OECD, 2020). While they primarily carry out tasks related to help with (instrumental) activities of daily living, in a small subset of countries, some of their tasks may be medical based, such as providing medications. In most countries, personal care workers comprise

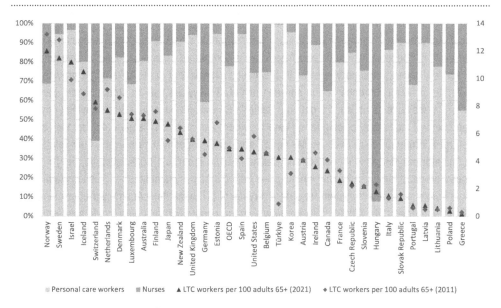

FIGURE 15.7 Composition of Care Workforce (Nurses vs. Personal Care Workers) and Total Number of Long-Term Care Workers (Nurses and Personal Care Workers) per 100 People Aged 65 and Over (2021 or Nearest Year)

Source: OECD Database (2023); OECD (2023); EU LFS

a larger share of the LTC workforce than nurses (Figure 15.7). The size of the care workforce also varies widely across countries, closely corresponding to the size (and demand) for formal service provision. The number of LTC workers per 100 people aged 65 and older ranges from as many as 12 in some of the Nordic countries (i.e., Norway, Sweden, and Iceland) where formal services are well-developed, accessible, affordable, and therefore widely used, to less than one in Greece, Poland, and Lithuania, where formal care delivery is less well-developed.

A common challenge faced by all countries is the growing shortage of care workers even if in some countries the share of LTC workers has increased over the last decade. This is partly due to an ageing of the workforce but also because professionals are leaving the sector due to poor working conditions, low pay, and limited professional development opportunities. This is primarily seen in institutional based care (Figure 15.8a), but less so in home-based care (Figure 15.8b), likely the result of investment and expansion of home-based care. Still, the growth in the number of older people with care needs has outpaced the growth of supply of LTC workers, raising concern that the care workforce will be insufficient to meet future demand for LTC.

Migrant care workers have gradually filled the labour shortages in the care sector, whether through regularised or unauthorised channels (Yeates, 2009). In a subset of countries, for instance in Austria, Germany and Mediterranean countries, live-in personal carers have presented an affordable option for middle-class families as an alternative and complement to family care (Schmidt et al., 2016; Di Rosa et al., 2012). These carers, often middle-aged women tending to hail from Eastern European countries,

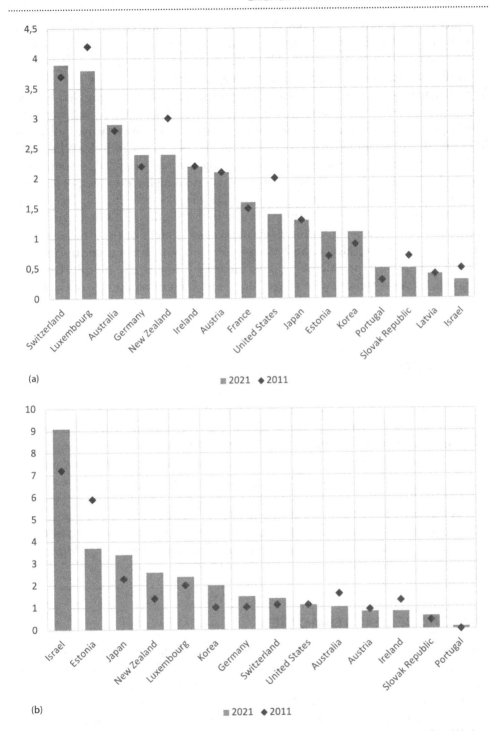

FIGURE 15.8 Full-Time Equivalent (a) Care Workers in Institutions and (b) Home-Based Care Workers across OECD Countries

Source: OECD Database (2023)

face precarious working conditions, long hours without breaks, low pay relative to local wages and limited support, calling for action to improve working conditions of all (migrant) care workers on a global level (King-Dejardin, 2019).

Finally, informal care – unpaid help and support provided by family and friends – forms the majority of LTC received by older adults, often filling the gaps left by inaccessible, unaffordable, and low-quality care services. The scope of informal care ranges quite substantially across countries, with nearly three in every five individuals in Denmark receiving informal care, versus around one in five in Italy. While at an initial glance, this is a seeming paradox given the strong family values and norms expected in Southern Europe, and therefore anticipated higher provision of informal care by family, prevalence of informal care receipt masks differences in intensity of care. More generous formal LTC provision, as in the Nordics, is likely to crowd out intensive family caregiving, while it encourages a lighter intensity of care, thus explaining the low prevalence, high intensity care in Southern European countries and conversely high prevalence of low intensity care in the Nordic countries (Verbakel, 2018). A trend towards formalising and supporting the role of the family in providing care as a means of sustainability and cost-containment has become evident across some countries in recent years (Ranci and Pavolini, 2015).

BOX 15.3 SUPPORTING INFORMAL CARERS IN THE UK

Over 5 million individuals provide informal care in the UK, amounting to £132 billion if this care was to be replaced by care workers (Buckner and Yeandle, 2015; Office for National Statistics, 2023). Policy dialogue surrounding informal caregiving has highlighted the need to support caregivers by ensuring their financial and social protection, providing respite care, and arranging health and psychological support for them. One crucial way to ensure that informal carers receive the support they need is to incorporate them into the needs assessment process of their care beneficiary, or to establish a separate needs assessment process for informal carers themselves. In the UK, there is an established process through which informal carers are entitled to request a needs assessment for themselves to inform their local council of the effects of caregiving on their physical and mental health and to subsequently receive support in the form of help, emotional support, additional information on benefits, etc (Carers UK, 2023).

FINANCING OF LONG-TERM CARE

The complex governance structures of LTC systems, often fragmented across different ministries and institutions, are reflected in the financing systems, too. The funding and organisation of LTC systems are scattered across healthcare, social care, and social protection systems, and at different levels, often separated based on the type of benefits. In most OECD countries, funding is primarily centralised and spent by either the central government or national social security fund, with a smaller share of financing being delegated to the regional or local level (de Biase and Dougherty, 2023). Revenue-raising methods also vary considerably across countries, with funds for LTC mostly raised through taxation, whether through general taxation or taxes ear-marked specifically for LTC. Tax-financed systems have the advantage of drawing from a large contribution base, thus spreading the risk of financial burden more thinly across society. A smaller subset of countries finance LTC primarily through compulsory contributions, typically through social insurance models, such as in Germany, Japan, the Netherlands, and Korea. While similar to tax-based systems in that they draw from a large contribution base, social insurance-based care systems have the disadvantage of being tied to labour income and are therefore subject to the sustainability and fluctuations of the labour force. Remaining countries employ a hybrid mixture of tax-based and contribution-based financing to cover LTC services.

Naturally, generosity and breadth of public coverage corresponds to higher levels of spending on LTC such as in northern Europe (i.e., Netherlands, Finland, Norway, Sweden, and Denmark). As the result of generous coverage of care needs and low out-of-pocket payments by users, in 2021, these countries publicly spent between 3.0 and 4.1 per cent of GDP on LTC (Figure 15.9). Recent years have seen a scaling back of eligibility for public benefits and services across the Nordic countries as a means for cost containment (Rostgaard et al., 2022). In stark contrast, the slow and limited development of services, or non-existence of services all together, has

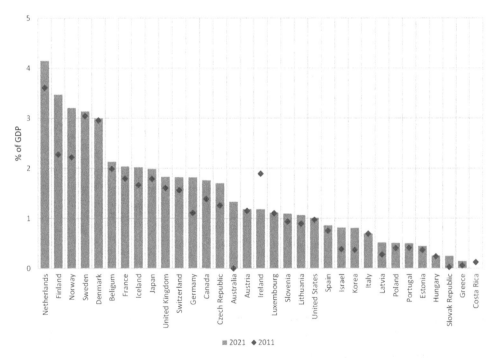

FIGURE 15.9 Total Public Expenditure on LTC (Health and Social Care) as Percentage of GDP (2021 versus 2011 or Nearest Year)

Source: OECD Database (2023)

Note: the graph includes all spending on long-term care, both for healthcare and social services.

kept expenditure on LTC low (below 0.5% of GDP) across several countries, concentrated among Southern and Eastern Europe (Greece, Slovak Republic, Hungary, Estonia Portugal, Poland, and Latvia). Despite this variation, nearly all countries have witnessed an upward adjustment of spending resulting from increases in care needs and demand for care, putting pressure on systems to adapt and accommodate the needs of older people. Projection models also indicate that public expenditure on LTC will continue to rise in decades to come as the result of demographic change and population ageing (DG ECFIN, 2021).

As means for limiting moral hazard (i.e., overconsumption of services due to limited risk or cost on care users) and keeping public expenditure in check, care users are typically required to contribute to their care fees through out-of-pocket payments (OOPs). These are frequently based on means-tests – dependent on the income and/or wealth of the individual or their family. Differences in spending are substantial across countries, often based on the level and scope of benefits and coverage, but also demand for services (Figure 15.10). Where coverage of LTC is generous, such

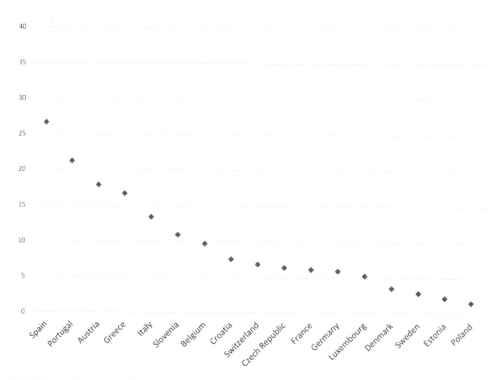

FIGURE 15.10 Average OOPs for Home Care Services as Percentage of Income (65+)

Source: Based on data of adults aged 65+ using home care services from the Survey on Health, Ageing and Retirement in Europe, wave 6 (2015)

Note: Out-of-pocket payments (OOPs) are operationalized as percentage of equivalized household income paid out of pocket for home care services, including help with personal care, domestic tasks, meals on wheels and other activities. Income is defined as equivalized household income, accounting for the size of households. Weighted results.

as in Denmark and Sweden, average OOPs required of individuals using care services are modest below 5% of household income. Limiting payments by care users, or structuring them dependent on an individual's means, ensures that individuals are protected from catastrophic payments, or from being financially burdened. The more limited public coverage of LTC is seen in countries where OOPs comprise a larger share of average income, such as in Spain, Portugal, Austria, Greece, and Italy, where payments amount to over 10% of household income. In a few select countries, where services are both limited and scarcely covered by public schemes, such as Estonia and Poland, OOPs also remain low. High out-of-pocket payments are a concern for individuals with care needs, as they are likely to correspond with reduced access to care due to affordability barriers.

BOX 15.4 ENSURING AFFORDABILITY OF LONG-TERM CARE

In the UK, LTC benefits are means-tested and available to either low-income individuals, or those that have exhausted most of their savings. As a result, individuals requiring residential care can be expected to pay on average 91% of the median disposable income out of pocket after public support has kicked in. For home care, individuals with moderate or severe care needs on average pay 35% of the median disposable income (OECD, n.d.). In comparison, universal systems such as the Netherlands, Sweden, and Denmark, employ relatively low ceilings on OOPs, particularly for lower-income beneficiaries, thus protecting individuals from substantial financial burden. In the Netherlands, out of pocket payments are very limited for low-income individuals, capped at €20 per month, resulting in a concentration of home care and residential care use among poorer individuals (Tenand et al., 2020). Such a system reduces the share of older adults in the Netherlands in relative income poverty after paying out-of-pocket payments to practically zero across both home and facility-based care (Oliveira Hashiguchi and Llena-Nozal, 2020).

CONCLUSIONS

International organisations such as the OECD, the WHO, the United Nations, and the European Union have promoted the realm of LTC needs on the global political agenda. Apart from a few forerunners, policies for integrated social and healthcare services, including LTC, are still limited to more developed welfare states. However, a rising number of countries are confronted with challenges to provide support to older persons in need of care and their families. This chapter shed light on some key aspects to be considered in constructing and developing LTC systems. This partly entails hard choices to be made starting from investing public expenditures in hitherto unpaid care provided mainly by women, to balancing the mixture between benefits in cash and in kind, as well as to better coordination between health and social care.

Over the past decades, policy, and practice in LTC have learned that person-centred and integrated community-based care must be the guiding principle for the development of LTC systems. This includes not only the acknowledgement of care as a social problem, which cannot be shouldered by individuals and families alone, but social investment that strengthens the continuity of care delivery in the community. Not least during the COVID-19 pandemic, it became obvious that the growing number of persons in need of LTC are among the most vulnerable in society – and that both the health and social care systems need to become better prepared to ensure the right support at the right time and the right place for this target group.

RESEARCH POINTS AND REFLECTIVE EXERCISES

- Reflect upon the reasons why long-term care is a late comer in social protection and why governments have started to introduce distinct policies to address long-term care as a social risk over the past decades. What would be next steps to overcome fragmentation of health and social care as well as formal and informal care delivery?
- List the different forms of financing long-term care services and discuss the advantages and inconveniences from different stakeholders' perspectives. Consider both the types of funding and their potential impact on inequalities (e.g., by consulting the chapter 'The long-term care financing problem' in Gori et al., 2016).
- Read the publications by Glendinning (2013; 2021) and analyse the changes in policy debates before and during/after the COVID-19 pandemic. You might want to deepen this analysis by consulting the website 'Resources to support community and institutional long-term care responses to COVID-19' (https://ltccovid.org).

ACKNOWLEDGEMENTS

This chapter is a product of research conducted in the Collaborative Research Center 1342 'Global Dynamics of Social Policy' at the University of Bremen. The Center is funded by the Deutsche Forschungsgemeinschaft (DFG, German Research Foundation) (project number 374666841 – SFB 1342) to J.F.

NOTE

1 With devolution from the late 1990s, health and social care became competencies of the four devolved nations of the UK, leading to diverging regulations and systems (Wright and Simpson, 2021). The 2014 introduction date for the UK refers to England as the largest UK nation.

REFERENCES

Buckner, L. and Yeandle, S. (2015). *Valuing Carers 2015*. London: Carers UK.

Burstow, P. (2018) The Care Act 2014. In A. Bonner (ed.), *Social Determinants of Health: An Interdisciplinary Approach to Social Inequality and Well-Being*. Bristol: Policy Press, 311–324.

Carers UK. (2023). Having a Carer's Assessment. Available at: www.carersuk.org/help-and-advice/practical-support/carers-assessment/ (Accessed: 2 November 2023).

Da Roit, B. and Gori, C. (2019). The Transformation of Cash-for-Care Schemes in European Long-Term Care Policies. *Social Policy and Administration*, 53 (4): 515–518. https://doi.org/10.1111/spol.12508

Da Roit, B. and Le Bihan, B. (2010) Similar and yet so Different: Cash-for-Care in Six European Countries' Long-Term Care Policies. *The Milbank Quarterly*, 88 (3): 286–309. https://doi.org/10.1111/j.1468-0009.2010.00601.x

de Carvalho, G. and Schmid, A. (2023). Global Historical Healthcare Systems Dataset (G2HSet): Technical Report and Codebook, SFB 1342 Technical Paper Series (15). Available at: www.socialpolicydynamics.de/f/c1fd574c3e.pdf (Accessed: 16 November 2023).

Department for Work and Pensions. (2023). DWP Benefits Statistics: February 2023. Available at: www.gov.uk/government/statistics/dwp-benefits-statistics-february-2023/dwp-benefits-statistics-february-2023#health-disability-and-care (Accessed: 3 November 2023).

Department of Health and Aged Care. (2023). Single Assessment System for Aged Care. Available at: www.health.gov.au/topics/aged-care/aged-care-reforms-and-reviews/single-assessment-system-for-aged-care (Accessed: 3 November 2023).

Di Rosa, M., Melchiorre, M. G., Luchetti, M. and Lamura, G. (2012). The Impact of Migrant Care Work in the Elder Care Sector: Recent Trends and Empirical Evidence in Italy, *European Journal of Social Work*, 15 (1): 9–27. https://doi.org/10.1080/13691457.2011.562034

Fischer, J., Sternkopf, M. and Rothgang, H. (2023). Covering A New Social Risk: The Introduction of Long-Term Care Systems Worldwide. In I. Mossig and H. Obinger (eds), *Mapping Global Dynamics of Social Policy*. Bremen: Collaborative Research Centre 1342 (SOCIUM SFB Working Papers, 25), 32–35.

Glendinning, C. (2013). Long-Term Care Reform in England: A Long and Unfinished Story. In C. Ranci and E. Pavolini (eds), *Reforms in Long-Term Care Policies in Europe: Investigating Institutional Change and Social Impacts*. New York: Springer, 179–197.

Glendinning, C. (2021). *ESPN Thematic Report on Long-Term Care for Older People. United Kingdom*. Luxembourg: European Commission.

Gori, C., Fernández, J. L. and Wittenberg, R. (2016). *Long-Term Care Reforms in OECD Countries: Successes and Failures*. Bristol: Policy Press.

Ilinca, S., Leichsenring, K. and Rodrigues, R. (2015). From Care in Homes to Care at Home: European Experiences with (De)institutionalisation in Long-Term Care (Policy Brief). Available at: www.euro.centre.org/publications/detail/420 (Accessed: 29 March 2023).

King-Dejardin, A. (2019). *The Social Construction of Migrant Care Work: At the Intersection of Care, Migration and Gender*. Geneva: International Labour Office.

Leichsenring, K., Nies, H. and Billings, J. (2013). *Long-Term Care in Europe – Improving Policy and Practice*. Basingstoke: Palgrave Macmillan.

National Health Service. (2022). Adult Social Care Statistics in England: An Overview: Table 3: Adults Receiving Long-Term Social Care Support from Local Authorities. Available at: https://digital.nhs.uk/data-and-information/publications/statistical/adult-social-care-statistics-in-england/an-overview (Accessed: 3 November 2023).

Office for National Statistics. (2023). Profile of the Older Population Living in England and Wales in 2021 and Changes Since 2011, 5 April. Available at: www.ons.gov.uk/peoplepopulationandcommunity/birthsdeathsandmarriages/ageing/articles/profileoftheolderpopulationlivinginenglandandwalesin2021andchangessince2011/2023-04-03#disability (Accessed: 24 October 2023).

Office for National Statistics. (2023). *Unpaid Care by Age, Sex and Deprivation*, England and Wales: Census 2021. Available at: www.ons.gov.uk/peoplepopulationandcommunity/healthandsocialcare/socialcare/articles/unpaidcarebyagesexanddeprivationenglandandwales/census2021 (Accessed: 2 November 2023).

OECD. (n.d.). Social Protection for Older People with Long-Term Care Needs. Available at: www.oecd.org/fr/sante/systemes-sante/social-protection-for-older-people-with-ltc-needs.htm (Accessed: 2 November 2023).

OECD. (2023). *Beyond Applause? Improving Working Conditions in LTC*. Paris: OECD Publishing.

OECD Database. (2023). Long-Term Care Resources and Utilisation (Expenditure, Recipients etc.). Available at: https://stats.oecd.org (Accessed: 30 October 2023).

OECD/European Commission. (2013). *A Good Life in Old Age? Monitoring and Improving Quality in Long-term Care*. Paris: OECD Health Policy Studies, OECD Publishing.

Oliveira Hashiguchi, T. C. and Llena-Nozal, A. (2020). *The Effectiveness of Social Protection for Long-Term Care in Old Age: Is Social Protection Reducing the Risk of Poverty Associated with Care Needs?* Paris: OECD Health Working Paper No. 117.

Pavolini, E. (2021). *Long-Term Care Social Protection Models in the EU*. Luxembourg: Publications Office of the European Union (European Social Policy Network – ESPN).

Prevolnik Rupel, V. (2022) *Slovenia Adopts the Long-Awaited Long-Term Care Act*. Brussels: ESPN (ESPN Flash Report 09). Available at: https://ec.europa.eu/social/BlobServlet?docId=25363&langId=en (Accessed: 31 October 2023).

Ranci, C. and Pavolini, E. (2015) Not all that Glitters is Gold: Long-Term Care Reforms in the Last Two Decades in Europe. *Journal of European Social Policy*, 25 (3): 270–285. https://doi.org/10.1177/0958928715588704

Ranci, C., Österle, A., Arlotti, M. and Parma, A. (2019). Coverage Versus Generosity: Comparing Eligibility and Need Assessment in Six Cash-for-Care Programmes. *Social Policy and Administration*, 53 (4): 551–566. https://doi.org/10.1111/spol.12502

Rothgang, H., Fischer, J., Sternkopf, M. and Frisina Doetter, L. (2021). The Classification of Distinct Long-Term Care Systems Worldwide: The Empirical Application of an Actor-Centered Multi-Dimensional Typology, SOCIUM SFB 1342 Working Papers (12). Available at: https://socialpolicydynamics.de/f/2483ea052c.pdf (Accessed: 8 July 2021).

Schmidt, A., Winkelmann, J., Rodrigues, R. and Leichsenring, K. (2016). Lessons for Regulating Informal Markets and Implications for Quality Assurance – The Case of Migrant Care Workers in Austria. *Ageing and Society*, 36 (4): 741–763. https://doi.org/10.1017/S0144686X1500001X

Tenand, M., Bakx, P. and Van Doorslaer, E. (2020). Equal Long-Term Care for Equal Needs with Universal and Comprehensive Coverage? An Assessment Using Dutch Administrative Data. *Health Economics*, 29 (4): 435–451. https://doi.org/10.1002/hec.3994

Theobald, H. and Ozanne, E. (2016). Multilevel Governance and its Effects on Long-Term Care Support. In C. Gori, J. L. Fernández and R. Wittenberg (eds), *Long-Term Care Reforms in OECD Countries: Successes and Failures*. Bristol: Policy Press, 271–292.

UN DESA. (2023). *Leaving No One Behind in an Ageing World. World Social Report 2023*. New York: United Nations Publications.

Verbakel, E. (2018) How to Understand Informal Caregiving Patterns in Europe? The Role of Formal Long-Term Care Provisions and Family Care Norms. *Scandinavian Journal of Public Health*, 46 (4): 436–447. https://doi.org/10.1177/1403494817726197

Wittenberg, R. (2016). Demand for Care and Support for Older People. In C. Gori, J. L. Fernández and R. Wittenberg (eds), *Long-Term Care Reforms in OECD Countries: Successes and Failures*. Bristol: Policy Press, 9–24.

WHO. (2015). *World Report on Ageing and Health*. Geneva: World Health Organization. Available at: http://apps.who.int/iris/bitstream/10665/186463/1/9789240694811_eng.pdf (Accessed: 10 August 2023).

WHO Euro. (2022). *Rebuilding for Sustainability and Resilience: Strengthening the Integrated Delivery of Long-Term Care in the European Region*. Copenhagen: WHO Regional Office for Europe.

Wright, S. and Simpson, M. (2021). Devolution and Social Policy. In H. Bochel and G. Daly (eds), *Social Policy*. Abingdon: Routledge, 90–110.

Yeates, N. (2009). *Globalizing Care Economies and Migrant Workers. Explorations in Global Care Chains*. Basingstoke: Palgrave Macmillan.

CHAPTER 16

Refugees and Migrants
Health Policies in OECD Countries

....

Floor Christie-de Jong

INTRODUCTION

Migration has been an integral part of society since the earliest days of civilisation. Migration is the process of moving from one place to another. The process of migration can severely impact migrants' health at multiple stages. Although globally the majority (96.4%) of people still live in the country in which they were born, and only one in 30 people are migrants (3.6%) (IOM, 2022a), an ever-increasing number of people are on the move, and migration has steadily increased in the last five decades. This chapter reviews global migration and proceeds to discusses the health of migrants and health inequalities given that health experiences evolve for migrants before, during and post migration. Migrants may come from countries affected by poverty and conflict, which may have impacted their access to healthcare already. The chapter also offers a critical comparison of health policies in OECD countries.

GLOBAL MIGRATION

There is no universally agreed definition of the term 'migrant,' who are a heterogeneous group, and include refugees, asylum seekers, as well as documented and undocumented economic migrants. Migration is the process of moving from one place to another. In many cases migrants do migrate in some form. However not all people who are referred to as 'migrants' do engage in migration, for example children born to migrants in their destination countries could be referred to as 'second generation migrants.' The International Organization for Migration (IOM) reported 128 million international migrants in 1990, 173 million in 2000, and 221 million in 2010. In 2021, the World Health Organization (WHO) estimated that there were 1 billion migrants globally, of whom 281 million international migrants, and approximately, 763 million were internal migrants (WHO, 2024).

DOI: 10.4324/9781003343608-18

Refugees are people who have been forced to flee their home country to escape conflict, violence, natural disaster, or persecution for reasons of race, religion, nationality, political stance, or association with a particular social group. The United Nations Refugee Agency (UNHCR) estimated mid-2023, that there were 110 million forcibly displaced people worldwide, of which 36.4 million were refugees; 62.5 million were internally displaced people; 6.1 million asylum seekers and 5.3 million other people were in need of international protection (UNHCR, 2023). Over half of all refugees derive from just three countries: Syrian Arab Republic (6.5 million), Afghanistan (6.1 million), and Ukraine (5.9 million). Of all refugees, 75% are hosted in low- and middle-income countries and 69% are hosted in neighbouring countries (UNHCR, 2023). The Islamic Republic of Iran and Türkiye host the largest refugee populations worldwide, 3.4 million each, followed by Germany with 2.5 million.

The UK presents considerably smaller numbers. In 2022, 81,130 asylum applications were made in the UK. Between 2004 and 2021, around 75% were refused at initial decision. At appeal, approximately 33% were upheld. Asylum seekers and refugees comprise 21% of all immigrants to the UK (UK Government, 2023). These numbers do not include more recent crises, such as the withdrawal from Afghanistan of British and US armed forces in 2021, the Russian invasion of Ukraine in 2022, or the Israeli–Palestinian conflict, which started in 2023. The International Organization for Migration estimates that the vast majority (65%) of international migrants are 'economic migrants' and are therefore workers or people seeking employment. Table 16.1 shows the top 10 destinations for international migrants, and 10 origins of international migrants in 2020 (IOM, 2022a).

The ability to migrate is often determined by policies and regulations that are impacted by one's nationality and visa access. Higher income countries generally have better visa access, while citizens of lesser income countries face more restrictions and at times their only option to migration are irregular migration pathways, increasing their vulnerability yet again. Migration is not uniform across the world

TABLE 16.1 Most Common Destinations and Host Countries for International Migrants in 2020

Most common destination countries	Most common origin
1. United States of America	1. India
2. Germany	2. Mexico
3. Saudi Arabia	3. Russian Federation
4. Russian Federation	4. China
5. United Kingdom	5. Syrian Arab Republic
6. France	6. Bangladesh
7. Canada	7. Pakistan
8. Australia	8. Ukraine
9. Spain	9. Philippines
10. Italy	10. Afghanistan

Source: IOM (2022a)

but is shaped by multiple factors, such as economic, geographical, and demographic. These factors assist the development of so called 'migration corridors', which are routes or pathways along which people might migrate. For example, the top three migration corridors are between (1) Mexico and the US, (2) Syrian Arab Republic and Türkiye, and (3) India and the Unites Arab Emirates. The first and third migration corridors mainly comprise economic migrants, but the second migration corridor mainly comprises refugees (McAuliffe and Triandafyllidou, 2021). Another popular route is the irregular migration corridor between the EU and Türkiye. Some migration corridors pose many more challenges for migrants, including dangerous and even fatal routes. Understanding trends and patterns relating to these migration corridors is vital to develop policies that can improve circumstances for migrants.

THE IMPACT UPON HEALTH

Migration is complex and the process of migration can severely impact migrants' health at multiple stages. Research provides evidence of health inequalities between native-born and migrant populations (Dourgnon et al., 2023). Health experiences evolve for migrants before, during and post migration. Migrants may come from countries affected by poverty and conflict, which may have impacted their access to healthcare already. Migrants may experience insufficient immunisation, and children may be at an increased risk of childhood preventable diseases, such as Measles, Rubella, Tetanus and Diphtheria and often lack immunisation records (WHO, 2021). Through the process of migration, overcrowded and poor living conditions and inadequate hygiene, migrants may also be at increased risk of communicable diseases, such as respiratory diseases, HIV/AIDS, Tuberculosis, and Hepatitis B. Migrants may also be at risk of inadequate or poor nutrition (WHO, 2021).

Non-communicable diseases may also be an issue. Engagement in preventative healthcare may be compromised, for example, uptake of cancer screening services has been found lower for migrant populations, compared with the general population, which again puts them at a higher risk (Lebano et al., 2020; Campbell et al., 2021; Nelson et al., 2021). Migrants have also been found to have poorer oral health and experience inequalities in sexual and reproductive health. WHO reports that refugee women face increased risks of unintended pregnancies, poor birth spacing, adverse pregnancy outcomes, higher rates of maternal death and morbidity, higher rates of postnatal depression, and increases in congenital abnormalities (WHO, 2021).

Mental health is a major health concern for migrants (WHO, 2021). Migrants may have been exposed to difficult situations coming from conflict areas or they may have suffered extreme poverty, significant factors that can affect mental health. Leaving homes behind, the loss of livelihood, and leaving possessions, as well as communities and social networks behind, are factors detrimental to mental health (Morgan and Shumba, 2023). During the migration journey, migrants may also have been exposed to stressful events and may be even in life-threatening situations in transit. Arriving in the country of destination, migrants may face more stress, for example due to uncertainty about their future, difficult migration processes, loneliness and isolation, or exposure to difficult occupational circumstances (WHO, 2021). Migrants have been found to face greater exposure to risky or harmful working conditions, which may impact their wellbeing (OECD, 2017).

Reduced health literacy, language and communication barriers and lack of understanding how to navigate the healthcare system, and experiences of discrimination are all variables that have been related to reduced access to healthcare in the host country (Lebano et al., 2020). Possibly due to lack of understanding of healthcare systems, migrants have been reported to make more use of emergency services as opposed to primary care than non-migrants (Lebano et al., 2020). There is a temporal element to migration, with decisions regarding migration returned to and reflected on in the future and throughout the life course (Czaika et al., 2021). However, key information, at the moment of decision making about the possibilities, and one's future, are uncertain and people lack control (Czaika et al., 2021).

The notion of 'choice' in migration is significantly complex. Presenting people as rational human beings who have a choice, or who do not have a choice, is problematic. However, the notion of migration as a choice by rational human beings, is often the basis of migration policy (Carling and Collins, 2018). Migration is a social determinant of health and refugees and migrants face barriers in accessing appropriate levels of healthcare, which are detrimental to health, and result in health inequalities (WHO, 2017). Countries differ in their migration policies and the type of healthcare they allow temporary migrants to access. Migration issues, such as achieving universal health coverage (UHC) and the promotion of a safe and secure working environment for all workers, including migrants, have been included in the UN 2030 Agenda for Sustainable Development (UN Sustainable Development Goals 3 and 8 (IOM, 2018). UHC that includes migrants is key and non-inclusion in UHC can form an important barrier to migrants in accessing healthcare, which can be detrimental to health and result in health inequalities.

COVID-19: INCREASING VULNERABILITY FOR MIGRANTS

The COVID-19 pandemic has highlighted migrant workers' vulnerability (Ullah et al., 2021) and there is evidence that migrant communities were disproportionally affected (Dourgnon et al., 2023). COVID-19 infection control policies led to unprecedented restrictions on global travel, as well as internal; and migration was significantly reduced. For example, in March 2020, to slow the spread of the virus, the Indian Government implemented a strict lockdown. In a country with 600 million internal migrants, this triggered a mass exodus on a scale never witnessed before (Saldanha et al., 2023). Migrants travelled to distant villages on foot, supporting or carrying family members, and some even died along their journey from heat exposure or accidents (Sumant and Patel, 2023; Saldanha et al., 2023).

In May 2020, 76% of all countries globally closed their borders completely, 23% partially, and only 5% had no travel restrictions (UNWTO, 2023). Some countries, including the UK, banned the entry of so called 'high risk of exposure to COVID-19' countries, which in 2022, included countries, such as Afghanistan, Yemen, and Venezuela (Public Health Scotland, 2022). These measures disrupted migration pathways and negatively impacted migrants. Travel restrictions, including visa disruptions, border restrictions or closures, no available flights, and quarantine measures, prevented some migrants from departing their country of origin, gain entry into transit or destination countries through formal routes, or to return home (IOM, 2022b). This included migrants who had planned to leave their country to work elsewhere, which had devastating global economic and social consequences. Migrants faced economic hardship and were not able look after their families financially, and livelihoods were lost. Some banks were closed and migrants who were still abroad, were not able to send their remittances home, which are vital to low-income countries.

Migrants not being able to travel and work, for example, in the agricultural sector, also had a disruptive consequence on global food supply chains (IOM, 2022a). Migrants were stranded due to travel restrictions and lived in overcrowded conditions with poor sanitation which made social distancing, personal hygiene, and self-isolation, difficult, such as locked down refugee camps and migrant labour camps. This left them at increased risk of COVID-19 infections (Mukumbang, 2020; Taylor and Azriel, 2023). Migrants who continued to work during the pandemic were often acclaimed as 'essential workers', often working at the front line in the health-care sector, or in low skilled jobs that could not be performed at home, and required physical proximity to other people, and put them at increased risk of COVID-19 infections (OECD, 2022).

Migrants, particularly those in low-skilled jobs such as domestic work, construction, and hospitality, faced job losses or reduced wages, again increasing their vulnerability. For example, domestic workers, composed of 80% women (IDWF, 2020), globally faced challenging circumstances. With families staying at home during the pandemic, the demand for domestic services, such as cleaning or childcare reduced. The International Labour Organization (ILO) estimated that 49.3% of domestic workers faced a reduction in hours of work, reduction in earnings, or job losses (IOM, 2022b). Some domestic workers also faced eviction from their homes (IDWF, 2020; Pandey et al., 2021). Domestic workers who lived with their employers faced heightened health and safety risk (Rosińska and Pellerito, 2022). They were asked to perform tasks that exposed them to COVID-19 and without adequate protection. Those who lived in with their employers also faced increased and uncompensated workloads, and additional risk of exploitation, gender-based violence, abuse, and increased isolation, as any physical contact with friends or peers was restricted and the pandemic exacerbated mental health issues for domestic workers (IDWF, 2020; Pandey et al., 2021).

Global travel restrictions also prevented people from leaving unstable countries, which put refugees and asylum seekers at risk of violence, abuse, persecution, and even death (IOM, 2022a). A reduction of asylum seekers arriving by air routes was witnessed in the UK in 2020 and 2021; instead, people risked dangerous routes and the number of people arriving in small boats increased significantly (UK Government, 2023). Greece tightened its borders and suspended asylum applications temporarily at the start of the pandemic, facing criticism from human rights organisations and advocacy groups (Reches, 2022). Germany, which pre-pandemic always applied an open-door policy, restricted travel in and out of the country. Although people were not stopped from seeking asylum, Germany operated stricter asylum-seeking processes, and altered some of their processes, for example, no in-person interviews were allowed (Reches, 2022). To control infection, mitigation measures were applied within asylum seekers centres, including social distancing measures.

Group activities, such as language courses or playgroups for children were all cancelled (Rast et al., 2023). Quarantine measures in asylum seeker centres were found to exacerbate the stressful circumstances people associated with migration and asylum seeking, and evoked feelings of imprisonment (Rast et al., 2023). However, a few countries proceeded to accommodate asylum seekers and refugees in this critical period. For example, asylum seekers who had been refugees, were provided with accommodation by the Home Office in the UK at the start of the pandemic. Portugal granted all asylum seekers and foreign-born migrants full citizenship at the start of the pandemic to remove structural barriers to accessing healthcare (Mukumbang, 2020).

HEALTH POLICIES RELEVANT TO MIGRANTS

It was with the help of migrants that many European states rebuilt their economies after the World War Two and migration has led to substantial interdependencies between countries. The period after the war could be perceived as the beginning of the welfare state in the UK and Western Europe. In the UK, the Beveridge Report in 1942 proposed a new type of welfare state, aimed at abolishing 'want', including a free health service, family allowances and social insurance, to help deal with periods of hardship and unemployment. In 1948, the National Health Service (NHS) was founded, and the UK was the first western country to offer free at the point of use medical care to the entire population.

Initially, there were no restrictions to accessing healthcare for migrants in the UK and there was no differentiation between migrants and citizens in accessing welfare benefits and public services offered (Römer, 2022). However, as in other OECD countries, welfare became restricted, and has been tied to migration status, and length of residency. Migrant welfare rights have been restricted through direct measures, but also through indirect measures. Direct restrictions refer to explicit policies that directly limit migrants' access to welfare benefits. Indirect restrictions, on the other hand, involve policies that may not target welfare benefits directly, but still effectively limit migrants' ability to access them (Vintila and Lafleur, 2020); for example, tying residency rights to employment, meaning migrants must have employment to maintain their legal status in the country, and prohibiting family reunification or the attainment of citizenship for recipients of welfare benefits. These policies are thus specific to migrants in that they rely on the defining feature of migrants' status limited residency rights-to exert control (Vintila and Lafleur, 2020). In a comparison of welfare benefits between OECD members from 1970 until 2018, it is apparent that, across all states, permanent migrants have more access rights to welfare benefits than temporary migrants, and across all years (Römer et al., 2021). This is particularly the case for refugees, who enjoy welfare rights like those granted to citizens in almost all countries (Römer, 2022). An exception would be Denmark, where political debates have significantly restricted migrant policies in the last decades (Vintila and Lafleur, 2020) and in 2019, the Danish Prime Minister declared that Denmark wanted 'zero asylum-seekers'.

In Denmark, refugees do have access to social welfare including healthcare. However, the extent and nature of the benefits, can be complex, with various programmes and requirements aimed at integration and self-sufficiency. Programmes can include language courses and activities intended to lead to employment, and where refugees take part in these programmes, financial support is offered (Jensen et al., 2011). Denmark was the first country to review refugees' residency status, with the aim of returning people to their home countries, if these are considered safe (Römer, 2022). Denmark has a universal healthcare system financed through taxes and it covers all persons registered with the National Register of Persons. Denmark has ratified several international conventions recognising the right to health care for all human beings, which includes asylum seekers, refugees, and other migrants. However, accessing healthcare for undocumented migrants is problematic and barriers to accessing healthcare remain for all other migrants too (Jensen et al., 2011).

Health policies for migrants and other related issues have become key elements of political discussions in OECD countries. However, there is a noticeable diversity in the policies of OECD countries regarding migration, encompassing aspects like social integration, housing, education, employment, welfare, and healthcare systems. Although European nations have shifted towards adopting universal healthcare systems, there are still variations in how inclusive these systems are towards migrants. These differences can have significant implications for the health outcomes of the migrant population (Dourgnon, et al., 2023). For instance, while Belgium, Czechia, France, Germany, Italy, and the Netherlands, provide primary and secondary care to undocumented migrants, Croatia, Cyprus, Finland, Greece, Hungary, Lithuania, Poland, Romania, Slovak Republic, Slovenia, and Spain grant only emergency care (da Costa Leite Borges and Guidi, 2018). In a review published in 2022, the authors stated that in 2004, in almost half of all countries in the EU, there were legal access barriers to the healthcare system, including in Austria, Denmark, Estonia, Finland, Germany, Hungary, Luxembourg, Malta, Spain and Sweden. Apart from Austria, asylum seekers only had access to emergency care. The authors state that these policies were reviewed in the context of the 2015 European refugee crisis. However, there is a gap in the literature and that this has not been systematically reviewed yet (Nowak et al., 2022).

The UK also introduced changes to NHS healthcare access for temporary migrants as part of a broader effort to control migration. As part of the Immigration Act (2014), the Immigration Health Surcharge (IHS) was introduced, which came into effect in April 2015. This surcharge requires non-European Economic Area (EEA) migrants staying in the UK for longer than six months to pay a fee for accessing NHS services, although certain services remained free, such as emergency services, and infectious disease treatment. The IHS must be paid in advance as part of the visa application process.

If the IHS payment is not completed, the visa application is denied. In 2015, the IHS was £200 per year. However, in February 2024, the IHS was raised to £1,035 per year. The IHS has raised over five billion pounds for healthcare spending (McKinney and Gower, 2024). Migrants already contribute to the NHS through regular taxes and therefore the IHS arguably represents double taxation for migrants. Asylum seekers and victims of human trafficking do not pay the IHS. The IHS was part of the government's aim to make the immigration system more selective, deter abuse, and reduce the burden on the NHS. However, critics argue that these measures could deter vulnerable and particularly undocumented migrants from accessing essential healthcare (Lilana and Van Ginneken, 2015). Denying undocumented migrants access to healthcare can result in greater economic burden on the health system later. Access to primary care is associated with lower costs of health services, with preventative healthcare, and with better health outcomes (da Costa Leite Borges and Guidi, 2018).

Article 12 of the United Nations' International Covenant on Economic, Social and Cultural Rights (ICESCR) establishes the right to the highest standard of health for everyone, emphasising equal health opportunities. This includes refugees, asylum seekers, and migrant workers, regardless of legal status. European human rights texts, though not explicitly stating health rights, suggest that access denial could breach fundamental rights. The European Social Charter explicitly grants medical assistance rights to irregular migrants. EU resolutions and directives support health rights for undocumented migrants, underlining the push for fair healthcare access. This reflects efforts to align national health policies with wider human rights obligations, recognising challenges in migrant health rights and healthcare access (da Costa Leite Borges and Guidi, 2018). Da Costa Leite Borges and Guidi (2018) present an interesting comparison between the UK and Italy, regarding access to healthcare for undocumented migrants.

The Italian and UK health systems have similar features: healthcare funding comes primarily from general taxation, rather than through social insurance. Both systems provide healthcare services free at the point of access for citizens or regular residents. Italian law recognises the right to health as a fundamental right, and therefore free access to healthcare is a constitutional guarantee, including for undocumented migrants. Although undocumented migrants are not allowed to register with the NHS, as an Italian citizen, undocumented migrants are entitled to register for a special card, which provides access to healthcare in the same conditions as Italian citizens or regular residents.

As a rule, emergency care, primary care (GP), preventive care (including vaccination, screening, and HIV prevention), prenatal, and maternity care (antenatal, birth and post-natal care), are offered free of charge. Although access to other types of care—such as secondary, rehabilitative, or chronic diseases treatment—is provided upon payment, fees can be waived, provided that undocumented migrants ask for an exemption from payment (da Costa Leite Borges and Guidi, 2018). The Italian health system is decentralised, meaning legislation regarding access to healthcare for undocumented migrants has been executed differently regionally, with some regions restricting and others extending rights (da Costa Leite Borges and Guidi, 2018).

In the UK, while there are policies and regulations in place to ensure access to healthcare services through the NHS for citizens and regular residents, Da Costa Leite Borges and Guidi (2018) state that the right to health is not specifically recognised as a fundamental constitutional right. Undocumented migrants do not have the same access to NHS services as citizens or regular residents if they are unable to provide evidence regarding their legal status. Although most services offered by the NHS to individuals regularly registered with the NHS are free at the point of delivery, undocumented migrants are considered overseas visitors. Therefore, the NHS is required to impose charges for any relevant services provided to anyone, not registered as a citizen, or regular resident. However, some services are exempt, and are offered free of charge, including accident and emergency care; family planning services (excluding termination of established pregnancy); diagnosis and treatment of specified infectious diseases like HIV, diagnosis, and treatment of sexually transmitted infections; and treatment required for physical or mental conditions resulting from torture, female genital mutilation, domestic or sexual violence (Matsuura, 2019).

THE MIPEX

The MIPEX, or Migrant Integration Policy index, is a comprehensive tool used to assess and compare migration integration policies across countries, developed by the Migration Policy group. The MIPEX measures eight areas of integration policies: (1) labour market mobility; (2) family reunification; (3) education; (4) political participation; (5) permanent residence; (6) access to nationality; (7) anti-discrimination; and (8) health. Each policy area is measured by a policy indicator, with each policy indicator measured by a score from 0 to 100, and the average score of the eight policy indicators form the MIPEX. The maximum of 100 is awarded when policies meet the highest standards for equal treatment. The top end of the MIPEX scale for health suggests that health systems are usually more 'migrant-friendly', with a strong commitment to equal rights and opportunities (Migration Policy Group, 2020). MIPEX scores for OECD countries based on 2019 data, are presented in Table 16.2.

The MIPEX score is interpreted along three dimensions:

1. Basic rights: Can migrants enjoy comparable rights as nationals e.g., equal rights to work, training, health, and non-discrimination?
2. Equal opportunities: Can migrants receive support to enjoy comparable opportunities as nationals e.g., targeted support in education, health, and political participation?
3. Secure future: Can migrants settle long-term and feel secure about their future in the country e.g., family reunification, permanent residence, and access to nationality (Migration Policy Group, 2020)?

TABLE 16.2 MIPEX and Health Indicator Scores for OECD Countries

OECD countries	Health	MIPEX 2019 (overall score with health)
1. Austria	81	46
2. Australia	79	65
3. Belgium	73	69
4. Canada	73	80
5. Chile	73	53
6. Colombia	Not available	Not available
7. Costa Rica	Not available	Not available
8. Czechia	61	50
9. Denmark	56	49
10. Estonia	29	50
11. Finland	67	85
12. France	65	56
13. Germany	63	58
14. Greece	48	46
15. Hungary	29	43
16. Iceland	54	56
17. Ireland	85	64
18. Israel	63	49
19. Italy	79	58
20. Japan	65	47
21. Korea	Not available	Not available
22. Latvia	31	37
23. Lithuania	31	37
24. Luxembourg	46	64
25. Mexico	42	51
26. Netherlands	65	57
27. New Zealand	83	77
28. Norway	75	69
29. Poland	27	40
30. Portugal	65	81
31. Slovak Republic	50	39
32. Slovenia	33	48
33. Spain	81	60
34. Sweden	83	86
35. Switzerland	83	50
36. Türkiye	69	43
37. United Kingdom	75	56
38. United States	79	73

Source: adapted from Migration Policy Group (2020)

Note: a score of 80–100 is favourable, 60–79 slightly favourable, 41–59 halfway favourable, 21–40 slightly unfavourable, 1–20 unfavourable, 0 critically unfavourable.

Reviewing Table 16.2, OECD countries that are perceived to offer a comprehensive approach to integration (average score 75/100) which fully guarantee equal rights and opportunities to migrants and citizens alike, are Finland, Sweden, Portugal, Belgium, Ireland, Canada, New Zealand, Australia, and the US. The United Kingdom scores with the Netherlands, Italy, Germany, and France as 'temporary integration-halfway favourable' (average score 57/100). The Migration Policy Group interprets that these countries provide immigrants with basic rights and equal opportunities, but not a secure future in the country. Policies in these countries promote the view of migrants as equals, but they also emphasise their status as foreigners rather than as potential citizens. Denmark, Austria, and Switzerland score 'halfway unfavourable' (average score 48/100), indicating that the countries only go halfway towards granting migrants with basic rights and equal opportunities and do not provide a secure future (Migration Policy Group, 2020).

How governments oversee migration policies has a significant impact on migrants' health and wellbeing. In countries with inclusive integration policies, migrants tend to have similar health outcomes to the general population. However, in countries with more restrictive policies, poorer health outcomes have been reported for migrants, compared with the general population, resulting in health inequalities (Dourgnon et al., 2023). To improve migrants' health outcomes, access to healthcare needs to be inclusive. The overall approach to migrant integration seems more of a determinant than any specific area of integration policy alone (Migration Policy Group, 2020). This highlights the importance of the 'Health in all Policies' approach, which is a strategy for public policy that recognises that health is influenced by policies and actions outside of the health sector and therefore advocates for incorporation of health into all policy-making process and across all sectors.

None of the OECD countries scored in the most unfavourable countries (average score 28/100) which includes China and Russia; however, Greece, Latvia, Lithuania, and Poland fell into the 'equality on paper-slightly unfavourable' category (average score of 39/100), which indicates that migrants do not enjoy equal opportunities. The Migration Policy Group states that this group of countries goes only halfway towards providing immigrants with basic rights and a secure future. Policies may encourage the public to see immigrants as subordinates, not equal and not potential citizens.

CONCLUSION

Migration is at an all-time high. Worse health outcomes and health inequalities have been reported for migrants. Migrants were disproportionally affected by COVID-19 and the pandemic highlighted their vulnerabilities. In addition to removing barriers to accessing healthcare, such as language and communication barriers, and ameliorating culturally appropriate access, overall global migration integration policies should be reviewed. In countries with inclusive integration policies, migrants tend to have better health outcomes than in countries with more restrictive policies, highlighting the importance of 'Health in All Policy' approach to improve migrants' health and wellbeing.

RESEARCH POINTS AND REFLECTIVE EXERCISES

- How do national healthcare policies in different countries impact migrants' access to healthcare? Consider different groups of migrants.
- Go to the Migration Integration Policy Index: www.mipex.eu Which country scores the worst, and which country scores the best on the MIPEX? Reflect on what that means.
- Considering the different categories in the MIPEX, discuss how the principle of 'Health in all Policies' approach could contribute to reducing health inequalities for migrants.

REFERENCES

Campbell, C., Sommerfield, T., Clark, G. R. C., Porteous, L. Milne, A. M., et al. (2021). COVID-19 and Cancer Screening in Scotland: A National and Coordinated Approach to Minimising Harm. *Preventive Medicine*, 151: 106606. https://doi.org/10.1016/J.YPMED.2021.106606.

Carling, J. and Collins, F. (2018). Aspiration, Desire and Drivers of Migration. *Journal of Ethnic and Migration Studies*, 44 (6): 909–926. https://doi.org/10.1080/1369183X.2017.1384134.

Czaika, M., Bijak, J. and Prike, T. (2021). Migration Decision-Making and Its Key Dimensions. *The ANNALS of the American Academy of Political and Social Science*, 697 (1), 15–31. https://doi.org/10.1177/00027162211052233

da Costa Leite Borges, D. and Guidi, C. F. (2018). Rights of Access to Healthcare for Undocumented Migrants: Understanding the Italian and British National Health Systems. *International Journal of Human Rights in Healthcare*, 11 (4): 232–243. https://doi.org/10.1108/IJHRH-01-2018-0006.

Dourgnon, P., Pourat, N. and Rocco, L. (2023). European Immigrant Health Policies, Immigrants' Health, and Immigrants' Access to Healthcare. *Health Policy*, 127: 37–43. https://doi.org/10.1016/J.HEALTHPOL.2022.12.012.

IDWF. (2020). The Impacts of COVID-19 on Domestic Workers and Policy Responses 1 May 2020. Available at: https://idwfed.org/en/covid-19/the-idwf/advocacy/idwf-policy-brief_final-eng.pdf (Accessed: 8 May 2020).

IOM. (2018). Migration and the 2030 Agenda: A Guide for Practitioners. Available at: https://publications.iom.int/books/migration-and-2030-agenda-guide-practitioners (Accessed: 1 March 2024).

IOM. (2022a). Interactive World Migration Report 2022. Available at: https://worldmigrationreport.iom.int/wmr-2022-interactive/ (Accessed: 1 March 2024).

IOM. (2022b). *The Impacts of Covid-19 on Migration and Migrants from a Gender Perspective*. Geneva: IOM.

Jensen, N. K., Norredam, M., Draebel, T., Bogic, M., Priebe, S., et al. (2011). Providing Medical Care for Undocumented Migrants in Denmark: What Are the Challenges for Health Professionals? *BMC Health Services Research*, 11 (1): 1–10. https://doi.org/10.1186/1472-6963-11-154.

Lilana, K. and Van Ginneken, E. (2015). Migrant Health: Restricting Access to the NHS for Undocumented Migrants Is Bad Policy at High Cost. *BMJ*, 350. https://doi.org/10.1136/BMJ.H3056.

Sumant, K. and Patel, A. B. (2023). The Death of Migrant Workers in India During the First Wave of COVID-19 Pandemic. *Mental Health and Social Inclusion*, ahead-of-print (ahead-of-print). https://doi.org/10.1108/MHSI-08-2023-0086.

Lebano, A., Hamed, S., Bradby, H., Gil-Salmerón, Durá-Ferrandis, E., et al. (2020). Migrants' and Refugees' Health Status and Healthcare in Europe: A Scoping Literature Review. *BMC Public Health*, 20 (1): 1–22. https://doi.org/10.1186/S12889-020-08749-8.

Matsuura, H. (2019). Exploring the Association Between the Constitutional Right to Health and Reproductive Health Outcomes in 157 Countries. *Sexual and Reproductive Health Matters*, 27 (1): 168–180. https://doi.org/10.1080/26410397.2019.1599653.

McAuliffe, M. and Triandafyllidou, A. (2021). World Migration Report 2022, International Organization for Migration. Available at: https://worldmigrationreport.iom.int/wmr-2022-interactive/ (Accessed: 2 February 2024).

McKinney, C. J. and Gower, M. (2024). The Immigration Health Surcharge, UK Parliament, House of Commons Library 2024. Available at: https://commonslibrary.parliament.uk/research-briefings/cbp-7274/ (Accessed: 2 February 2024).

Migration Policy Group. (2020). Migration Integration Policy Index 2020. Available at: www.mipex.eu/political-participation (Accessed: 25 February 2024).

Morgan, J. and Shumba, C., (2023). Armed Conflict and Children's Mental Health. In V. La Placa and J. Morgan (eds), *Social Science Perspectives on Global Public Health*. London: Routledge, 129–139.

Mukumbang, F. C. (2020). Are Asylum Seekers, Refugees and Foreign Migrants Considered in the COVID-19 Vaccine Discourse? *BMJ Global Health*, 5 (11): e004085. https://doi.org/10.1136/BMJGH-2020-004085.

Nelson, M., Patton, A., Robb, K., Weller, D. Sheikh, A., et al. (2021). Experiences of Cervical Screening Participation and Non-Participation in Women from Minority Ethnic Populations in Scotland. *Health Expectations*, 24 (4): 1459–72. https://doi.org/10.1111/HEX.13287.

Nowak, A. C., Namer, Y. and Hornberg, C. (2022). Health Care for Refugees in Europe: A Scoping Review. *International Journal of Environmental Research and Public Health*, 19 (3). https://doi.org/10.3390/IJERPH19031278.

OECD. (2017). Migrants' Well-Being: Moving to a Better Life? Available at: https://doi.org/10.1787/HOW_LIFE-2017-7-EN (Accessed: 5 January 2024).

OECD. (2022). The Unequal Impact of COVID-19: A Spotlight on Frontline Workers, Migrants and Racial/Ethnic Minorities - OECD. 2022. Available at: https://read.oecd-ilibrary.org/view/?ref=1133_1133188-lq9ii66g9w&title=The-unequal-impact-of-COVID-19-A-spotlight-on-frontline-workers-migrants-and-racial-ethnic-minorities (Accessed: 5 January 2024).

Pandey, K., Parreñas, R. S. and Sabio, G. S. (2021). Essential and Expendable: Migrant Domestic Workers and the COVID-19 Pandemic. *American Behavioral Scientist*, 65 (10), 1287–1301. https://doi.org/10.1177/00027642211000396

Public Health Scotland. (2022). Fit for Travel. Available at: www.fitfortravel.nhs.uk/news/newsdetail.aspx?id=24163# (Accessed: 10 January 2024),

Rast, E., Perplies, C., Biddle, L. and Bozorgmehr, K. (2023). Between Care and Coercion: Asylum Seekers' Experiences With COVID-19 Containment and Mitigation Measures in German Reception Centres. *International Journal of Public Health*, 68. https://doi.org/10.3389/ijph.2023.1605230.

Reches, D. (2022). Complying with International and Regional Law During the Pandemic - Asylum Seekers and COVID-19 Emergency Measures in EU Member States Germany and Greece. *Social Sciences and Humanities Open*, 6 (1): 100370. https://doi.org/10.1016/J.SSAHO.2022.100370.

Römer, F. (2022). Differentiation of Welfare Rights for Migrants in Western Countries From 1970 to Present. In. F. Nullmeier, D. González de Reufels and H. Obinger (eds.) *International Impacts on Social Policy: Global Dynamics of Social Policy*. Cham: Palgrave Macmillan, 501–513.

Römer, F., Harris, E., Henninger, J. Missler, F., Böhme, M., et al. (2021). The Migrant Social Protection Data Set (MigSP) Technical Report. Available at: https://doi.org/10.26092/elib/2043 (Accessed: 21 January 2024).

Rosińska, A. and Pellerito, E. (2022). Pandemic Shock Absorbers: Domestic Workers' Activism at the Intersection of Immigrants' and Workers' Rights. *IMISCOE Research Series*, 123–144. https://doi.org/10.1007/978-3-030-81210-2_7.

Saldanha, K., D'Cunha, C. and Kovick, L. (2023). India's Internal Migrants and the First Wave of COVID-19: The Invisibility of Female Migrants. *Asian Journal of Social Science*, 51 (2): 116–122. https://doi.org/10.1016/J.AJSS.2023.02.001.

Taylor, M. and Levin Azriel, I. (2023). Games Without Frontiers - Covid Living in Refugee Camps. *Interiors in the Era of Covid-19*, 10: 127–38. https://doi.org/10.5040/9781350294257.CH-010.

UK Government. (2023). Asylum Statistics - House of Commons Library. Available at: https://commonslibrary.parliament.uk/research-briefings/sn01403/ (Accessed: 1 February 2024).

Ullah, A. K. M., Nawaz, F. and Chattoraj, D. (2021). Locked Up Under Lockdown: The COVID-19 Pandemic and the Migrant Population. *Social Sciences and Humanities Open*, 3 (1): 100126. https://doi.org/10.1016/J.SSAHO.2021.100126.

UNHCO. (2023). Refugee Data Finder. Available at: www.unhcr.org/refugee-statistics/ (Accessed 1 February 2024).

United Nations World Tourism Organization. (2023). The End of COVID-19-Related Travel Restrictions – Summary of Findings from the COVID-19-Related Travel Restrictions Reports. Available at: https://doi.org/10.18111/9789284424320. (Accessed 1 February 2024).

Vintila, D. and Lafleur, J. M. (2020). Migration and Access to Welfare Benefits in the EU: The Interplay between Residence and Nationality. *IMISCOE Research Series*, 1–32. https://doi.org/10.1007/978-3-030-51241-5_1.

WHO. (2017). Migration and Health: Key Issues. Euro.Who.Int. Available at: www.euro.who.int/en/health-topics/health-determinants/migration-and-health/migrant-health-in-the-european-region/migration-and-health-key-issues (Accessed 1 February 2024).

WHO. (2021). Common Health Needs of Refugees and Migrants: Literature Review. Geneva. 2021. Available at: www.who.int/publications/i/item/9789240033108 (Accessed: 1 February 2024).

WHO. (2024). Essential Knowledge Health and Migration. Available at: www.who.int/tools/refugee-and-migrant-health-toolkit/essential-knowledge-health-and-migration# (Accessed: 3 February 2024).

CHAPTER 17

Loneliness

....

Julia Morgan and Vincent La Placa

INTRODUCTION

Loneliness has been identified as a significant global public health issue (La Placa and Morgan, 2023; Morgan and La Placa, 2023). This global concern about loneliness has been highlighted by the World Health Organization (WHO, 2023a), who launched a new Commission on Social Connection to address the issue. In the United Kingdom and Japan, ministers for loneliness have been appointed, whose remits are to implement strategies to increase social connectedness. This chapter will define loneliness and discuss the impact of loneliness on health and wellbeing. The chapter's second half will then explore loneliness among young people across OECD countries and include a focus on loneliness interventions used globally.

DEFINING LONELINESS

On average, reported loneliness increased in OECD countries from 8–15% between 2003–2018. The largest increases were witnessed in the Slovak Republic, Australia, and Iceland. Japan, however, witnessed a significant decrease over this period (OECD, 2021a). Loneliness has been defined as 'the unpleasant experience that occurs when a person's network of social relations is deficient in some important way, either quantitatively or qualitatively' (Perlman and Peplau, 1981). It is, thus, a subjective feeling about the gap between an individual's desired levels of social contact and the actual level of social contact. This means an individual can feel lonely and simultaneously have many friends as it is a subjective and personal evaluation. Definitions of loneliness, however, are often multidimensional.

Emotional loneliness, for example, occurs when an individual perceives that they lack the relationship provisions of close emotional attachments, including emotional support, affection, and intimacy. Emotional loneliness encompasses emotions around not being close to others, lacking acquaintances, who are highly familiar with an individual, and adequately understand the person in question, and who are

DOI: 10.4324/9781003343608-19

often present in times of need. Social loneliness is more linked to social integration and lacking people to communicate with. It occurs when an individual perceives that he or she does not possess the relationship provisions of a network of relationships, including social integration and belongingness. Social loneliness involves emotions around not being connected to others, lacking individuals to spend time with and enjoy adequate communication and friendships, and a sense of belonging. Existential loneliness, on the other hand, focuses on a perceived disconnection from society and from others generally (Mansfield et al., 2019). It has been described as a sense of 'nothingness' (Ettema et al., 2010), a separation 'related to the nature of existence' and a lack of meaning in life (van Tilburg, 2021: e336). Research has explored existential loneliness in relation to end of life care and severe illnesses (Boston et al., 2011; Tarbi and Meghani, 2019).

Loneliness may also be defined as a 'distressing' feeling which accompanies the perception that an individual's social needs are not adequately met by the quantity or especially the quality of one's social relationships (Hawkley and Cacioppo, 2010). An individual may experience loneliness as a temporary phenomenon, which is a result of a particular situation, for example, the COVID-19 lockdown, or as chronic condition more generally (Alam et al., 2023). Age UK (2015) argue that similarly, loneliness is often used interchangeably with the concept of 'isolation' but that the latter, is more concerned with an external/quantitative phenomenon, which can affect subjective feelings of loneliness, such as disconnection from, for instance, families and services. Donbavand (2020) argues that the structure of modern society is responsible for loneliness as opposed to, for example, individual circumstances and subjective interpretations. Traditional societies were historically characterised by uniformity, commonalities, and integration into a wider set of experiences and interactions.

However, modern societies allocate individuals to various specialised groups and interests, based on, for instance, specialised work and economic roles, which are smaller, and relations less intense, than in societies characterised by more homogeneity. Individuals become immersed within a diminishing number of groups, networks, and social circles, and experiences, with individuals outside their specialised environments, limiting contact with the wider society. Structural processes of modernity, independent of individual agency and subjective experience, are a significant contribution to social isolation and personal loneliness as a result. La Placa and Oham (2019) and La Placa and Morgan (2023) have argued that while loneliness can be conceptualised as affected by and constructed through wider determinants, it is also most effectively perceived as a symbolic and discursive social construction, albeit constructed within social and community constraints. Loneliness is a social, relational, and subjective phenomenon, and often separate, from, for instance, the physical reality of social isolation and objective phenomena; and as such, the study of loneliness, is distinct from, for example, psychological, and biomedical studies of mental health and stress, which often dominate the theoretical frameworks, through which it is often defined and theorised (La Placa and Oham, 2019).

IMPACT OF LONELINESS ON HEALTH AND WELLBEING

Feelings of loneliness are a phenomenon that is a universal lived experience which is significant to health, wellbeing, and quality of life. Loneliness has implications for global health and social care services as it often results in earlier and increased use of costly health and social care services. For example, lonely people are more likely to visit their general practitioner (GP) and to use other health services, due to enhanced issues with physical and mental health. While Geller et al. (1999) argue that loneliness is often a predictor of accidents and emergencies, often independent of chronic illness.

Social connectedness has been highlighted as an important social determinant of health (Holt-Lunstad, 2022) and loneliness, or a lack of social connectedness, can have important impacts on health and wellbeing. While many individuals may feel lonely at some time or other, it is often a temporary feeling which, while distressing, goes away. Chronic loneliness, however, has been shown to be associated with a range of mental health issues including depression (Qualter et al., 2010; Ladd and Ettekal, 2013; Qualter et al., 2013), long-term stress (Segrin et al., 2018), anxiety (Vanhalst et al., 2013), and suicidal ideation (Schinka et al., 2013). Moreover, chronic loneliness has been implicated in physical health conditions, including an increased risk of dementia (Salinas et al., 2022) and increases in cardiovascular diseases, strokes, obesity, diabetes, and pulmonary issues (Petitte et al., 2015). Furthermore, chronic loneliness has been found to be associated with increases in mortality and morbidity (House et al., 1988; Holt-Lunstad et al., 2015) and has been shown to contribute to health inequalities between socio-economic groups (Meisters et al., 2021).

These concerns about the impact of loneliness on health and wellbeing has led to the introduction of loneliness strategies in both the UK and in Japan. In 2018, the UK Government introduced its strategy to combat loneliness (Department for Digital, Culture, Media and Sport, 2018a). This strategy was based on recommendations from the Jo Cox Commission on Loneliness (2017) and led to the appointment of Tracey Crouch as ministerial lead for loneliness and the announcement of funding of £20 million to support organisations to tackle loneliness and build more socially connected communities. The strategy focused on reduction of stigma and increasing conversations about loneliness including the introduction of Loneliness Awareness Week and campaigns such as 'Let's Talk Loneliness', and 'Better Health: Every Mind Matters'. It also aimed to improve and build the evidence base on loneliness to identify interventions which could be implemented; and to ensure that policy makers across departments considered the importance of social connectedness when designing policy. In relation to building the evidence base the recent review of the loneliness strategy (Department for Digital, Culture, Media and Sport, 2023a) identified numerous ways in which the research base could be strengthened including more information around how loneliness impacts on different groups, such as those with disabilities, those of different ages, and sexual minorities; the use of more robust research designs such as longitudinal population studies to explore how circumstances interact over time; as well as more research on the relationship between mental health and loneliness.

In relation to policy, the Scottish Government introduced its strategy to tackle social isolation and loneliness and build stronger social connections (2018) and put emphasis on the role of all government departments in reducing loneliness including health and social care, the fire service, and the building of safer communities. The Welsh Government (2020) also put emphasis on infrastructure, including planning, housing, and transport to support social connectedness and highlighted the importance of 'government action across a range of policy areas'. Japan, because of concerns about more recent rates of loneliness and suicide, created a cabinet post, in 2021, to reduce loneliness, with Tetsushi Sakamoto being appointed as the first Minister for Loneliness and Isolation. Since then, the Government has passed the 'Act on Promotion of Policy for Loneliness and Isolation', which comes into effect on 1 April 2024. The Act outlines the importance of devising priority plans, at both national and local government level, to tackle loneliness, including more support for research into loneliness to provide evidence for interventions and policy. The Act led to the setting up of a 'Headquarters for Promotion of Measures for Loneliness and Isolation' within the Cabinet Office as a special agency to co-ordinate policies around loneliness and priority plans. Membership of the Headquarters would include representation from across government including the Minister of Education, Culture, Sports, Science and Technology, the Minister of Health, Labour and Welfare and the Minister of Agriculture, Forestry and Fisheries.

YOUNG PEOPLE AND LONELINESS

Increasing evidence indicates that younger people may be experiencing loneliness at higher rates than other age groups. This was found in a global survey of 237 countries, islands, and territories (Barreto et al., 2021), in the USA (Cigma, 2018; 2020; Weissbourd et al., 2021), in New Zealand (Ministry of Social Development, 2016), in the Netherlands (Franssen et al., 2020), in Denmark (Lasgaard et al., 2016) and in England (Office for National Statistics, 2018a). The Community Life Survey (Department for Digital, Culture, Media and Sport, 2018b; 2019; 2020; 2021; 2023b) in England shows that for the years 2017–2022, younger people aged 16–24 years old had the highest rates of feeling often/always lonely closely followed by those in the age range 25–34 years old.

These rates remained stable across the five years for 25–34 years old but have increased slightly for 16–24-year-olds from 8% feeling often/always lonely in 2017–2018 to 10% in 2021–2022. What is apparent from the Community Life Survey, is that loneliness follows a U-shaped trajectory, which tends to be highest among younger people, decreasing towards middle-age, and then starting to increase again for those aged 75+. While the COVID-19 pandemic led to increases in 'lockdown loneliness' for younger people (Baarck et al., 2021; Weissbourd et al., 2021; Office for National Statistics, 2021), the research above indicates that the trends for elevated levels of loneliness among younger people were already evident before the lockdown. Interestingly, some research has also indicated that even older people report, retrospectively, that they felt lonelier when they were younger (Hammond, 2018).

However, these findings have not consistently been found with a meta-analysis based on European data (Surkalim et al., 2022) and a survey across Europe (Baarck et al., 2021) finding that older people were more likely to be lonely. These conflicting findings may be a result of differences in the measurement of loneliness, how the data was collected (for example, the use of online surveys, which may preclude participation for some groups) and possible heterogeneity in loneliness between countries with some possibly reporting more loneliness. For example, in relation to the last point, it may be the case that more individualistic societies report higher loneliness than more collectivist societies (Barreto et al., 2021) and this may explain some of the differences between countries. However, having said that some indictors (WHO, 2023b) show the opposite with 12.7% of adolescents in the African region and 14.4% in the Eastern Mediterranean region (traditionally perceived as more collectivist societies) reporting feeling lonely compared to 5.3% in the European region.

Loneliness can impact some young people more than others. Research in England indicates that for children aged 10 to 15 years old, loneliness was more likely to be reported if the children received free school meals, lived in a city, reported low satisfaction with their health and low satisfaction with their relationships with family and friends (Office for National Statistics, 2018b). For those aged between 16 to 24 years old, women were more likely than men to report feeling lonely, as were young people with a long-term illness or disability, and those living in single adult households (Office for National Statistics, 2018b). Other research in the UK found that those who were unemployed (Matthews et al., 2018), those who left home to attend university (Vasileuiou et al., 2019), LGBTQI+ young people, and those who felt a lower sense of belonging in their community were more likely to feel lonely (Marquez et al., 2023). While, in the Netherlands ethnic minorities were more likely to feel lonely (Franssen et al., 2020) and in the US, Mexican youth who were immigrants, were more likely to report feeling lonely than Mexican youth who were born in the USA (Polo and Lopez, 2009).

FACTORS THAT INCREASE LONELINESS FOR YOUNG PEOPLE

The factors which have contributed to the higher levels and increased intensity of loneliness among young people have been explained with recourse to both wider social determinants and in the more personal and subjective dimensions. However, both wider social determinants affect personal and subjective responses to and the causes of loneliness and vice versa. Both facilitate and constrain how young people feel and respond to loneliness across their lives. To illustrate the roles of wider determinants, Sagan (2018) has argued that loneliness is principally begot through the pre-eminence of neoliberalism which permeates current formations of capitalism. Neoliberal philosophy and policies increasingly lead to restructuring of social and economic relations, which creates a fracturing of social relations and networks, which encourages separation and atomisation of individuals. This leads to higher rates of mental illness, for instance, as individuals find themselves increasing alone and separated from significant others as collective groups and institutions decline.

Sagan (2018) also emphasises the process of Globalisation and its tendencies to homogenise and cause similar experiences across the globe. Imrie (2018) contends that increasing global urbanisation is a key social and structural determinant of loneliness, where depleted infrastructure and networks curtail opportunities and options to develop relationships with other groups and individuals. As a solution to loneliness, and the negative health and wellbeing outcomes, associated with it, Imrie (2018), posits urban developments which can encourage communication and assist in creation of urban spaces, where individuals can more easily connect in meaningful ways. Moreover, some research has demonstrated that 'urban greening' and the introduction of green spaces into urban areas may reduce loneliness (Astell-Burt et al., 2022).

On a more personal and subjective level, young people face various unpredictable situations around puberty, schooling, finding friends, becoming adults, and finding a partner, and individuation from family (Morgan and La Placa, 2023) which seemingly form part of the life course of a young individual, and which require reflections around how to respond and what actions to assume (but which also occur within wider social circumstances). These are often dependent upon different behavioural drivers such as social cognitions, attitudes, experiences, and motivations (produced through positive and negative experiences throughout life). This can be compounded by the complex and potentially risky decisions young people often face in their daily lives, such as education, leaving home, career choices, and starting a family. Fardghassemi and Joffe (2022), in their study of deprived areas in London, argue that transitions between life stages such as breakups, loss of significant others, and transitory stages associated with education and employment are perceived to cause loneliness. They also ascertained that perceptions around inability to express oneself authentically; feelings around not being understood; lack of face-to-face social interaction and care from others; and perceptions of life as a 'rat race' were of significance.

In Finland, loneliness was associated with social transitions, group differences, social expectations, and negative self-image (Sundqvist and Hemberg, 2021). Children and young people may also experience loneliness due to an inability to socialise and mix with friends in and outside of educational settings as they proceed to become adults, which can lead to depression. Verity et al. (2021), in their study based on the perspectives of children in Italy and Belgium, highlighted conflict with others, and the school environment as being potential triggers for loneliness. Achterberg et al. (2020) in their meta-analysis of the literature, found that young people with depression experience loneliness as an unyielding distance between themselves and others. Non-disclosure of depression, and the detrimental nature of it, also perpetuates loneliness and depression. Achterberg et al. (2020) posits that approaches to tackling this issue might include assisting young people to communicate more about their depression to, for instance, trusted friends, and educating their social networks in navigating responses to support them.

However, risk and complexity not only play out on a personal level with younger people potentially more at risk of loneliness, but because they are constructed by and responded to across situations, often at a societal level, perceived as beyond their control (Morgan and La Placa, 2023). This often includes changes in the ways in which younger people relate to one another, including the usage of social media, as well as social, political, and economic changes, such as increases in the gig economy and the cost of living and housing crises. Fardghassemi and Joffe (2022) found, for example, that social media contributed to loneliness because of 'fake' representations, where posts gave the impression that others were having 'an exciting time' even though the young people, themselves, knew that this was not always the case. All these experiences can precipitate perceptions of their circumstances and environments as insurmountable, unpredictable, and unsafe, to be navigated in isolation, and with little support from others. Stigma around loneliness can often mean that young people do not seek assistance, or share their experiences, which compounds loneliness (Shah and Househ, 2023).

The COVID-19 pandemic not only impacted physical health, and mortality rates, but also impacted wellbeing (Mareike et al., 2022). Younger people experienced some of the most significant declines in mental health, social connectedness, and life satisfaction in 2020 and 2021, as well as disruption to employment and study, which exacerbated insecurity. Data from OECD countries also demonstrates young people experienced the highest rates of anxiety and depression, both earlier and later, in the pandemic (OECD, 2021b). Since its outbreak in 2020, most OECD countries implemented, for instance, lockdowns, travel bans, and reverted to remote work, and schooling, resulting in reduced social interaction and enhanced social isolation, which increased loneliness (OECD, 2021b). However, the impact of COVID-19 on young people's loneliness and mental health in the long-term is still up for debate and as stated earlier, some evidence indicates that loneliness for young people was on the rise before the pandemic.

INTERVENTIONS: YOUNG PEOPLE AND LONELINESS

When considering the design and implementation of loneliness interventions for young people, it is of course, important to bear in mind the definitions of loneliness, for example, the difference between emotional and social loneliness mentioned above. The complexity of loneliness experiences means that it is possible to feel lonely in one regard, but not in another. For instance, someone may be feeling lonely regarding relations with parents but not with friends, or to feel either socially or emotionally lonely. Also of significance is the interconnecting risk factors of loneliness, both personal and subjective, but also the wider social determinants which impact. For example, at an individual level, behavioural drivers, personality, cognitions, and psychological health may assume significance. It is also important to focus upon relationships, including those with parents, but also a range of parental attachments, and parenting styles (La Placa and Corlyon, 2016). Consideration of relations within communities and neighbourhoods, as well as those with peers and friendship networks, are also important, given its links to, for instance, accumulation of social capital.

Given the divergent durations and types of loneliness, and the various personal and social determinants, which contribute to it, it is unlikely that a one size fits all approach would suffice and assist all young people in mitigating and reducing feelings of loneliness. However, research suggests that types of loneliness interventions can be categorised into three main themes. These are on the tertiary, secondary, and primary levels (see Table 17.1).

TABLE 17.1 Types and Characteristics of Loneliness Interventions

Type of intervention	Characteristics of intervention
Tertiary	These interventions primarily aim to prevent individuals from becoming lonely and, for instance, target younger individuals in schools and educational settings. Schools are often perceived as an important settings-based intervention – for example, 'Promoting Alternative Thinking Strategies' (PATHS) comprises lessons on, for example, reducing and mitigating shyness and maintaining friendships, and awareness of emotions, as well as teaching children about positive social behaviours, to enhance belonging and integration into the school environment.
Secondary	These interventions target vulnerable young individuals, for example, those with long-term illnesses or who are at risk of bullying. For instance, interventions which promote friendships between adolescents have been shown to halve the risk of developing depression over six to 12 months (Hill et al., 2015).
Primary	These interventions target individuals and groups who currently experience loneliness. The aim is to reduce and mitigate loneliness but also to reduce its impact on physical and psychological health. Often these interventions promote enhanced opportunities for social contact through group and community work but also comprise more intensive one-to-one individual interventions. These intervention types may often focus upon social skills development in, for example, schools and universities. For instance, Ellard et al. (2023) found that group and community-based interventions in universities, which increase social interaction, encouraged students to spend more time with others, for example, through playing sports, or participating in creative exercises, reduced loneliness, and increased social connectedness and belonging. These interventions often foster a protective mechanism against developing poor mental health (Hawkley and Cacioppo, 2010). These interventions may also seek to address maladaptive social cognitions through targeted individual counselling and support. For instance, some young individuals who experience loneliness have maladaptive social cognitions meaning, for example, that they interpret 'neutral' situations as more ominous or belligerent, and therefore, have higher expectations of quicker rejection. Lonely young people can also find it difficult to disengage from social threats. To mitigate this, cognitive approaches can reduce loneliness by teaching young people to redirect their attention away from perceived threatening social information. Similarly, cognitive behavioural therapy (CBT) that targets mistaken social cognitions has been demonstrated to be highly effective in reducing loneliness in young people.

These types of interventions can similarly comprise interventions identified as 'direct' interventions, (Mann et al., 2017; La Placa and Oham, 2019) which specifically aim at reducing individual feelings of loneliness. These encompass counselling approaches to reduce maladaptive patterns of thinking, training in social skills, support to access new opportunities for social contact, and involvement in community-based groups. For example, the UK Local Government Association (2018) has identified 'structural enablers', people, and organisations, which foster individuals to engage with, and support one other. 'Indirect' interventions refer to more structural determinants and efforts to enhance individuals' wellbeing and mitigate loneliness. These could, for example, include attempts to lessen inequalities and reduced opportunities, when devising interventions, with a structural impact. These can, for instance, assume design of services such as transport, technology, spatial planning, and housing, which make it easier for communities to coalesce, in, for example, urban planning (La Placa and Oham, 2019).

CONCLUSION

Loneliness is a considerable public health issue across OECD countries and can impact people of all ages and may induce significant physical, mental, and social outcomes. However, some groups are more at risk of loneliness than others. More population based research is required on the elements that put some individuals and groups at increased risk of experiencing loneliness, whether the changes in loneliness were principally the result of alterations in the quality or the quantity of people's social interactions, and whether those differed across subpopulations, such as students, sexual minorities, and younger people or according to socio-economic status, ethnicity, gender and health or disability status. This could assist in further development of more effective social policy, support, and interventions to increase peoples' social interaction or to enhance the quality of their close relationships.

RESEARCH POINTS AND REFLECTIVE ACTIVITIES

- Discuss the impact of COVID 19 on loneliness and mental health.
- Read the following (Barreto et al., 2022; Department for Digital, Culture, Media and Sport, 2023c) and reflect upon how stigma can impact on loneliness and ways in which stigma can be reduced.
- Research the progress that has been made to date in reducing loneliness (for example, Department for Digital, Culture, Media and Sport, 2023d) and discuss what more needs to be done to reduce loneliness.

REFERENCES

Achterbergh, L., Pitman, A., Birken, M., Pearce, E., Sno, H., et al. (2020). The Experience of Loneliness Among Young People with Depression: A Qualitative Meta-Synthesis of the Literature. *BMC Psychiatry*, 415. https://doi.org/10.1186/s12888-020-02818-3

Age UK. (2015). *Promising Approaches to Reducing Loneliness and Isolation in Later Life*. London: Age UK.

Alam, I., Khayri, E., Podger, T. A. B., Aspinall, C., Fuhrmann, D., et al. (2023). A Call for Better Research and Resources for Understanding and Combatting Youth Loneliness: Integrating the Perspectives of Young People and Researchers. *Eur Child Adolesc Psychiatry*, 32 (3): 371–374. https://doi.org/10.1007/s00787-022-02127-y

Astell-Burt, T., Hartig, T., Gusti Ngurah Edi Putra, I., Walsan, R., Dendup, T., et al. (2022). Green Space and Loneliness: A Systematic Review with Theoretical and Methodological Guidance for Future Research. *Science of The Total Environment*, 847. https://doi.org/10.1016/j.scitotenv.2022.157521.

Barreto, M., van Breen, J., Victor, C., Hammond, C., Eccles, A., et al. (2022). Exploring the Nature and Variation of the Stigma Associated with Loneliness. *Journal of Social and Personal Relationships*, 39 (9): 2658–2679. https://doi.org/10.1177/02654075221087190

Barreto, M., Victor, C., Hammond, C., Eccles, A., Richins, M.T., et al. (2021). Loneliness Around the World: Age, Gender, and Cultural Differences in Loneliness. *Personality and Individual Differences*, 169. https://doi.org/10.1016/j.paid.2020.110066.

Boston, P., Bruce, A. and Schreiber, R. (2011). Existential Suffering in the Palliative Care Setting: An Integrated Literature Review. *Journal of Pain and Symptom Management*, 41 (3): 604–618. https://doi.org/10.1016/j.jpainsymman.2010.05.010

Cigma. (2018). Cigma US Loneliness Index. Available at: www.multivu.com/players/English/8294451-cigna-us-loneliness-survey/docs/IndexReport_1524069371598-173525450.pdf (Accessed: 25 January 2024).

Cigma. (2020). Loneliness and the Workplace. 2020 US Report. Available at: https://legacy.cigna.com/static/www-cigna-com/docs/about-us/newsroom/studies-and-reports/combatting-loneliness/cigna-2020-loneliness-report.pdf (Accessed: 25 January 2024).

Department for Digital, Culture, Media and Sport. (2018a). A Connected Society: A Strategy for Tackling Loneliness – Laying the Foundations for Change. Available at: www.gov.uk/government/publications/a-connected-society-a-strategy-for-tackling-loneliness (Accessed: 15 February 2024).

Department for Digital, Culture, Media and Sport. (2018b). Community Life Survey: 2017–18. Available at: https://assets.publishing.service.gov.uk/media/5b76b131ed915d14f4404b75/Community_Life_Survey_2017-18_statistical_bulletin.pdf (Accessed: 15 February 2024).

Department for Digital, Culture, Media and Sport. (2019). Community Life Survey 2018–19. Available at: https://assets.publishing.service.gov.uk/media/5d3874fee5274a400da42ec7/Community_Life_Survey_2018-19_report.pdf (Accessed: 16 February 2024).

Department for Digital, Culture, Media and Sport. (2020). Community Life Survey 2019/20 – Wellbeing and Loneliness. Available at: www.gov.uk/government/statistics/community-life-survey-201920-wellbeing-and-loneliness (Accessed: 16 February 2024).

Department for Digital, Culture, Media and Sport. (2021). Community Life Survey 2020/21 – Wellbeing and Loneliness Available at: www.gov.uk/government/statistics/community-life-survey-202021-wellbeing-and-loneliness (Accessed: 17 February 2024).

Department for Digital, Culture, Media and Sport. (2023a). Tackling Loneliness Evidence Review: Executive Summary. Available at: www.gov.uk/government/publications/tackling-loneliness-evidence-review/tackling-loneliness-evidence-review-summary-report (Accessed: 17 February 2024).

Department for Digital, Culture, Media and Sport. (2023b). Community Life Survey 2021/22: Wellbeing and Loneliness Available at: www.gov.uk/government/statistics/community-life-survey-202122/community-life-survey-202122-wellbeing-and-loneliness (Accessed: 17 February 2024).

Department for Digital, Culture, Media and Sport. (2023c). Loneliness Stigma Rapid Evidence Assessment (REA). Available at: www.gov.uk/government/publications/research-exploring-the-stigma-associated-with-loneliness/loneliness-stigma-rapid-evidence-assessment-rea (Accessed: 18 February 2024).

Department for Digital, Culture, Media and Sport. (2023d). Tackling Loneliness Annual Report March 2023: The Fourth Year. Available at: www.gov.uk/government/publications/loneliness-annual-report-the-fourth-year/tackling-loneliness-annual-report-march-2023-the-fourth-year?dm_i=21A8,894YO,FM9TNZ,XWBSS,1 (Accessed: 18 February 2024).

Donbavand, S. (2020). A Simmelian Theory of Structural Loneliness. *Journal of the Theory of Social Behaviour*, 51 (1): 72–86. doi:101111/jtsb.12263

Ellard, O. B., Dennison, C. and Tuomainen, H. (2023). Review: Interventions Addressing Loneliness Among University Students: A Systematic Review. *Child and Adolescent Mental Health*, 28 (4): 512–523. https://doi.org/10.1111/camh.12614

Ettema, E. J., Derksen, L. D. and van Leeuwen, E. (2010). Existential Loneliness and End-of-Life Care: A Systematic Review. *Theoretical Medicine and Bioethics*, 31 (2): 141–169. doi:10.1007/s11017-010-9141-1

Baarck, J., Balahur-Dobrescu, A., Cassio, L.G., D`hombres, B., Pasztor, Z., et al. (2021). *Insights From Surveys and Online Media Data, EUR 30765 EN*. Luxembourg: Publications Office of the European Union.

Fardghassemi, S. and Joffe, H. (2022). The Causes of Loneliness: The Perspective of Young Adults in London's Most Deprived Areas. *PLoS One*, 17 (4): e0264638. https://doi.org/10.1371/journal.pone.0264638.

Franssen, T., Stijnen, M., Hamers, F. and Schneider, F. (2020). Age Differences in Demographic, Social, and Health-Related Factors Associated with Loneliness Across the Adult Life Span. (19–65 Years): A Cross-Sectional Study in the Netherlands. *BMC Public Health*, 20 (1): 1118. https://doi.org/10.1186/s12889-020-09208-0

Geller, J., Janson, P., McGovern, E. and Valdini, A. (1999). Loneliness as a Predictor of Hospital Emergency Department Use. *Journal of Family Practice*, 48 (10): 801–804. www.jfponline.com/pages.asp?aid=2697

Hammond, C. (2018). The Surprising Truth About Loneliness. Available at: www.bbc.com/future/article/20180928-the-surprising-truth-about-loneliness (Accessed: 22 December 2023).

Hawkley, L. C. and Cacioppo, J. T. (2010). Loneliness Matters: A Theoretical and Empirical Review of Consequences and Mechanisms. *Ann Behav Med*, 40 (2): 218–227. https://doi.org/10.1007/s12160-010-9210-8.

Hill, E. M., Griffiths, F. E. and House, T. (2015). Spreading of Healthy Mood in Adolescent Social Networks. *Proceedings of the Royal Society B: Biological Sciences*, 282 (1813): Article 20151180. https://doi.org/10.1098/rspb.2015.1180

Holt-Lunstad, J. (2022). Social Connection as a Public Health Issue: The Evidence and a Systemic Framework for Prioritizing the 'Social' in Social Determinants of Health. *Annu Rev Public Health*, 43: 193–213. https://doi.org/10.1146/annurev-publhealth-052020-110732

Holt-Lunstad, J., Smith, T. B., Baker, M., Harris, T. and Stephenson, D. (2015). Loneliness and Social Isolation as Risk Factors for Mortality: A Meta-Analytic Review. *Perspect Psychol Sci*, 10 (2): 227–237. https://doi.org/10.1177/1745691614568352

House, J. S., Landis, K. R. and Umberson, D. (1988). Social Relationships and Health. *Science*, 241: 540–545. https://doi.org/10.1126/science.3399889

Imrie, R. (2018). 'The Lonely City': Urban Infrastructure and the Problem of Loneliness. In O. Sagan and E. D. Miller (eds), *Narratives of Loneliness: Multidisciplinary Perspectives from the 21st Century*. London: Routledge, 140–152.

Jo Cox Commission on Loneliness. (2017). Combatting Loneliness One Conversation at a Time: A Call to Action. Available at: www.ageuk.org.uk/globalassets/age-uk/documents/reports-and-publications/reports-and-briefings/active-communities/rb_dec17_jocox_commission_finalreport.pdf (Accessed: 18 February 2024).

Ladd, G. W. and Ettekal, I. (2013). Peer-Related Loneliness Across Early to Late Adolescence: Normative Trends, Intra-Individual Trajectories, and Links with Depressive Symptoms. *Journal of Adolescence*, 36: 1269–1282. https://doi.org/10.1016/j.adolescence.2013.05.004

La Placa, V. and Corlyon, J. (2016). Unpacking the Relationship Between Parenting and Poverty: Theory, Evidence and Policy. *Social Policy and Society*, 15 (1): 11–28. https://doi.org/10.1017/S1474746415000111

La Placa, V. and Oham, C. (2019). Loneliness and Young People Experiencing Mental Health Difficulties: Evidence and Further Research. *PEOPLE: International Journal of Social Sciences*, 5 (2): 1024–1039. https://dx.doi.org/10.20319/pijss.2019.52.10241039

La Placa, V. and Morgan, J. (2023). Global Public Health and Loneliness. In V. La Placa and J. Morgan (eds), *Social Science Perspectives on Global Public Health*. London: Routledge, 189–197.

Lasgaard, M., Friis, K. and Shevlin, M. (2016). 'Where Are All the Lonely People': A Population-Based Study of High-Risk Groups Across the Life Span. *Soc Psychiatry Psychiatr Epidemiol*, 51 (10): 1373–1384. https://doi.org/10.1007/s00127-016-1279-3.

Local Government Association. (2018). *Loneliness: How Do You Know Your Council is Actively Tackling Loneliness?* London: The Local Government Association.

Mann, F., Bone, J. K., Lloyd-Evans, B., Frerichs, J., Pinfold, V., et al. (2017). A Life Less Lonely: The State of the Art in Interventions to Reduce Loneliness in People with Mental Health Problems. *Soc Psychiatry Psychiatr Epidemiol*, 52 (6): 627–638. https://doi.org/10.1007/s00127-017-1392-y

Mansfield, L., Daykin, N., Meads, C., Tomlinson, A., Gray, K., et al. (2019). A Conceptual Review of Loneliness Across the Adult Life Course (16+ Years) Synthesis of Qualitative Studies. Available at: https://whatworkswellbeing.org/wp-content/uploads/2020/02/V3-FINAL-Loneliness-conceptual-review.pdf (Accessed: 15 December 2023).

Mareike, E., Niederer, D., Werner, A. M., Czaja, S. J., Mikton, C., et al. (2022). Loneliness Before and During the COVID-19 Pandemic: A Systematic Review with Meta-Analysis. *American Psychologist*, 77 (5): 660–677. https://doi.org/10.1037/amp0001005.

Marquez. J., Goodfellow, C., Hardoon, D., Inchley, J., Leyland, A. H., et al. (2023). Loneliness In Young People: A Multilevel Exploration of Social Ecological Influences and Geographic Variation. *J Public Health (Oxf)*, 45 (1): 109–117. https://doi.org/10.1093/pubmed/fdab402.

Matthews, T., Danese, A., Caspi, A., Fischer, H. L., Goldman-Mellor, S., et al. (2018). Lonely Young Adults in Modern Britain: Findings from an Epidemiological Cohort Study *Psychological Medicine*, 49 (2): 268–277. https://doi.org/10.1017/S0033291718000788

Meisters, R., Putrik, P., Westra, D., Bosma, H., Ruwaard, D., et al. (2021). Is Loneliness an Undervalued Pathway Between Socio-Economic Disadvantage and Health? *International Journal of Environmental Research and Public Health*, 18 (19): 10177. https://doi.org/10.3390/ijerph181910177

Ministry of Social Development. (2016). *The Social Report 2016*. Available at: www.socialreport.msd.govt.nz/social-connectedness/loneliness.html (Accessed: 18 February 2024)

Morgan, J. and La Placa, V. (2023). Loneliness is a Major Public Health Problem and Young People are Bearing the Brunt of it, The Conversation. Available at: https://theconversation.com/loneliness-is-a-major-public-health-problem-and-young-people-are-bearing-the-brunt-of-it-218391 (Accessed: 5 January 2024).

OECD. (2021a). All the Lonely People: Education and Loneliness Trends Shaping Education, Spotlight 23. Available at: www.oecd-ilibrary.org/docserver/23ac0e25-en.pdf?expires=1708016056&id=id&accname=guest&checksum=DDA4FE3B5175F4A1BE87251B959C8C1D (Accessed: 15 February 2024).

OECD. (2021b). *Covid-19 and Well-being: Life in the Pandemic*. Paris: OECD Publishing. https://doi.org/10.1787/1e1ecb53-en

Office for National Statistics. (2018a). Loneliness - What Characteristics and Circumstances are Associated with Feeling Lonely? Available at: www.ons.gov.uk/peoplepopulationandcommunity/wellbeing/articles/lonelinesswhatcharacteristicsandcircumstancesareassociatedwithfeelinglonely/2018-04-10 (Accessed: 18 January 2024).

Office for National Statistics. (2018b). Children's and Young People's Experiences of Loneliness: 2018. Available at: www.ons.gov.uk/peoplepopulationandcommunity/wellbeing/articles/childrensandyoungpeoplesexperiencesofloneliness/2018 (Accessed: 18 January 2024).

Office for National Statistics. (2021). Mapping Loneliness During the Coronavirus Pandemic. www.ons.gov.uk/peoplepopulationandcommunity/wellbeing/articles/mappingloneliness duringthecoronaviruspandemic/2021-04-07 (Accessed: 18 January 2024)

Perlman, D. and Peplau, L. A. (1981). Towards a Social Psychology of Loneliness. In S. Duck and R. Gihour (eds), *Personal Relationships in Disorder*. London: Academic Press, 31–56.

Petitte, T., Mallow, J., Barnes, E., Petrone, A., Barr, T., et al. (2015). A Systematic Review of Loneliness and Common Chronic Physical Conditions in Adults. *The Open Psychology Journal*, 8 (2): 113–132. https://doi.org/10.2174/1874350101508010113

Polo, A. J. and Lopez, S. R. (2009). Culture, Context, and the Internalizing Distress of Mexican American Youth. *Journal of Clinical Child and Adolescent Psychology*, 38 (2): 273–285. https://doi.org/10.1080/15374410802698370

Qualter, P., Brown, S. L., Munn, P. and Rotenberg, K. J. (2010). Childhood Loneliness as a Predictor of Adolescent Depressive Symptoms: An 8-Year Longitudinal Study. *Eur Child Adolesc Psychiatry*, 19: 493–501 https://doi.org/10.1007/s00787-009-0059-y

Qualter, P., Brown, S. L., Rotenberg, K. J., Vanhalst, J., Harris, R. A., et al. (2013). Trajectories of Loneliness: Predictors and Health Outcomes. *Journal of Adolescence*, 36: 1283–1293. https://doi.org/10.1016/j.adolescence.2013.01.005

Sagan, O. (2018). Narratives of Loneliness and Mental Health in a Time of Neoliberalism. In O. Sagan and E. D. Miller (eds), *Narratives of Loneliness: Multidisciplinary Perspectives from the 21st Century*, London: Routledge, 89–100.

Salinas, J., Beiser, A. S., Samra, J. K., O'Donnell, A., DeCarli, C.S., et al. (2022). Association of Loneliness with 10-year Dementia Risk and Early Markers of Vulnerability for Neurocognitive Decline. *Neurology*, 98 (13): e1337–e1348. https://doi.org/10.1212/WNL.0000000000200039

Schinka, K. C., van Dulmen, M. H. M., Mata, A. D., Bossarte, R. M. and Swahn, M. (2013). Psychosocial Predictors and Outcomes of Loneliness Trajectories from Childhood to Early Adolescence. *Journal of Adolescence*, 36: 1251–1260. https://doi.org/10.1016/j.adolescence.2013.08.002.

Scottish Government. (2018). A Connected Scotland: Our Strategy for Tackling Social Isolation and Loneliness and Building Stronger Social Connections. Available at: www.gov.scot/publications/connected-scotland-strategy-tackling-social-isolation-loneliness-building-stronger-social-connections/pages/4/(Accessed: 15 February 2024).

Segrin, C., McNelis, M. and Pavlich, C. A. (2018). Indirect Effects of Loneliness on Substance Use through Stress. *Health Communication*, 33 (5): 513–518. https://doi.org/10.1080/10410236.2016.1278507

Shah, H. A. and Househ, M. (2023). Understanding Loneliness in Younger People: Review of the Opportunities and Challenges for Loneliness Interventions. *Interact J Med Res*, 12: e45197. https://doi.org/10.2196/45197

Sundqvist, A. and Hemberg, J. (2021). Adolescents' and Young Adults' Experiences of Loneliness and their Thoughts About its Alleviation. *International Journal of Adolescence and Youth*, 26 (1): 238–255. https://doi.org/10.1080/02673843.2021.1908903

Surkalim, D. L., Luo, M., Eres. R, Gebel, K., van Buskirk, J., et al. (2022). The Prevalence of Loneliness Across 113 Countries: Systematic Review and Meta-Analysis. *BMJ*, 376. https://doi.org/10.1136/bmj-2021-067068

Tarbi, E. C. and Meghani, S. H. (2019). A Concept Analysis of the Existential Experience of Adults with Advanced Cancer. *Nursing Outlook*, 67 (5): 540–557. https://doi.org/10.1016/j.outlook.2019.03.006

Vanhalst, J., Goossens, L., Luyckx, K., Scholte, R. H and Engels, R. C. (2013). The Development of Loneliness from Mid-to Late Adolescence: Trajectory Classes, Personality Traits, and Psychosocial Functioning. *Journal of Adolescence*, 36 (6): 1305–1312. https://doi.org/10.1016/j.adolescence.2012.04.002

van Tilburg, T. G. (2021). Social, Emotional, and Existential Loneliness: A Test of the Multidimensional Concept. *The Gerontologist*, 61 (7): e335–e344. https://doi.org/10.1093/geront/gnaa082

Vasileuiou, K., Bernett, J., Barreto, M., Vines, J., Atkinson, M., et al. (2019). Coping with Loneliness at University: A Qualitative Interview Study with Students in the UK. *Mental Health and Prevention*, 13: 21–30. https://doi.org/10.1016/j.mhp.2018.11.002

Verity, L., Schellekens, T., Adam, T., Sillis, F., Majorano, M., et al. (2021). Tell Me About Loneliness: Interviews with Young People About What Loneliness Is and How to Cope with It. *International Journal of Environmental Research and Public Health*, 18 (22): 11904. https://doi.org/10.3390/ijerph182211904

Weissbourd, R., Batanova, M., Lovison, V. and Torres, E. (2021). Loneliness in America: How the Pandemic Has Deepened an Epidemic of Loneliness and What We Can Do About It. Available at: https://static1.squarespace.com/static/5b7c56e255b02c683659fe43/t/6021776bdd04957c4557c212/1612805995893/Loneliness+in+America+2021_02_08_FINAL.pdf (Accessed: 15 December 2023).

Welsh Government. (2020). Connected Communities: A Strategy for Tackling Loneliness and Social Isolation and Building Stronger Social Connections. Available at: www.gov.wales/sites/default/files/publications/2020-02/connected-communities-strategy-document.pdf (Accessed: 15 February 2024).

WHO. (2023a). WHO Launches Commission to Foster Social Connection. Available at: www.who.int/news/item/15-11-2023-who-launches-commission-to-foster-social-connection (Accessed: 15 December 2023).

WHO. (2023b). WHO Commission on Social Connection. Available at: https://uploads.guim.co.uk/2023/11/15/CSC_-_Slide_Deck_-_June_2023_(1)_(1).pdf (Accessed: 16 December 2023).

CHAPTER 18

Conclusion

Comparative Perspectives on Health and Social Care Policy and Practice across OECD Countries

....

Vincent La Placa and Julia Morgan

As was mentioned in Chapter 1, health and social care are vital in provision of transparency and equitability across societies and a significant part of welfare provision across OECD countries. Health and social care can refer to an array of activities, structures of organisation, and systems, which support health, wellbeing, needs, care, and quality of life, for adults and children, which can occur in a range of settings including prisons, hospitals, and schools. Health and social care conventionally occur in the home, community or in residential care facilities and can be formally provided through a range of private, statutory, or voluntary organisations, or informally provided through an individual's family, and community, as well as trained healthcare professionals. Indeed, the book indicates strongly that health and social care and welfare is a consistent and recognised feature of the OECD, with spending significantly increasing since the 1950s/1960s. This is due to the need to provide services to a host of different populations with diverse needs and recognition of the role of the State in providing services, although this is increasingly changing, as is posited below.

The book also makes discernible another emerging three key themes which are in important in the study of health and social care across the OECD:

1. All OECD countries are subject to increasingly important global developments which affect approaches to health and social care, for example, ageing populations, health and social inequalities, the need to diversify and expand the workforce, and wider structural configurations of globalisation and inter-dependence.
2. While there is a trend and convergence towards increasing expenditure upon health and social care, this is accompanied by a dual convergence towards, for instance, marketisation, and diversity in provision of health and social care.

DOI: 10.4324/9781003343608-20

3. Health and social care research, policy and practice, requires adaptation to increasing complexity and change, and in an era of increasing competition for resources.

Interestingly, all OECD countries are subject to increasingly significant global developments, which affect health and social care approaches, and which increasingly impinge upon specifically national considerations (Chapters 2 and 3). While OECD welfare regimes can be located within specific typologies (Chapter 2) with different approaches, they currently display a convergence and homogenisation of approaches and systems, often the result of a globalisation of events and processes, impinging upon all OECD countries and systems. As was mentioned in Chapter 2, Globalisation represents processes whereby rapid development and expansions of a network of independencies and connections, across politics, economics, culture, and technology intensify, and require greater global responses, as developments in one area of the globe affect others.

For instance, the COVID-19 pandemic had substantial consequences for health and social care systems with significant demands to create more resilient systems across the OECD, which can respond to global health developments (OECD, 2023). This includes consideration around health inequalities (Chapter 5) including for specific populations such as those imprisoned (Chapter 12) and those who experience homelessness (Chapter 8), population movement and migration (Chapter 16), workforce expansion and digitalisation (Chapter 15) (digital infrastructure is increasingly important to system performance across the globe); and new responses to emerging global concerns around, for instance, wellbeing, as distinct from traditional concepts of health (Chapter 4) and growing global evidence around the phenomenon and negative effects of loneliness (Chapter 17) as global social developments often make experiences of the latter more intense.

The need to respond rapidly to ageing populations is a core global concern, as are the choices around providing care for ever increasing numbers of older people, with less resources due to economic dislocation, caused by fiscal contraction and the global pandemic (Chapters 13 and 15). These emerging concerns demand that all OECD countries focus upon development of systems which can minimise the negative consequences of global crises, recover as speedily as possible, and adapt to become more effective in performance and preparedness (OECD, 2023). However, as Chapter 2, also argues, OECD countries can continue to harness control and discretion over policies and expenditure (and as the COVID-19 pandemic demonstrated, even this was characterised by differing degrees of success and outcomes).

Nevertheless, this argument also needs to be counterbalanced by increasing evidence around 'de-globalisation' (La Placa and Knight, 2023) and 'de-risking' (Chapter 2), the tendency to focus upon the greater risks of global interdependence, especially the role of supply chains, and international co-operation around health and social care. The global pandemic demonstrated the risks of over-reliance on other areas of the globe, for instance, personal protective equipment (PPE), and ventilators, among other things, including COVID-19 vaccinations (Mundy, 2022). International trade did shore up increases in availability of vaccines and medical devices later in the pandemic, but reliance upon supply chains, now perceived as unreliable, can compromise assessment of future risk and national responses to disease management and health and social care services. As a result, resilient health and social care supply chains are a key determinant in global approaches within all OECD countries, adapting to the need for flexibility and agility in supplying medicine and services.

The evidence across the book also indicates a trend and convergence towards increasing expenditure upon health and social care, due to greater diversity in, for instance individual need and service delivery; but this is accompanied by a shift towards enhanced marketisation and diversity in provision of health and social care, as opposed to the traditional collective approaches, for example, typical of post-war social democratic regimes (Chapter 2). Greater expenditure is encouraged through adaption of health and social care systems to effectively respond to future shocks and increased spending on prevention and digital and technology infrastructures. However, as mentioned, increasingly ageing populations, and lower birth rates, are pressuring all OECD countries to consider the future effects upon the health and care of an older population, and the complex medical and social care requirements which will result from this (as well as end of life care) (Chapters 13 and 15).

Current economic difficulties and pressures to enhance expenditure on older populations is likely to mean spending reductions in other areas, for example, young people (Chapter 17) or with disabilities (Chapter 11). Furthermore, such pressures are likely to increase interest in more diverse provision and less state intervention, as a result. Marketisation, for instance, often entails a system where relations and behavioural drivers are compelled by competition and profit, and where private and voluntary organisations often assume more significance than the state. Such processes characterise the Anglo Saxon/Liberal regimes referred to in Chapter 2. This is driven partly by neoliberal ideologies (Chapters two and four), but also the need to locate ways of delivering services, which can also innovate and diversify- for example, in the UK, NHS providers may subcontract services to another provider to help manage demand or improve efficiency, where demand is high, and the state struggles to provide the service.

The aim is to capitalise on the benefits of competition through providing effective quality services efficiently and is often perceived as effective in meeting ever increasing demand without the need to significantly reduce services or cap expenditure. Indeed, much of the increased expenditure across the OECD is achieved through these diversification processes and is increasingly used in the more Nordic/ social democratic states (Chapter 2), demonstrating convergence around increased long-term expenditure, but by and through, non-state activities. Nevertheless, as was argued in Chapter 3, this needs to be balanced by the fact that one of the key driving forces behind current debates about reform and expenditure is the continued desire to attempt to achieve some means of universal coverage without people facing financial hardship, (and despite trends towards markets and diversity in provision).

Finally, the book demonstrates the requirement of health and social care research, policy, and practice, to respond to increasing change and complexity, driven by the above, and the evidence provided throughout the book. For example, demographic factors, changes in the size, age structure, and burden of ill health, income effects and other cost pressures, (which encompass technological advances and increasing relative prices) demand innovative methods to model projected health and social care expenditure pressures (Chapter 3) and needs assessments to enhance wellbeing and adapt services (Chapter 4). Newly emerging issues such as domestic violence (Chapter 9), public health and criminal justice approaches to drug and alcohol use (Chapter 10) and loneliness and isolation (Chapter 17) demand more insight and evidence around public health trends and risk factors, outcomes of service use, and public health interventions, patterns of care, as well as costs and use.

Simultaneously, more insight will be required as to the qualitative experiences of, for instance, service use, and effectiveness of various models of partnerships (Chapter 6) including the centring of service user involvement (Chapter 7) in systems development. This needs to be conducted across all areas of the health and social care systems across the OECD, especially given the noted drive and convergence of developments in information technology and increasing emphasis on productivity and competitiveness; and the need to avoid research approaches, which are too over reliant upon totalisation of systems, negate individual experiences and needs, and lead to 'one size fits all' type policies and discourses (La Placa and Knight, 2023). This will foster approaches, based upon evidence-based research, to join up, and coordinate policy across the OECD, despite differences in how individual countries define, fund, and coordinate health and social care (Chapter 3). For example, the OECD Framework and Scorecard for People-Centred Health Systems identifies crucial dimensions of people-centredness for health systems and benchmarks the progress individual countries make towards a more people-centred approach to health (OECD, 2021).

These policies are deemed necessary and perceived in the light of wider global and social determinants, such as health inequalities, effects of the global pandemic, and the convergence of systems towards increasing expenditure and diversity of provision, beyond traditional statist approaches, whether we agree with the latter or not. The integration of health and social care services into wider welfare policies; the emergence of new priorities and interest, and the shift towards convergence and diversity simultaneously, makes it an exciting time to develop and compare health and social care policy and practice, whichever area one currently works within.

REFERENCES

La Placa, V. and Knight, A. (2023). Globalisation and Global Public Health. In V. La Placa and J. Morgan (eds), *Social Science Perspectives on Global Public Health*. London: Routledge, 17–28.

Mundy, C. (2022). Safeguarding Healthcare Supply Chains Post-Pandemic. Available at: www.hsj.co.uk/hsj-partners/safeguarding-healthcare-supply-chains-post-pandemic/7033618.article (Accessed: 23 February 2024).

OECD. (2020). *A Systemic Resilience Approach to Dealing with Covid-19 and Future Shocks, OECD Policy Responses to Coronavirus (COVID-19)*. Paris: OECD Publishing.

OECD. (2021). Health for the People, By the People: Building People-Centred Health Systems. Available at: www.oecd-ilibrary.org/sites/c259e79a-en/index.html?itemId=/content/publication/c259e79a-en (Accessed: 23 February 2024).

OECD. (2023). *Ready for the Next Crisis? Investing in Health System Resilience, OECD Health Policy Studies*. Paris: OECD Publishing.

Index

Printed in the United States
by Baker & Taylor Publisher Services